PSYCHIATRIC NURSING DIAGNOSES

A Comprehensive Manual of Mental Health Care

Janyce G. Dyer, RN, DNSc, CS
Assistant Professor
Psychiatric Mental Health Nurse Practitioner Graduate Program
Health and Community Systems Department
School of Nursing, University of Pittsburgh
Pittsburgh, Pa.

Sheila M. Sparks, RN, DNSc, CS
Assistant Professor, School of Nursing
Georgetown University
Washington, D.C.

Cynthia M. Taylor RN, MS, CS, CNAA
Independent Nurse Consultant
Former Chief Operating Officer
Suburban Hospital
Bethesda, Md.

Springhouse Corporation
Springhouse, Pennsylvania

Staff

Executive Director, Editorial
Stanley Loeb

Senior Publisher
Matthew Cahill

Art Director
John Hubbard

Senior Editor
Michael Shaw

Clinical Manager
Cindy Tryniszewski, RN, MSN

Editors
Marcia Andrews, Judd L. Howard, Richard Koreto, Judith Lewis, Pat Wittig

Copy Editors
Cynthia C. Breuninger (manager), Lewis Adams, Priscilla DeWitt, Jennifer George Mintzer

Designers
Stephanie Peters (associate art director), Lesley Weissman-Cook (book designer), Joseph Daniel Fiedler (cover illustrator), Donald G. Knauss

Typography
Diane Paluba (manager), Elizabeth Bergman, Joyce Rossi Biletz, Phyllis Marron, Robin Mayer, Valerie L. Rosenberger

Manufacturing
Deborah Meiris (director), Pat Dorshaw (manager), Anna Brindisi, T.A. Landis

Production Coordinator
Patricia McCloskey

Editorial Assistants
Maree DeRosa, Beverly Lane, Mary Madden

Indexer
Janet Hodgson

Printed in the United States of America.

PND-021296

A member of the Reed Elsevier plc group

Library of Congress Cataloging-in-Publication Data

Dyer, Janyce G.
  Psychiatric nursing diagnoses: a comprehensive manual of mental health care / Janyce G. Dyer, Sheila M. Sparks, Cynthia M. Taylor.
    p.   cm.
  Includes bibliographical references and index.
  1. Psychiatric nursing.   2. Nursing diagnosis.
I. Sparks, Sheila M.   II. Taylor, Cynthia M.   III. Title.
  [DNLM: 1. Mental Disorders—nursing.
2. Nursing Diagnosis. WY 160 D996p 1994]
RC440.D94   1994
610.73′68—dc20
DNLM/DLC   94-36038
ISBN 0-87434-757-2   CIP

Contents

Contributors

ADULT MENTAL HEALTH

Donna Anderson, RN, MSN, Clinical Nurse Specialist, Allegheny Neuropsychiatric Institute, Oakdale, Pa.

Leslie Nield Anderson, RN, PhD, Assistant Professor, Yale University School of Nursing; Psychiatric Consultation Liaison Nurse Specialist, Yale-New Haven (Conn.) Hospital

Cynthia A. Belonick, RN,C, MSN, Clinical Nurse Specialist, Institute of Living, Hartford (Conn.) Hospital's Mental Health Network

Marianne D. Borelli, RN, PhD, Assistant Professor, School of Nursing, Georgetown University, Washington, D.C.

Elizabeth A. Burggraf, RN, BSN, Teaching Assistant, School of Nursing, Georgetown University, Washington, D.C.

Cynthia Flynn Capers, RN, PhD, Associate Professor and Director of Undergraduate Programs, School of Nursing, La Salle University, Philadelphia

Lynne Hutnik Conrad, RN,C, MSN, Perinatal Clinical Nurse Specialist, Albert Einstein Medical Center, Philadelphia

Mari D'Onofrio, RN, MSN, Medical-Psychiatric Clinical Specialist, West Haven (Conn.) VA Medical Center-Yale University Clinical Campus, New Haven, Conn.

Nancy Endler, RN, MSN, CS, Mental Health Liaison Nurse Specialist, Suburban Hospital, Bethesda, Md.

Priscilla Goral, RN,C, MSN, Clinical Nurse Specialist, Department of Veterans Affairs Medical Center, Fayetteville, N.C.

Randolph E. Gross, RN, MS, Clinical Nurse Specialist, Memorial Sloan-Kettering Cancer Center, New York

Kathleen Hammill, RN, MSN, CRNP, Instructor, Psychiatric Mental Health Nurse Practitioner Graduate Program, Health and Community Systems Department, School of Nursing, University of Pittsburgh

Maryanne Lachat, RN, PhD, Clinical Assistant Professor, School of Nursing, Georgetown University, Washington, D.C.

Stephen B. Leder, PhD, Associate Professor, Department of Surgery, Section of Otolaryngology, Yale University School of Medicine; Co-Director, Communication Disorders Center, Yale-New Haven (Conn.) Hospital

Margaret Lunney, RN, PhD, CS, Associate Professor, Hunter-Bellevue School of Nursing, Hunter College of the City University of New York

Janet Interrante Makover, RN, MA, CNAA, Program Instructor, Yale University School of Nursing; Associate Director of Nursing, Connecticut Mental Health Center, New Haven

Renee A. Milligan, RN,C, PhD, Assistant Professor, School of Nursing, Georgetown University, Washington, D.C.

Patricia Pearson, RN, CS, MS, Nurse Clinician, Suburban Hospital, Bethesda, Md.

Linda C. Pugh, RN,C, PhD, Assistant Professor, School of Nursing, The Johns Hopkins University, Baltimore

Joan B. Riley, RN, MSN, Clinical Instructor, School of Nursing, Georgetown University, Washington, D.C.

Rosemarie Satyshur, RN, DNSc, Assistant Professor, School of Nursing, The Catholic University of America, Washington, D.C.

Christina Bond Sokoloff, RN, MS, CS, Gerontological Clinical Nurse Specialist, Senior Care Concepts, Woonsockett, RI

Carol Taylor, RN, MSN, CSFN, Assistant Professor of Nursing, Research Scholar, Center for Clinical Bioethics, Georgetown University, Washington, D.C.

Nancy R. Tommasini, RN, MSN, CS, Assistant Professor, Yale University School of Nursing; Psychiatric Consultation Liaison Nurse Specialist, Yale-New Haven (Conn.) Hospital

Margaret Wicks, RN, CS, MA, Psychiatric Nurse Specialist, Suburban Hospital, Bethesda, Md.

CHILD AND ADOLESCENT MENTAL HEALTH

Regina Devine, RN, MS, Nurse Clinician, Suburban Hospital, Bethesda, Md.

Jennifer Dooling, RN, BSN, Independent Nurse Consultant, Columbia, Mo.

Jean Farley, RN, MS, Clinical Instructor, School of Nursing, Georgetown University, Washington, D.C.

Carole Logan Kuhns, RN, PhD, Assistant Professor, Department of Public Policy, Georgetown University; Project Director, National Resource Center for Health Safety and Child Care, Washington, D.C.

Alison L. Moriarty, RN, PNP, MSN, Pediatric Nurse Practitioner, Adolescent Clinic, Yale-New Haven (Conn.) Hospital Program Instructor, School of Nursing, Yale University

Carolyn M. Yurick, RN, MSN, Nurse Education Clinician for the Child Psychiatry Inpatient Program; Adjunct Faculty, School of Nursing, Psychiatric Mental Health, University of North Carolina at Chapel Hill

GERIATRIC MENTAL HEALTH

Mary Burke, RN, DNSc, ANP, Assistant Professor, Coordinator, Gerontology Program, School of Nursing, Georgetown University, Washington, D.C.

Karen Kelleher, RN, MS, CS, Director, Mental Health Services, Suburban Hospital, Bethesda, Md.

Teresa Lien-Gieschen, RN,C, MS, CNP, Nurse Practitioner, Department of Internal Medicine, VA Medical Center, Richmond, Va.

Marjorie A. Maddox, RN, PhD, ARNP, ANP-C, Associate Professor, School of Nursing, University of Louisville; Adult Nurse Practitioner, Nurse Clinic, St. William Adult Day Center, Louisville, Ky.

Ruth Anne McCormick, RN, DNSc, Clinical Assistant Professor, School of Nursing, Georgetown University, Washington, D.C.

Preface

All nurses need expertise in psychiatric and mental health care. After all, skillfully tending to a patient's psychological and social needs isn't specialized care, it's simply good nursing.

We've written *Psychiatric Nursing Diagnoses* as a comprehensive guide to mental health care for the entire profession, from the student to the advanced practitioner. Here's why:

- Caring effectively for any patient requires looking at both psychological and physiologic aspects of health. Patients who seek help for cardiovascular or GI complaints, for example, may need to be assessed for anxiety, depression, or social isolation.
- Many people with psychiatric disorders live in the community. You may encounter them in a hospital or primary care facility. Not only do these patients have tremendous psychological and social needs, but they also have a range of medical problems.
- Rapid social, economic, and scientific changes are pushing nurses to the front lines of mental health care delivery. Numerous factors, such as the need to lower health care costs, a better understanding of the biological aspects of mental illness and advances in drug therapy, higher rates of psychiatric disturbances in the general population, and increased awareness of substance abuse, domestic violence, sexual abuse, and other social ills, are expanding the role nurses play.

Whether you work in a hospital, primary care facility, mental health institution, nursing home, or home health care service, you must be able to:
- assess psychological, physiologic, and social needs
- develop an effective plan of care
- write measurable patient outcomes
- perform interventions to achieve those outcomes.

Psychiatric Nursing Diagnoses will help you meet these goals. It's the only comprehensive psychiatric nursing book organized by the nursing process. Each plan of care has been written and reviewed by leading nurse clinicians, educators, and researchers and is complete and can be used independently to avoid wasting valuable time searching for additional information.

Unfortunately, many care planning manuals don't address the realities of clinical practice today. In contrast, this manual covers many of the difficult and controversial issues facing nurses: care of patients with acquired immunodeficiency syndrome, domestic violence, substance abuse, law and ethics in health care, and more.

At the heart of the book are more than 130 plans of care; each includes the following features:
- ***Diagnostic statement.*** Each diagnostic statement is comprised of a label approved by the North American Nursing Diagnosis Association and, in most cases, a related etiology.

- **Definition.** This section offers a brief explanation of the diagnosis.
- **Assessment.** Comprised of parameters to use when collecting data to validate the diagnosis, this section of *Psychiatric Nursing Diagnoses* features expanded assessment guidelines that include neurologic, biological, and psychological parameters as well as family assessment guidelines.
- **Defining characteristics.** This section lists clinical findings that, when grouped together, confirm the diagnosis. For diagnoses that express the possibility of a problem, such as "high risk for injury," this section is titled *Risk factors*. Keep in mind that not all defining characteristics need to be present for a diagnosis to be valid. Defining characteristics should be individualized to accurately characterize the patient's clinical picture.
- **Associated disorders.** Selected examples of medical and psychiatric problems commonly associated with the nursing diagnosis are listed in this section. Note that all psychiatric disorders have been updated to reflect the latest *Diagnostic and Statistical Manual of Mental Disorders (DSM-IV)* terminology.
- **Patient outcomes.** Written in measurable behavioral terms, these outcomes contain realistic goals for resolving or ameliorating the patient's health problem. They are organized according to time frame and patient acuity (initial, interim, and discharge).
- **Interventions and rationales.** This section provides specific activities you can carry out to help attain patient outcomes. Each intervention lists a specific rationale, highlighted in *italic*

type. Rationales receive typographic emphasis because they form the premise for every nursing action. Interventions are also arranged according to time frame and patient acuity (initial, interim, or discharge) to make it easy to correlate patient outcomes with the appropriate interventions.
- **Evaluation statements.** This list of statements describes changes in the patient's behavior or condition that demonstrate goal achievement. The statements are useful when documenting care and when determining whether or not patient outcomes have been achieved.
- **Documentation.** This section lists critical topics to include in your documentation — for example, patient perceptions, status, and response to treatment as well as nursing observations, interventions, and goal attainment. Using this information as a reference will help you write the clear, concise documentation required to meet professional nursing standards.

You will also find that many plans of care can be adapted to meet special clinical or learning needs. There are many plans of care for working with patients' families, as well as for helping staff members cope with difficult situations. You'll also find a section devoted to geriatric mental health in addition to sections on adult, child, and adolescent mental health. Also included are numerous plans for helping patients in acute care settings cope with the emotional effects of medical illnesses. These plans may be of special value to nurses and students interested in the emerging field of psychiatric consultation and liaison nursing.

Psychiatric Nursing Diagnoses also contains several useful appendices that will help you locate psychiatric and mental health nursing diagnoses for virtually every clinical situation. Use these appendices as tools to develop your nursing diagnoses. You will find that there is no easier way to make accurate nursing diagnoses.

We express our sincere appreciation to the nurses who contributed to the book. Their vast experience and commitment to quality patient care make it an invaluable reference. Special thanks go to the Springhouse editorial staff — in particular, Michael Shaw, for his diligence, good humor, and attention to detail.

Finally, we dedicate this book to our patients. In this age of increasing technology and cost containment, the true essence of nursing — patient care — deserves the attention and expertise of each of us in the nursing profession.

Janyce G. Dyer, RN, DNSc, CS
Sheila M. Sparks, RN, DNSc, CS
Cynthia M. Taylor, RN, MS, CS, CNAA

Psychiatric Care and the Nursing Process

Nurses in all health care settings are taking on greater responsibility for providing psychiatric and mental health care. Consider the following trends:
- Psychiatric patients are moving out of specialty institutions into ambulatory care settings, long-term care facilities, and hospitals.
- Growing numbers of children and adolescents suffer from depressive disorders and substance abuse.
- Elderly patients live longer with chronic medical illness, commonly accompanied by severe emotional stress.
- Cost limits on psychiatric treatment are forcing emotionally distressed patients to seek help in outpatient and primary health care settings.
- According to one study, 40% of patients in all health care settings suffer from identifiable psychiatric disorders, such as phobias, alcohol dependence, and major depressive disorders.

Meeting the complex needs of patients with psychiatric and emotional disturbances requires a comprehensive approach to care, based on the nursing process. The cornerstone of clinical nursing, the nursing process is a systematic method for taking independent nursing action. Knowing how to apply this process is especially important in psychiatric care. Because you are frequently in the best position to develop a close, long-term relationship with the patient, you are the most capable of assessing his emotional and mental health care needs and identifying appropriate interventions.

Steps in the nursing process include:
- assessing the patient's problems
- forming a diagnostic statement
- identifying expected outcomes
- creating a plan of care to achieve expected outcomes
- implementing the plan or assigning others to implement it
- evaluating the plan's effectiveness.

ASSESSMENT

In the assessment stage, you will gather information from the patient's history, physical examination, and laboratory and diagnostic tests to determine his psychological and medical status.

When performing a psychiatric assessment, consider all aspects of the patient's functioning: biological, psychological, and social. All these affect the development and course of psychiatric illness and the patient's overall quality of life.

Even if a patient's specific problems in one area of functioning appear to dominate, be sure to perform a complete assessment. For example, in addition to identifying a schizophrenic patient's disordered thought processes, you should also assess him for possible physiologic complications of illness, including impaired skin integrity, malnutrition, fluid and electrolyte imbalance, or sexually transmitted diseases. Alternatively, you may need to assess a cardiac patient on a medical-surgical unit for depression or suicidal thoughts.

Individualizing your assessment
Psychiatric and mental health assessment must be tailored to the patient's individual needs. For example, the assessment of a patient who is under emotional stress because of a pending divorce will be different than one for a patient who complains vaguely of memory impairment, reports severe headaches, and is unable to follow a logical thought sequence.

In *Psychiatric Nursing Diagnoses*, assessment parameters are written in a standardized but flexible format. This will help you individualize your assessment based on the patient's history, his current problem, and any other relevant facts.

Taking the health history
A complete history provides the following information about a patient:
- demographic data for the patient and family
- the patient's chief complaint or concern
- the history of the present illness (or current health status)
- past psychiatric illness
- personal and developmental history
- family history
- social history
- general medical history
- cultural beliefs and practices that may affect health care outcomes.

To establish rapport, begin by asking the patient about himself; for example, what kind of work he does or what he's studying in school. Rather than "grill" the patient, use a conversational tone to convey warmth and your genuine interest in learning about him.

Determining the chief complaint
Sometimes the patient's chief complaint will be explicit ("I've been feeling very depressed."). Other times it may be vague ("I don't know why I'm here; my family brought me.") and will require follow-up questions.

Getting sufficient detail
Ask the patient to describe his experiences as specifically as possible. For example, if the patient reports hearing voices, ask when and where the problem started, how often he hears voices, whether they're male or female, and what happens just before he hears them. To observe his thought patterns (and reveal problems), try to get him to talk for 5 minutes, uninterrupted.

Continue to ask specific questions to help the patient focus on his problem. For example, if the patient asserts that voices are telling him to harm himself, ask, "When did you first hear these voices? Who was with you at the time? Where did this occur? What else was happening in your life? Have you told your family or friends about these voices? Have the voices led you to seek treatment before? Do you recognize any of these voices? Do you hear these voices as we speak?" and so forth. In addition, use sources, such as family members, medical records, or other health care professionals, to validate the patient's history.

Dealing with difficult topics
Don't avoid potentially embarrassing or threatening questions. Topics such as sexual experiences, drug and alcohol abuse, delusions and hallucinations, and suicidal thoughts may be particularly difficult to discuss. If the patient seems angry or offended, explain that these questions are necessary to complete a thorough history. The subject of suicide can be raised with such questions as, "Have you ever thought that life is not worth living?" or "Have you ever thought about taking your own life or killing yourself?"

Finally, give the patient an opportunity to ask questions. His questions usually tell much about what he's thinking and reflect his major concerns.

Performing a family assessment
Completing a family assessment is essential in psychiatric and mental health nursing. Family health history, communication patterns, roles and responsibilities, family resources, family members' perceptions of problems, and family stressors are important pieces of information for developing a comprehensive plan of care. Involving family members in the treatment plan will help them cope effectively with the challenges of caring for the patient.

Documenting health history data
Be sure to record assessment data in an organized fashion so the information will be meaningful to everyone involved in the patient's care. If possible,

use a hospital-provided patient questionnaire or computerized checklist. Your assessment will be easier if you ask the history questions in the same order every time. With experience, you'll know which questions to ask in specific patient situations. (See *Documenting your assessment,* page 4.)

The patient's health history becomes part of a permanent written record and serves as a subjective database that you and other members of the interdisciplinary team use to monitor the patient's progress.

Performing a physical examination
The physical examination provides objective data that may help to confirm or rule out suspicions raised during the health history interview.

Examination techniques
The most common approaches to a total systematic physical assessment are the head-to-toe and the major-body-systems methods. The head-to-toe method examines all parts of one body region before progressing to the next lower region. Proceed from left to right within each region to make symmetrical comparisons. The major-body-systems method systematically examines each body system in priority order or in a predesignated sequence. Both methods provide a logical, organized framework for collecting physical assessment data.

Chief complaint
When appropriate, consider planning your physical examination around the patient's chief complaint or concern. Begin by examining the most important body system or region. For ex-

Documenting your assessment

These guidelines, followed routinely, help ensure the accuracy of your documentation of the initial assessment.
- Document your findings as soon as possible after you take the health history and perform the physical examination.
- Document your assessment away from the patient's bedside. Jot down only key points while you're with the patient.
- Print or write legibly in ink.
- Be concise, specific, and exact when you describe your assessment findings.
- Answer every question on an assessment form. If a question doesn't apply to your patient, write "N/A" or "not applicable" in the space.
- If you delegate the job of filling out some sections of the form, remember that you must review the information and validate it to make sure it is correct.
- Directly quote the patient or family member who gave you information if you fear that summarizing it will lose some of the meaning.
- When recording a symptom, always report the behavioral indicator. For example, "Patient exhibits delusions of grandeur, as evidenced by the statement, 'I am Julius Caesar, Emperor of Rome.'"
- Record negative and positive findings. Note the absence of symptoms that other data indicate may be present. For example, if a patient reports recurrent periods of overwhelming fear of losing control and going crazy, ask him if he also experiences other common symptoms of a panic attack: palpitations, shortness of breath, nausea, chills or hot flashes, and feelings of derealization or depersonalization. If he answers "no," document the absence of these symptoms.
- Go back to the patient or other source to clarify or validate information that seems incomplete or inaccurate.
- Maintain the confidentiality of information documented in the patient's record. Remember, you have a legal and ethical responsibility to protect the patient's right to privacy.
- Demonstrate accountability for your assessment by signing your name to the areas you've completed.

ample, if the patient reports difficulty concentrating, begin with a neurologic assessment. This will help you identify priority problems promptly and reassure the patient that you are paying attention to his primary reason for seeking health care.

NURSING DIAGNOSIS

According to the North American Nursing Diagnosis Association (NANDA), a nursing diagnosis is a "clinical judgment about individual, family, or community responses to actual or potential health problems or to life processes." In other words, a nursing diagnosis describes a patient problem that can be addressed within the scope of nursing practice. It expresses your professional evaluation of the patient's clinical status, his emotional and social well-being, his responses to illness and treatment, and his nursing care needs. A nursing diagnosis may describe actual or potential health problems.

Developing a diagnosis

To formulate a nursing diagnosis, you must evaluate the essential assessment information. The following questions will help you zero in on appropriate diagnoses in psychiatric and mental health nursing:

- What are the patient's signs and symptoms?
- Which assessment findings are abnormal for the patient?
- Is the patient experiencing a psychiatric or medical emergency that must be addressed before his long-term psychological needs can be considered?
- How do particular behaviors affect the patient's emotional and physical well-being?
- What strengths or weaknesses does the patient have that affect his emotional or physical well-being?
- How does the patient's environment affect his health and emotional well-being?
- If the patient has a medical illness, how does he respond to it? How does it interfere with other aspects of his functioning? Does he want to improve his state of health?
- How does the patient deal with emotional distress? Does he express a desire for increased happiness, fulfillment, or social contact or for decreased anxiety or depression?
- What kinds of relationships does the patient have with his family and with other members of the community?
- What does the patient perceive as his greatest needs?

- Can the patient problems I've identified be treated by nursing interventions?
- Do I need to gather any other information for my diagnosis?

Writing a nursing diagnosis

Whenever possible, use terminology recommended by NANDA. NANDA diagnostic headings, combined with a "related to" statement, provide a clear picture of the patient's needs. Many NANDA diagnoses, from *Anxiety* to *Violence, high risk for: Self-directed*, are ideally suited to address a variety of psychosocial needs.

"Related to" statements describe factors that contribute to the development or continuation of the diagnosis. They may include environmental, physiologic, psychological, sociocultural, or spiritual circumstances identified during your analysis of assess-ment data.

Psychiatric Nursing Diagnoses includes more than 130 diagnostic labels with "related to" statements. These nursing diagnoses address the full range of needs encountered in psychiatric and mental health nursing. While you may want to individualize labels to more accurately reflect your patient's specific circumstances, the broad variety of alphabetically arranged examples will make it easy for you to locate an appropriate nursing diagnosis. (See *Case study: Developing a nursing diagnosis,* page 6.)

Here are a few examples of the diagnostic statements you'll find in this book:

- Anxiety related to obsessive-compulsive behavior

Case study: Developing a nursing diagnosis

The following case study provides an example of using assessment findings to formulate a nursing diagnosis in psychiatric care.

Peter Jones, age 31, was taken unconscious to the hospital by ambulance. His father reports that he found his son unresponsive in bed this morning. He adds that his son has been in treatment for "emotional problems" for the past 5 years but that he "has never seen him like this." He also explains that Peter has been taking "tranquilizers for his nerves" for some time, and that recently the dosage has been increased. Mr. Jones then shows you a bottle of chlorpromazine hydrochloride.

Nursing assessment

You initially assess the patient's vital signs: temperature, 106° F (41° C); pulse rate, 134 beats per minute; respiratory rate, 29 to 30 breaths per minute; blood pressure, 150/100 mm Hg.

You also note that Peter is mute, with rigid muscles and some posturing of his limbs. Because of Peter's signs and symptoms, his psychiatric and medication history, and your observations, your physical examination focuses on his cardiovascular, neurologic, genitourinary, musculoskeletal, integumentary, and respiratory systems. The doctor also orders the following laboratory tests: drug toxicology screen; serum creatine kinase, electrolyte, and blood urea nitrogen levels; complete blood count; and arterial blood gas values.

Formulation of the diagnosis

Results of the physical examination show catatonia with severe muscle rigidity, hypertension, diaphoresis, tachypnea, tachycardia, hyperpyrexia, dehydration, urinary incontinence, and incoherence. Laboratory tests show an elevated white blood cell count, elevated serum creatine kinase enzyme levels, and metabolic acidosis.

Given these findings and the patient's health history, you make a nursing diagnosis of *Ineffective thermoregulation related to neuroleptic malignant syndrome.* (See page 248 for the associated nursing plan of care.) Once you address Peter's immediate physiologic needs, you will assess him further to explore underlying emotional issues.

- Coping, family: Potential for growth related to marital conflict
- Coping, ineffective individual related to psychiatric disturbance
- Injury, high risk for related to use of restraints
- Personal identity disturbance related to history of sexual abuse
- Social isolation related to dysfunctional interpersonal relations
- Thought process alteration related to neuropsychiatric manifestations of AIDS

NANDA and the DSM-IV

Published by the American Psychiatric Association, the *Diagnostic and Statistical Manual of Mental Disorders,* Fourth edition *(DSM-IV),* is a standard interdisciplinary psychiatric diagnostic system designed to be used by all members of the mental health care team. The manual includes a complete description of psychiatric disorders and other conditions and describes diagnostic criteria that must be met to support each diagnosis. It provides codes for the classification of mental disorders; these codes are used by insurance companies to determine reimbursement for psychiatric services. (See DSM-IV *and multiaxial assessment,* page 8.) In *Psychiatric Nursing Diagnoses,* all psychiatric disorders listed in the associated disorders section of each plan of care conform to *DSM-IV* terminology.

The *DSM-IV* has many important features:
- It allows for interdisciplinary collaboration.
- It uses a descriptive, phenomenologic approach rather than a theoretical psychiatric orientation.
- It provides a level of diagnostic specificity appropriate for specialty practice.

Nursing diagnoses provide an excellent framework for addressing patient care issues that evolve from *DSM-IV* diagnoses. For example, a patient may be diagnosed with paranoid-type schizophrenia. You're not going to be able to develop nursing interventions that will cure him of schizophrenia. But you can use nursing diagnoses to address many problems related to schizophrenia that are clearly within the domain of nursing practice — problems such as self-care deficits, social isolation, role performance alteration, thought process alteration, ineffective family coping, and high risk for self-directed violence.

The American Nurses Association's *Standards of Psychiatric and Mental Health Nursing Practice* (1994) clearly acknowledges the importance of both *DSM-IV* and NANDA nursing diagnoses in psychiatric nursing practice.

OUTCOME IDENTIFICATION

During this phase of the nursing process, you will identify expected outcomes — realistic, measurable, patient-focused goals based on the patient's nursing diagnoses. Expected outcomes serve as the basis for evaluating the effectiveness of your nursing interventions.

In *Psychiatric Nursing Diagnoses,* outcomes are organized into three categories, based on the time frame and patient acuity:
- *Initial outcomes:* top-priority goals that must be met as soon as possible to secure the patient's welfare or stabilize his condition
- *Interim outcomes:* goals that continue for the duration of the patient's care
- *Discharge outcomes:* goals that the patient should meet by discharge and goals that he should meet thereafter to ensure continuity of care.

Writing outcome statements
Always use a specific action verb that focuses on the patient's behavior when documenting an expected outcome statement. For example, begin with *demonstrates, verbalizes,* or *states* to give members of the health care team clear guidelines for evaluating the patient's progress.

When writing outcomes, identify a target time by which the outcome should be achieved. Make sure the goal time frames are appropriate and realistic. Be flexible enough to adjust the date if the patient needs more time to respond to the intervention or to incorporate new behaviors into his lifestyle. Consult with the patient and

DSM-IV and multiaxial assessment

The *Diagnostic and Statistical Manual of Mental Disorders,* Fourth edition *(DSM-IV),* is the most important reference for diagnosing and classifying mental disorders. The manual provides a complete description of each disorder and specifies symptoms that must be present to support a diagnosis. It lists the current numeric codes for most mental disorders.

In the *DSM-IV* multiaxial assessment system, the patient is evaluated on five axes, each of which refers to a different domain of information that may help you plan treatment and predict outcome. The multiaxial assessment system is comprehensive; it covers mental disorders and general medical conditions, psychosocial and environmental problems, and levels of functioning that might be overlooked if assessment focused on a single problem. The five axes are:

- Axis I: Clinical disorders and other conditions that may be the focus of clinical attention
- Axis II: Personality disorders and mental retardation
- Axis III: General medical conditions
- Axis IV: Psychosocial and environmental problems
- Axis V: Global assessment of functioning.

Understanding components of the multiaxial system

To use the multiaxial assessment system effectively, you must understand its components.
- Axes I and II include all the mental disorders in the *DSM-IV* and represent psychological functioning.
- Axis III is used to assess general medical conditions that are potentially relevant to understanding or managing the patient's mental disorder; it represents physical functioning.
- Axis IV is used to report psychosocial and environmental problems that may affect the diagnosis, treatment, and prognosis of mental disorders (Axes I and II).
- Axis V is used to assess overall level of functioning. Axes IV and V combined represent a patient's social functioning.

The multiaxial system encourages consideration of biological, psychological, and social factors and recognition of all the related functions of an individual, which is essential to psychiatric nursing.

family members about outcomes to help ensure their participation in care.

The following are examples of outcome statements you will find in *Psychiatric Nursing Diagnoses*:

- Patient discusses feelings and behaviors related to phobia and phobic triggers.
- Patient consumes at least _____ calories daily.
- Patient cooperates with psychiatric evaluation and attends teaching sessions, individual and family counseling, and appropriate support group.
- Patient engages in conversation and activities with his family, caregivers, and other support people.
- Patient expresses understanding of goals of hospitalization and treatment.
- Child participates in activities appropriate for his age and developmental stage.
- Patient's family members and spouse or companion express understanding that acquired immunodefi-

ciency syndrome is a disease, not a punishment.
- Patient indicates through gestures, behavior, writing, or speaking that he is coming to terms with his impaired speech.

PLANNING

Planning involves four stages:
- assigning priorities to the nursing diagnoses
- establishing expected outcomes (goals)
- selecting appropriate nursing actions (interventions)
- documenting the nursing diagnoses, expected outcomes, and nursing interventions in the plan of care.

Prioritize interventions based on the patient's clinical status. For example, if a patient exhibits suicidal behavior, you'll need to take measures to maintain his safety before helping him to differentiate effective and ineffective coping strategies.

Plan of care

The nursing plan of care refers to a written plan of action designed to help you deliver quality patient care. It includes relevant nursing diagnoses, expected outcomes, and nursing interventions. It usually forms a permanent part of the patient's health record.

Benefits of writing a plan of care

A plan of care that's well conceived and properly written helps decrease the risk of incomplete or incorrect care by:
- giving direction
- providing continuity of care

- establishing communication between you and nurses on other shifts, other members of the interdisciplinary care team, and your patient.

You may write your plan of care from scratch or you may use a computer-generated form or customized standard plan. Some health care facilities use protocols or critical paths that give sequential instructions for treating specific problems. Nearly all care-planning formats include space in which to document the nursing diagnoses, expected outcomes, and nursing interventions and, in many hospitals, you may also document assessment data and discharge planning.

Write your plan of care in concise, specific terms that other health care team members can follow. Because the patient's problems and needs will likely change, you'll have to review your plan frequently and modify it when necessary. (See *Guidelines for writing the plan of care,* page 10.)

Care planning for students

Writing a plan of care helps students understand the nursing process and improve writing skills. More importantly, it shows how to apply classroom and textbook knowledge to practice. Longer than standard plans, the student plan progresses, step-by-step, from assessment to evaluation. However, some schools model the student plan of care on the plan used by the affiliated hospital, adding a space for the scientific rationale for each nursing intervention.

Guidelines for writing the plan of care

These tips will help you write a plan of care that is accurate and useful.
- Write your patient's plan of care in ink. It's part of the permanent record. Sign your name.
- Be specific. Don't use vague terms or generalities. Later, they'll puzzle you and others.
- Never use abbreviations that may be confused with other similar ones.
- Take time to review all your assessment data before you select an approach for each problem. (*Note:* If you can't complete the initial assessment, immediately note "insufficient data" on your records.)
- Write a specific patient outcome for each problem or need you identify, and record a target date for its completion.
- Avoid setting an initial goal that's too high to be achieved. For example, suppose the newly admitted patient has trouble communicating with others and reports being isolated from social contact for many years. Your eventual goal may be to encourage him to participate in group activities; however, several preliminary patient outcomes must be achieved before he will be ready for group activity.
- Correlate nursing interventions with your outcomes, keeping in mind the time frame for care and patient acuity. Initial interventions should focus on patient monitoring and the immediate priorities of patient care. Interim interventions should focus on nursing measures to continue patient progress once initial goals have been achieved. Discharge interventions should focus on what to teach the patient and family before discharge, referrals for follow-up care, or ongoing monitoring requirements.
- Make each nursing intervention specific.
- Make sure nursing interventions match the resources and capabilities of staff members.
- Be creative when you write your patient's plan of care; include a drawing of an innovative procedure if it will make your directions more specific. Use the information in *Psychiatric Nursing Diagnoses* as a starting point; then individualize your plan based on your patient's circumstances and your own knowledge, talents, and experiences.

IMPLEMENTATION

During this phase, you put your plan of care into action, using your nursing interventions to help the patient cope with psychological and social problems and meet his health care needs. When coordinating implementation, you may seek help from other caregivers, the patient, and the patient's family. (See *Nursing interventions: Four types.*)

Examples of interventions commonly used in psychiatric and mental health nursing include:
- assessing and monitoring (for example, recording vital signs or conducting a Mini–Mental Status Examination)
- taking steps to ensure the patient's safety (for example, removing any sharp objects from his room if he is at risk for suicide)
- monitoring the effects of psychotropic medications

Nursing interventions: Four types

The list below groups interventions performed in psychiatric mental health nursing into four types.

- *Individual interventions:* Measures carried out to meet the mental health care needs of individual patients. Examples include monitoring the effects of prescribed drugs (some advanced practice nurses may have the authority to prescribe drugs), patient teaching, implementing cognitive and behavioral strategies, interpersonal counseling, social skills training, and helping the patient with activities of daily living.
- *Family interventions:* Measures carried out on behalf of the patient's spouse, children, relatives, or partner. Examples include therapy, counseling, teaching, demonstrating techniques for caring for the patient, or helping family members improve coping skills.
- *Group interventions:* Measures performed to meet the needs of group members. Examples include conducting group therapy, encouraging expression of feelings in a group setting, and facilitating group interaction.
- *Staff interventions:* Measures carried out to help staff members deal with issues surrounding patient care, such as responding to manipulative behavior or grieving for terminally ill patients. Examples include group therapy, individual counseling, and referral to a psychiatric clinical nurse specialist.

- helping the patient to be more comfortable and assisting him with activities of daily living
- managing the environment (for example, controlling noise to help reduce sensory overload)
- actively listening to the patient's concerns, always being careful to maintain a nonjudgmental attitude
- role-modeling appropriate behaviors
- providing food and fluids or skin care, if needed
- teaching, counseling, and aiding psychotherapy
- setting limits on self-destructive behavior
- using restraints, if necessary, and making sure all legal and safety precautions are carefully observed
- conducting family, group, or individual therapy
- referring the patient to appropriate agencies or services

- seeking assistance from other staff members or resources to help meet the patient's needs.

Documenting interventions

Implementation isn't complete until you've documented each intervention, the time it occurred, the patient's response, and any other pertinent information. Remember that each entry must relate to a nursing diagnosis.

EVALUATION

In this phase of the nursing process, you assess your plan's effectiveness by answering such questions as the following:

- How has the patient progressed in terms of the plan's projected outcomes?
- Does the patient have new needs?
- Does the plan of care need revision?

Steps in the evaluation process

Include the patient, family members, and other health care professionals in the evaluation. Use the plan of care's expected outcomes as your evaluation criteria. Collect information from all available sources and include your own observations. Compare the patient's response to nursing interventions to the evaluation criteria, and consider the following questions:

- Did the patient meet the plan of care's outcome criteria?
- Has his condition improved, deteriorated, or stayed the same?
- Were the nursing diagnoses accurate?
- Have the patient's nursing needs been met?
- Which nursing interventions should I revise or discontinue?
- Why did the patient fail to meet some goals (if applicable)?
- Should I reorder priorities? Revise goals and outcome criteria?

Analyze your findings and modify the plan of care as needed.

The evaluation statements included in each plan of care in *Psychiatric Nursing Diagnoses* provide a guide to documenting the evaluation phase of the nursing process. For example, if the patient is at risk for suicide, appropriate evaluation statements might read, "Patient makes commitment not to act upon suicidal thoughts" and "Patient does not harm self while in hospital."

Continue to reevaluate every step in the nursing process for as long as you care for the patient. Due to the complex nature of psychiatric and emotional problems, patients may need a stable therapeutic relationship over a long period of time. Always remain nonjudgmental and open to the possibility of patient recovery throughout the care process.

PART ONE

ADULT MENTAL HEALTH

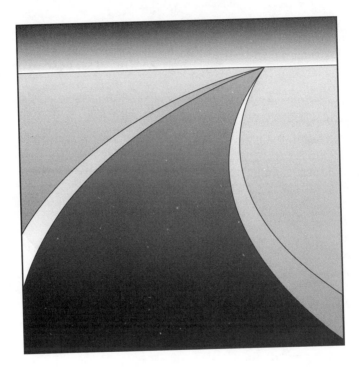

Adjustment impairment

related to loss of control

DEFINITION

Poor coping resulting from a change in health status and increased dependence on others

ASSESSMENT

Cultural status
- *Demographics:* age, sex, level of education, occupation, nationality, race, ethnic group
- *History:* beliefs, values, and attitudes about health and illness; health customs, practices, and rituals
- *Diagnostic test:* Cultural Assessment Guide

Family status
- *History:* marital status, family role, coping patterns
- *Diagnostic test:* Family Genogram

Psychological status
- *History:* self-esteem and self-image, functional ability, independence level, problem-solving and decision-making skills, anxiety level, statements indicating perceived locus of control, behaviors related to anticipated loss of control

Self-care status
- *Observation:* functional ability (muscle tone, size, and strength; range of motion; coordination), daily activities (dressing, grooming, bathing, toileting, and hygiene)

DEFINING CHARACTERISTICS
- Aggressive behavior
- Agitation
- Anxiety
- Apathy
- Fear of losing control over self and situation
- Increased dependence on others
- Refusal to comply with treatment
- Unrealistic expectations of self or others
- Withdrawal from social activity

ASSOCIATED DISORDERS

Acquired immunodeficiency syndrome, anxiety, cancer, cerebrovascular accident, diabetes mellitus, dependent personality disorder, major depressive disorder

EXPECTED OUTCOMES

Initial outcomes
- Patient participates in health care regimen.
- Patient participates in planning care.
- Patient discusses fear of losing control.

Interim outcomes
- Patient accepts help with daily activities.
- Patient accepts help making daily decisions.
- Patient reports decreased anxiety.

Discharge outcomes
- Patient seeks help from others.
- Patient reports increased acceptance of change in health status.
- Patient identifies ability to maintain control over various aspects of his life.

INTERVENTIONS AND RATIONALES

Initial interventions
- Encourage the patient to participate in planning care *to increase his sense of control.*
- Encourage him to express his feelings about loss of control *to convey to him unconditional acceptance and positive regard.*

Interim interventions
- Help the patient identify and contact sources of assistance *to foster his ability to accept help.*
- Help the patient identify parts of his life where he can maintain control *to reduce his feelings of powerlessness and increase his involvement with a team effort.*

Discharge interventions
- Provide the opportunity for others with similar health problems to speak with the patient, companion, or family *to foster a support network and to provide a role model for the patient.*
- Help the patient identify his capabilities and point out aspects of his life where he remains in control *to foster a sense of mastery and empowerment.*

EVALUATION STATEMENTS

Patient:
- identifies at least two areas in which he can maintain control.
- demonstrates the ability to cope with changes in health status.
- identifies support network for help after discharge.

DOCUMENTATION
- Results of diagnostic tests
- Patient's verbal and nonverbal expressions about loss of control
- Patient's ability to participate in care
- Patient's improved coping strategies
- Evaluation statements.

Anxiety
related to obsessive-compulsive behavior

DEFINITION

Feeling of threat or danger to self arising from an unidentifiable source

ASSESSMENT

Cultural status
- *Demographics:* age, sex, level of education, occupation, nationality, race, ethnic group
- *History:* beliefs, values, and attitudes about health and illness; health customs, practices, and rituals
- *Diagnostic test:* Cultural Assessment Guide

Family status
- *History:* marital status, family composition, family roles
- *Family communication:* style and quality of communication, methods of conflict resolution
- *Physical and emotional needs:* family's ability to meet patient's physical and emotional needs
- *Family health history:* bipolar disorder, depression, suicide, schizophre-

nia, mental retardation, substance abuse, stress-related illness, non-psychiatric illness
- *Diagnostic tests:* Family Genogram, Family Assessment Device

Psychological status
- *Current illness:* precipitating events; evidence of acting out behavior; alcohol or drug abuse
- *Signs and symptoms:* withdrawal; lack of eye contact; aggressiveness; changes in appetite, energy level, personal hygiene, self-image, self-esteem, sleep pattern, sexual drive, competence
- *Childhood development:* birth order, reactions to illness, losses through separation or death, developmental milestones, intelligence quotient, personality traits, school performance, relationships with peers, social interactions, experience of being nurtured, maladaptive, ritualistic, or antisocial behaviors
- *Adolescent development:* involvement in church, synagogue, or clubs; recreational interests; relationship with parents, authority figures, or therapists; sexual activities; academic and social comfort and performance; level of independence; ability to connect emotionally with other people
- *Adult development:* level of independence; sexual behavior; educational, military, and occupational histories; dating and marital history; spirituality; reactions to illness and disability; hobbies and recreational activities; quantity and quality of support systems
- *Diagnostic tests:* Brief Psychiatric Rating Scale, Hamilton Rating Scale for Depression, Behavioral Checklist, Minnesota Multiphasic Personality Inventory, Social Adjustment Scale, Wechsler Adult Intelligence Survey, Yale-Brown Obsessive Compulsive Scale, National Institute of Mental Health Global Obsessive Compulsive Scale

Cardiovascular status
- *History:* cardiovascular disease, exercise patterns, use of caffeine
- *Physical examination:* general observations, vital signs, precordial inspection, carotid and apical pulse rates, normal and extra heart sounds
- *Signs and symptoms:* palpitations, syncope, dyspnea, chest pain, fatigue
- *Laboratory tests:* complete blood count and differential
- *Diagnostic tests:* electrocardiography, echocardiography

Gastrointestinal status
- *History:* alcohol use, medications
- *Physical examination:* abdominal inspection, palpation and auscultation, stool characteristics, bowel sounds
- *Signs and symptoms:* abdominal pain, nausea, vomiting, belching, gagging, change in appetite, weight change, constipation, diarrhea
- *Laboratory tests:* gastric analysis, serum electrolyte levels, urinalysis
- *Diagnostic tests:* upper GI series, barium enema, computed tomography scan of abdomen, magnetic resonance imaging of abdomen, barium swallow

Neurologic status
- *History:* usual sleep pattern; energy level after sleep; rest and relaxation patterns; use of caffeine, alcohol, amphetamines, sedatives

- *Mental status:* appearance and attitude, level of consciousness, motor activity, thought and speech, mood and affect, perceptions, orientation, memory, general information, calculations, capacity to read and write, visual-spatial ability, attention span, abstraction, judgment and insight
- *Physical examination:* motor and sensory function, reflexes, tardive dyskinesia or other adverse drug effects
- *Signs and symptoms:* restlessness, tremors, paresthesia, paresis, numbness and tingling, tics, fasciculation, short-term memory loss
- *Laboratory tests:* drug toxicology, thyroid function
- *Diagnostic tests:* Folstein Mini-Mental Health Status Examination, lumbar puncture, electroencephalography, magnetic resonance imaging

Nutritional status
- *History:* usual exercise pattern, typical daily food intake
- *Medical conditions:* nutritional deficiencies, obesity or cachexia, anorexia, bulimia
- *Physical examination:* height, weight
- *Signs and symptoms:* weight loss or gain, nausea and vomiting, fainting, pallor, irritability
- *Laboratory tests:* serum albumin and total protein levels

Respiratory status
- *History:* tobacco use, exposure to occupational hazards, medications
- *Physical examination:* skin color, temperature, and turgor; color of lips and nails; symmetry of chest expansion; rate, depth, and pattern of respirations; auscultation and percussion of lung fields; tracheal position; palpation for thoracic excursion and fremitus
- *Signs and symptoms:* dyspnea, cough
- *Laboratory tests:* arterial blood gas levels
- *Diagnostic tests:* pulmonary function studies, ventilation-perfusion scan

Self-care status
- *Observation:* functional ability (muscle tone, size, and strength; range of motion; coordination), daily activities (dressing, grooming, bathing, toileting, and hygiene)
- *Diagnostic tests:* Functional Ability Scale, Self-Care Assessment Tool

DEFINING CHARACTERISTICS

- Attempt to suppress unwanted thoughts, which worsens anxiety
- Excessive criticism of others
- Excessive inner control, demonstrated by moralistic attitude, frequent "I should" statements, and a negative perception of pleasurable activity
- Excessive self-restraint, demonstrated by caution, deliberation, pensiveness, grave appearance, neatness, frugality, emotional distance with little affect
- Expression of hostility through ritualistic behavior
- Inability to say no to requests from others
- Indecision, insecurity
- Interpersonal relationships characterized by alternating periods of closeness and distance
- Physiologic symptoms of anxiety, such as palpitations, nausea, hot and cold flashes, dizziness, dry mouth, diaphoresis

- Recognition that behavior is irrational despite compulsion to perform ritualistic behaviors
- Repetitive actions or rituals, such as obligatory hand washing, touching, counting; more elaborate ceremonies performed in an exact order
- Repetitive, unwanted thoughts
- Speech filled with facts and details
- Stubbornness

ASSOCIATED DISORDERS

Affective disorders, anorexia nervosa, anxiety disorders, bulimia nervosa, obsessive-compulsive disorder, paraphilia, schizophrenia, substance abuse, Tourette's disorder

EXPECTED OUTCOMES

Initial outcomes
- Patient's ritualistic behavior doesn't produce harmful effects.
- Patient reduces the amount of time spent each day on obsessive and ritualistic behavior.
- Patient performs activities of daily living.

Interim outcomes
- Patient expresses feelings of anxiety as they occur.
- Patient expresses anger in socially acceptable ways.
- Patient makes fewer attempts to exert control over self and environment.

Discharge outcomes
- Patient copes with stress without excessive obsessive-compulsive behavior.
- Patient forms a relationship without excessive dependence or aloofness.

- Patient begins to develop self-esteem.

INTERVENTIONS AND RATIONALES

Initial interventions
- Understand your own feelings toward the patient *to prevent prejudices from interfering with treatment.* Be aware that anxiety causes the patient's problem and accept his need to obsess or ritualize, *to minimize his guilt feelings.*
- Don't attempt to thwart ritualistic behavior. *Forcing the patient to change his behavior can lead to panic and, possibly, psychosis.*
- If rituals interfere with nutrition, place the patient on a feeding schedule *to promote health and prevent indecisiveness about meals.*
- If the patient practices washing or "picking" rituals, take steps, such as providing hand lotion and rubber gloves, bandaging his hands, and trimming his fingernails, *to prevent skin breakdown.*
- If needed, set consistent limits on self-destructive behavior *to promote the patient's physical safety. Consistent limits will help keep the patient from vacillating.*
- Allow the patient ample time to perform ritualistic activity, within reasonable limits, *to reduce his anxiety.*
- Don't attempt to reason with the patient about his obsession. *The patient already recognizes the irrationality of his symptoms. Your explanations may worsen his feelings of inadequacy.*
- Avoid initiating discussion of the patient's ritual behavior or criticizing it

to avoid further damage to his already low self-esteem.

▪ Change the patient's environment as little as possible, and explain any necessary changes *to avoid increasing anxiety and causing a greater need for compulsive behaviors.*

▪ Provide simple structured tasks requiring concentration *to help the patient organize his free time.*

▪ Tell the patient what to do rather than ask him, *to relieve him of decision-making anxieties and limit the time devoted to repetitive thinking.*

▪ Approach the patient in a caring way. For example, you might say, "I've noticed you've made your bed three times today; that must be very tiring for you." *This demonstrates that you are aware of the patient's behavior and his feelings.*

Interim interventions

▪ Encourage the patient's open expression of emotions *to help him cope effectively with feelings that usually remain repressed.*

▪ When possible, preempt ritual behavior by helping the patient meet psychological needs that are motivating this behavior. For example, if the patient seeks attention through ritual behavior, ignore the ritual but pay ample attention to him at other times. *This may help him realize that gains can be achieved without ritual behavior. If ignored, negative behavior is less likely to be repeated.*

▪ Teach relaxation techniques *to counteract anxiety.*

▪ Teach assertiveness skills. *Learning to say no to other people's demands can help the patient manage anger.*

▪ Tell the patient about possible biological and neuroendocrine causes of obsessive-compulsive symptoms *to help him avoid guilt and embarrassment caused by assuming that his symptoms represent unresolved psychological conflicts.*

▪ Support family members' or a companion's efforts to cope with the patient's obsessive-compulsive symptoms *to allay their anxiety as well as the patient's.*

Discharge interventions

▪ When the patient is ready to overcome ritual behavior, assist in setting goals for limiting unwanted behavior *to help motivate him to change.*

▪ Promote the patient's self-esteem by encouraging participation in activities, beginning with simple objectives and praising his efforts. *Feelings of accomplishment increase his sense of worth and decrease anxiety, thus decreasing the need for rituals.*

▪ When possible, help the patient channel ritualistic behavior into constructive outlets, such as writing, painting, or physical activity, *to develop his self-esteem.*

▪ Confirm that the patient understands his medication, including indication, dosage, adverse effects, contraindications, habituation and withdrawal symptoms, and follow-up care. *Participation in his own care, as an informed and responsible adult, increases his independence and self-esteem.*

▪ Refer family members and the patient to a support group *for continued learning and support.*

▪ Encourage continued therapy *to retain gains and prevent relapse.*

EVALUATION STATEMENTS

Patient:

- doesn't harm himself.
- shows less evidence of ritualized behavior and reports that obsessive thoughts are less frequent.
- performs daily toileting efficiently, unhampered by distracting rituals.
- eats at least 80% of meals without being distracted by obsessive thoughts or rituals.
- achieves 6 to 8 hours of uninterrupted sleep each night.
- maintains intact and supple skin.
- expresses anxiety.
- voices anger or expresses it through writing, painting, recreation, physical activity, or other healthy outlets.
- participates in hobbies or other diversional activities.
- uses problem-solving skills, maintains balance of work and play, and displays well-balanced use of psychological defense mechanisms.
- demonstrates less perfectionism and decreases moralizing.
- appears relaxed and assertive, thinks and behaves moderately, and exhibits greater affect.

DOCUMENTATION

- Observations of ritualistic behavior
- Statements indicating obsessive thoughts
- Nursing interventions
- Patient's response to nursing interventions
- Patient's ability to accept less control over self and environment
- Patient's achievement of mutually established goals
- Evaluation statements.

Anxiety

related to phobic reactions

DEFINITION

Feeling of threat or danger to self arising from an unidentifiable source

ASSESSMENT

Cultural status

- *Demographics:* age, sex, level of education, occupation, nationality, race, ethnic group
- *History:* beliefs, values, and attitudes about health and illness; health customs, practices, and rituals
- *Diagnostic test:* Cultural Assessment Guide

Psychological status

- *Current illness:* level of anxiety, use of escape-avoidance behaviors, use of defense mechanisms, alcohol or drug abuse
- *Signs and symptoms:* withdrawal; lack of eye contact; aggressiveness; changes in appetite, energy level, personal hygiene, self-image, self-esteem, sleep pattern, sexual drive; periods of excessive crying
- *Childhood development:* birth order, reactions to illness, losses through separation or death, developmental milestones, intelligence quotient, personality traits, school performance, relationships with peers, experience of being nurtured, maladaptive behaviors
- *Adolescent development:* involvement in church, synagogue, or clubs; recreational interests; relationship

with parents, authority figures, or therapists; sexual activities; academic and social comfort and performance; level of independence; ability to connect emotionally with other people
- *Adult development:* level of independence; social activities; sexual behavior; academic, military, and occupational histories; spirituality; reactions to illness and disability; hobbies and recreational activities; quantity and quality of support systems
- *Diagnostic tests:* Brief Psychiatric Rating Scale, Hamilton Rating Scale for Depression, Behavioral Checklist, Minnesota Multiphasic Personality Inventory, Social Adjustment Scale, Wechsler Adult Intelligence Survey, Spielberger State-Trait Anxiety Inventory

Family status
- *History:* marital status, family composition, family roles
- *Family communication:* style and quality of communication, methods of conflict resolution
- *Physical and emotional needs:* family's ability to meet patient's physical and emotional needs
- *Family health history:* bipolar disorder, depression, suicide, schizophrenia, mental retardation, substance abuse, stress-related illness, medical illness
- *Diagnostic tests:* Family Genogram, Family Assessment Device

Cardiovascular status
- *History:* cardiovascular disease
- *Physical examination:* general observations, vital signs, precordial inspection, carotid and apical pulse rates, normal and extra heart sounds

- *Signs and symptoms:* palpitations, syncope, dyspnea, chest pain, fatigue, exercise patterns, use of caffeine
- *Laboratory tests:* complete blood count and differential
- *Diagnostic tests:* electrocardiography, echocardiography

Gastrointestinal status
- *History:* smoking, alcohol use, medications
- *Physical examination:* abdominal inspection, palpation and auscultation, stool characteristics, bowel sounds
- *Signs and symptoms:* abdominal pain, nausea, vomiting, belching, gagging, change in appetite, weight change, constipation, diarrhea
- *Laboratory tests:* gastric analysis, serum electrolyte levels, urinalysis
- *Diagnostic tests:* upper GI series, barium enema, computed tomography scan of abdomen, magnetic resonance imaging of abdomen, barium swallow

Neurologic status
- *History:* usual sleep pattern; energy level after sleep; rest and relaxation patterns; use of caffeine, alcohol, amphetamines, sleeping aids
- *Mental status:* appearance and attitude, level of consciousness, motor activity, thought and speech, mood and affect, perceptions, orientation, memory, general information, calculations, capacity to read and write, visual-spatial ability, attention span, abstraction, judgment and insight
- *Physical examination:* motor and sensory function, reflexes, tardive dyskinesia or other adverse effects of medication

- *Signs and symptoms:* restlessness, tremors, paresthesia, paresis, numbness and tingling, tics, fasciculation, short-term memory loss
- *Laboratory tests:* drug toxicology, thyroid function
- *Diagnostic tests:* Folstein Mini-Mental Health Status Examination, lumbar puncture, electroencephalography, magnetic resonance imaging

Nutritional status
- *History:* usual exercise pattern, typical daily food intake
- *Medical conditions:* nutritional deficiencies, obesity or cachexia, anorexia, bulimia
- *Physical examination:* height, weight
- *Signs and symptoms:* weight loss or gain, nausea and vomiting, fainting, pallor, irritability
- *Laboratory tests:* serum albumin and total protein levels

Respiratory status
- *History:* tobacco use, exposure to occupational hazards, medications
- *Physical examination:* skin color, temperature, and turgor; color of lips and nails; symmetry of chest expansion; rate, depth, and pattern of respirations; auscultation and percussion of lung fields; tracheal position; palpation for thoracic excursion and fremitus
- *Signs and symptoms:* dyspnea, cough
- *Laboratory tests:* arterial blood gas analysis
- *Diagnostic tests:* pulmonary function studies, ventilation-perfusion scan

Self-care status
- *Observation:* functional ability (muscle tone, size, and strength; range of motion; coordination), daily activities (dressing, grooming, bathing, toileting, and hygiene)
- *Diagnostic tests:* Functional Ability Scale, Self-Care Assessment Tool

DEFINING CHARACTERISTICS

- Agoraphobia
- Behavior meant to escape or avoid feared event (reclusiveness, avoidance)
- Depersonalization
- Feelings of weakness or failure and low self-esteem
- High anxiety when confronting feared situation, object, or activity
- Impaired social, occupational, educational, and marital functioning
- Obsessive tendencies
- Panic attacks
- Physical symptoms, such as palpitations, restlessness, decreased concentration, muscle tension, irritability, sleep disturbances, and GI problems, when confronting feared object
- Recognition of irrationality of behavior
- Social phobias (such as fear of public speaking or urinating in public toilet)
- Specific phobias (such as snakes, airplanes, fire)
- Use of drugs and alcohol to promote relaxation of phobic reactions

ASSOCIATED DISORDERS

Acute stress disorder, anorexia nervosa, generalized anxiety disorder, panic disorder, posttraumatic stress disorder, schizophrenia, social phobia, specific phobia, substance abuse, thyroid disease

EXPECTED OUTCOMES

Initial outcomes
- Patient identifies situations that precipitate phobic reactions.
- Patient connects life events to current problems with anxiety.
- Patient discusses feelings and behaviors related to phobia and phobic triggers.

Interim outcomes
- Patient verbalizes understanding of the biological and psychological components of phobic illness.
- Patient sets limits on phobic behavior, when ready.
- Patient develops more effective coping behaviors.
- Patient exhibits less guilt and anxiety related to phobias.

Discharge outcomes
- Patient maintains autonomy and independence without being handicapped by phobic behavior.
- Patient verbalizes understanding of medications, and importance of continued therapy or treatment.
- Patient agrees to comply with ongoing medication and follow-up care.

INTERVENTIONS AND RATIONALES

Initial interventions
- Communicate to the patient your acceptance of him and his phobic behavior *to avoid forcing him to change before he is ready and causing him to panic.*

- Review the results of the patient's history, laboratory tests, physical examination, and observations of his behavior *to detect possible physiologic causes of anxious and phobic symptoms.*
- Evaluate the patient's suicide potential. *The phobic patient's withdrawal, further depression, anxiety, and frustration may lead to suicidal thoughts or attempts.*
- Provide for the patient's safety and comfort and monitor fluid and food intake *to keep his phobias from further interfering with his health.*
- No matter how ridiculous the patient's phobia appears, do not trivialize it. *To the patient, this behavior is a vital coping mechanism, and a superficial pep talk or ridicule can worsen his situation.*
- Reassure the patient who perceives his own behavior as silly that the behavior serves as a way of coping with anxiety *to help him feel better about himself.*
- Don't let the patient withdraw completely, but encourage small steps to overcome fear by interaction with a supportive family member or friend *to avoid isolation.*
- Give the patient a chance to ventilate feelings *to reduce his tendency to suppress or repress feelings.*
- Explore "triggers" that precipitate the patient's phobic reactions and anxiety and their impact on his life *to help him understand his illness.*
- Develop an individualized program of care with a multidisciplinary treatment team *to find the most effective treatment for the patient's phobia. Some phobias respond well to medications; others, to cognitive or behavioral approaches.*

Interim interventions

- Tell the patient about possible bio-chemical and neuroendocrine causes of phobias *to help him avoid guilt and embarrassment related to the common assumption that phobias represent unre-solved psychological conflicts.*
- Encourage the patient's participa-tion in treatments, but do not force in-sight. *Challenging the patient may ag-gravate him or cause him to panic.*
- Help the patient set limits on his phobic behavior when he's ready. Al-low the patient to be afraid, *to show that fear is simply a feeling, neither right nor wrong.* Discuss openly with him the consequences of fear and anx-iety in his life *to encourage him to take steps to manage his own problem.*
- Encourage the patient not to run away when afraid *to help him learn that fear can be faced and managed.*
- Teach the patient cognitive and be-havioral management strategies, such as interrupting thoughts and behav-iors that usually result in a panic at-tack (distraction), challenging nega-tive thoughts, and focusing on the time-limited nature of panic attacks and on the "here and now," *to help the patient develop strategies for controlling panic attacks.*
- Teach the patient relaxation tech-niques (guided imagery, deep breath-ing, muscle relaxation) and desensiti-zation techniques (gradual exposure to phobic stimulus) *to help the patient assume self-control and a sense of mas-tery over panic attacks.*

Discharge interventions

- Help the patient develop his own techniques for dealing with fears *to es-tablish alternatives to escape or avoid-ance behaviors.*
- Offer positive feedback about the pa-tient's progress *to help him appreciate his accomplishments.*
- Suggest that the patient and family members become involved in support groups, such as the Anxiety Disorders Association of America, *for continued learning and support.*
- Confirm that the patient under-stands his medication, including the indication, dosage, adverse effects, contraindications, habituation, with-drawal symptoms, and follow-up care. *Participation in his own care as an in-formed and responsible adult increases the patient's independence and self-esteem.*
- Encourage continued therapy *to re-tain gains made during hospitalization and prevent relapse.*

EVALUATION STATEMENTS

Patient:
- demonstrates reduced physical symptoms of anxiety, improved con-centration, and reduced preoccupa-tion with fears.
- discusses possible relationship be-tween anxiety and past and present ex-periences.
- lists stressors that trigger a panic re-action.
- limits phobic behavior, when ready.
- participates in relaxation, cognitive, behavioral, and desensitization thera-pies and learns to better manage stress, health, and responsibilities.
- makes decisions and shows greater independence.
- decreases behavior that limits spon-taneous activity.

DOCUMENTATION

- Diagnostic test results
- Observations of phobic reactions
- Nursing interventions to reduce anxiety and increase coping
- Patient's response to nursing interventions
- Patient's preferred methods for limiting phobic reactions
- Evaluation statements.

Anxiety

related to situational crisis

DEFINITION

Feeling of threat or danger to self arising from fear of death or disability

ASSESSMENT

Cultural status

- *Demographics:* age, sex, level of education, occupation, nationality, race, ethnic group
- *History:* beliefs, values, and attitudes about health and illness; health customs, practices, and rituals
- *Diagnostic test:* Cultural Assessment Guide

Psychological status

- *Current illness:* level of anxiety, use of escape-avoidance behaviors, use of defense mechanisms, alcohol or drug abuse
- *Signs and symptoms:* withdrawal; lack of eye contact; aggressiveness; changes in appetite, energy level, personal hygiene, self-image, self-esteem, sleep pattern, sexual drive; periods of excessive crying
- *Childhood development:* birth order, reactions to illness, losses through separation or death, developmental milestones, intelligence quotient, personality traits, school performance, relationships with peers, experience of being nurtured, maladaptive behaviors
- *Adolescent development:* involvement in church, synagogue, or clubs; recreational interests; relationship with parents, authority figures, or therapists; sexual activities; academic and social comfort and performance; level of independence; ability to connect emotionally with other people
- *Adult development:* level of independence; social activities; sexual behavior; academic, military, and occupational histories; spirituality; reactions to illness and disability; hobbies and recreational activities; quantity and quality of support systems
- *Diagnostic tests:* Brief Psychiatric Rating Scale, Hamilton Rating Scale for Depression, Behavioral Checklist, Minnesota Multiphasic Personality Inventory, Social Adjustment Scale, Wechsler Adult Intelligence Survey, Spielberger State-Trait Anxiety Scale

Family status

- *History:* marital status, family composition, family roles
- *Family communication:* style and quality of communication, methods of conflict resolution
- *Physical and emotional needs:* family's ability to meet patient's physical and emotional needs
- *Family health history:* bipolar disorder, depression, suicide, schizophrenia, mental retardation, substance

abuse, stress-related illness, medical illness
- *Diagnostic tests:* Family Genogram, Family Assessment Device

Cardiovascular status
- *History:* cardiovascular disease
- *Physical examination:* general observations, vital signs, precordial inspection, carotid and apical pulse rates, normal and extra heart sounds
- *Signs and symptoms:* palpitations, syncope, dyspnea, chest pain, fatigue, exercise patterns, use of caffeine
- *Laboratory tests:* complete blood count and differential
- *Diagnostic tests:* electrocardiography, echocardiography

Gastrointestinal status
- *History:* smoking, alcohol use, medications
- *Physical examination:* abdominal inspection, palpation and auscultation, stool characteristics, bowel sounds
- *Signs and symptoms:* abdominal pain, nausea, vomiting, belching, gagging, change in appetite, weight change, constipation, diarrhea
- *Laboratory tests:* gastric analysis, serum electrolyte levels, urinalysis
- *Diagnostic tests:* upper GI series, barium enema, computed tomography scan of abdomen, magnetic resonance imaging of abdomen, barium swallow

Neurologic status
- *History:* usual sleep pattern; energy level after sleep; rest and relaxation patterns; use of caffeine, alcohol, amphetamines, sleeping aids

- *Mental status:* appearance and attitude, level of consciousness, motor activity, thought and speech, mood and affect, perceptions, orientation, memory, general information, calculations, capacity to read and write, visual-spatial ability, attention span, abstraction, judgment and insight
- *Physical examination:* motor and sensory function, reflexes, tardive dyskinesia or other adverse effects of medication
- *Signs and symptoms:* restlessness, tremors, paresthesia, paresis, numbness and tingling, tics, fasciculation, short-term memory loss
- *Laboratory tests:* drug toxicology, thyroid function
- *Diagnostic tests:* Folstein Mini-Mental Health Status Examination, lumbar puncture, electroencephalography, magnetic resonance imaging

Nutritional status
- *History:* usual exercise pattern, typical daily food intake
- *Medical conditions:* nutritional deficiencies, obesity or cachexia, anorexia, bulimia
- *Physical examination:* height, weight
- *Signs and symptoms:* weight loss or gain, nausea and vomiting, fainting, pallor, irritability
- *Laboratory tests:* serum albumin and total protein levels

Respiratory status
- *History:* tobacco use, exposure to occupational hazards, medications
- *Physical examination:* skin color, temperature, and turgor; color of lips and nails; symmetry of chest expansion; rate, depth, and pattern of respirations; auscultation and percussion

of lung fields; tracheal position; palpation for thoracic excursion and fremitus
- *Signs and symptoms:* dyspnea, cough
- *Laboratory tests:* arterial blood gas analysis
- *Diagnostic tests:* pulmonary function studies, ventilation-perfusion scan

Self-care status
- *Observation:* functional ability (muscle tone, size, and strength; range of motion; coordination), daily activities (dressing, grooming, bathing, toileting, and hygiene)
- *Diagnostic tests:* Functional Ability Scale, Self-Care Assessment Tool

DEFINING CHARACTERISTICS

- Altered communication, such as pressured speech, blocking, flood of talk, stammering, rumination, argumentative or demanding remarks
- Fear of future or of death
- Impaired attention, concentration, or short-term memory
- Impaired functioning in social roles
- Lack of awareness
- Inability to make decisions
- Little or no family support
- Mood changes, such as increased irritability, anger, apprehension
- Orientation lapses, including a distorted sense of time and place
- Perceptions changes, such as hypervigilance and reduced perceptual field
- Physiologic responses, such as increased heart rate, increased blood pressure, rapid breathing, inhibited salivation, tightened muscle tone, dilated pupils, increased blood glucose

level, cold skin and extremities, increased alertness
- Presence of any chronic or terminal medical condition
- Selective inattention, focus on scattered details, inability to problem solve, increased distractibility, impaired ability to follow directions, repetitive questioning
- Sensory changes, such as decreased hearing, fixed vision, decreased pain perception
- Sympathetic nervous system activation; for example, increases in epinephrine level, pulse rate, blood pressure, respirations, and body temperature, as well as skin vasoconstriction, diaphoresis, dry mouth, urinary urgency, loss of appetite, decreased circulation to digestive system, increased glucose production by liver

ASSOCIATED DISORDERS

Any hospitalized patient, but most often patients with conditions requiring surgery, diseases that threaten self-concept, treatments that use high-technology devices or techniques, or newly diagnosed chronic or terminal diseases; also, a devastating situational crisis or medical illnesses, such as acquired immunodeficiency syndrome, acute myocardial infarction, acute respiratory failure, adult respiratory distress syndrome, anemia, congestive heart failure, hyperthyroidism, malignant neoplasms, pulmonary embolism

EXPECTED OUTCOMES

Initial outcomes
- Patient states feelings of anxiety.

- Patient identifies factors that elicit anxious behaviors.
- Patient maintains normal sleep and nutritional patterns.
- Patient discusses activities that tend to decrease anxious behaviors.

Interim outcomes

- Patient engages in conversation and activities with family, caregivers, and other support people.
- Patient copes with threat of anxiety by being involved in decisions about care.
- Patient demonstrates fewer physical symptoms of anxiety.
- Patient practices progressive relaxation techniques twice daily.
- Patient begins to gain self-control over anxiety through an increased understanding of its causes.

Discharge outcomes

- Patient copes with current medical situation without demonstrating severe signs of anxiety.
- Patient obtains referrals to appropriate community resources.

INTERVENTIONS AND RATIONALES

Initial interventions

- Maintain awareness and sensitivity to the threat experienced by the patient *to recognize, respect, and cope with his emotions and behaviors.*
- Organize your work to spend as much time as possible with the patient *to allay his fears of being neglected or forgotten.*
- Remain with the patient during severe anxiety. *Anxiety may be related to his fear of being left alone.*

- Give the patient clear, concise explanations of any treatment or care *to avoid information overload that may impair his cognitive abilities.*
- Make no demands on the patient *to avoid eliciting the anxious patient's characteristic hostile response to such demands.*
- Identify and reduce as many environmental stressors (often individuals) as possible *to allay the anxiety caused by lack of trust in the environment.*
- Thoroughly attend to the patient's physical needs *to reassure him and demonstrate that his needs will continue to be met.*
- Provide nutritious, regular meals *to encourage healthy eating patterns and to prevent nutrition deficiencies that further exacerbate the patient's illness.*
- Promote sleep with comfort measures (warm bath, back rub, quiet presence of significant person) *to help the patient relax and get restful sleep.*
- Provide medication as prescribed for sleep *to assist the patient in relaxing when anxiety is severe and sleep is disturbed.*
- Listen attentively to the patient's verbally expressed feelings *to allow him to identify anxious behaviors and discover the source of anxiety.*
- Determine the patient's level of knowledge about his situation *so you can correct any misconceptions.*
- Provide the patient with opportunities to discuss reasons for anxiety. *Without assistance, some patients will not be able to express their fears of disability or dying. By drawing the patient out in conversation, you allow communication to proceed at his pace.*

- Have the patient state what activities he finds comforting and encourage them *to give him a sense of control.*

Interim interventions
- When possible, include the patient in decisions about his care *to build his confidence in his own abilities and reduce anxious behaviors.*
- Support family members' or a companion's efforts to cope with the patient's anxious behavior *to allay their anxiety as well as the patient's.*
- Allow extra visiting periods with family members, if this seems to allay the patient's anxiety, *to allow him and family members to support each other according to their abilities and at their own pace.*
- Involve the family in joint planning and decision making with the patient *to foster trust between the patient and family.*
- Provide regular periods of supportive therapy in which the patient can explore thoughts, feelings, and beliefs *to gain insight into the source of anxiety.*
- Teach the patient relaxation techniques to be performed at least every 4 hours, such as guided imagery, progressive muscle relaxation, and meditation. *These measures can restore psychological and physical equilibrium by decreasing autonomic response to anxiety.*
- Provide the patient with an opportunity to discuss feelings and beliefs with others who are experiencing similar problems *to reassure him that he is not alone and reinforce learning from others.*

Discharge interventions
- Support the patient's efforts to improve his coping skills *to increase potential for further adaptive behaviors.*
- Refer the patient to community or professional mental health resources *to provide ongoing mental health assistance.*

EVALUATION STATEMENTS

Patient:
- experiences normal sleep patterns and appetite.
- reports feelings of anxiety.
- describes anxiety-inducing situations.
- engages in conversation and activities with family, caregivers, and other support people.
- makes appropriate care-related decisions.
- states at least two ways to eliminate or minimize anxious behaviors.
- demonstrates progressive relaxation exercises.
- practices relaxation exercises a specified number of times each day.
- experiences fewer physical symptoms associated with anxiety.
- reports being able to cope with current situation without experiencing severe anxiety.

DOCUMENTATION

- Patient's statements of anxious feelings
- Patient's perceptions of reasons for anxiety
- Observed physical signs of anxiety
- Nursing interventions to reduce patient's anxiety

- Patient's response to nursing interventions
- Patient behaviors and statements that indicate increased control of anxiety
- Family's willingness to participate in patient's care
- Evaluation statements.

Body image disturbance

related to a change in appearance

DEFINITION

Negative self-perception in which an alteration in body image adversely affects the patient's psychosocial function

ASSESSMENT

Cultural status
- *Demographics:* age, sex, level of education, occupation, nationality, race, ethnic group
- *History:* beliefs, values, and attitudes about health and illness; health customs, practices, and rituals
- *Diagnostic test:* Cultural Assessment Guide

Family status
- *Marital status*
- *Family roles:* formal and informal roles, role performance, degree of family agreement on each member's role, interrelationships of roles
- *Family communication:* style and quality of communication, methods of conflict resolution
- *Developmental stage of family:* relationships between members, how fam-

ily adapts to change, shifts in responsibility, changes in problem-solving skills
- *Family subsystems:* how family alliances affect individual members and family as a unit
- *Physical and emotional needs:* ability of family to meet patient's physical and emotional needs, disparities between patient's needs and family's willingness or ability to meet them
- *Coping patterns:* major life events, meaning of life events to each family member, usual coping patterns, perception of effectiveness of coping patterns
- *Family health history:* presence of medical illness
- *Diagnostic tests:* Family Environment Scale, Family Adjustment Device, Family Genogram

Musculoskeletal status
- *Physical examination:* range of motion of all joints; joint and muscle symmetry; muscle size, strength, and tone
- *Signs and symptoms:* pain; falls; joint swelling, stiffness, movement difficulty, deformity, dislocation, inflammation, swelling, contracture, subluxation; muscle atrophy, weakness, tenderness; masses
- *Diagnostic tests:* Functional Mobility Scale, Muscle Strength Scale

Psychological status
- *Current illness:* changes in appetite, energy level, motivation, personal hygiene, self-perception, self-esteem, sleep pattern, sexual drive
- *Psychiatric history:* presence of psychiatric disorder, age of onset, impact

on functioning, type of treatment, patient's response to treatment
- *Developmental history:* higher education, occupation and job changes, dating and marital history, hobbies and recreational activities, spirituality, reaction to illness or disability
- *Diagnostic test:* Hamilton Rating Scale for Depression

Self-care status
- *History:* presence of neurologic, sensory, or motor impairment; ability to carry out voluntary and social activities; coping skills
- *Observation:* functional ability (muscle tone, size, and strength; range of motion; coordination), daily activities (dressing, grooming, bathing, toileting, and hygiene)
- *Diagnostic tests:* Functional Ability Scale, Self-Care Assessment Tool

Sexuality status
- *History:* contraceptive practices; attitudes toward sex; sexual preference, desire, or responsiveness; previous and usual sexual response patterns; menstrual history
- *Medications:* oral contraceptives, sedatives, tranquilizers, estrogen
- *Physical examination:* penis, scrotum, testicles (male patient); vulva, urethra, Skene's and Bartholin's glands, vaginal discharge (female patient)
- *Signs and symptoms:* decreased or increased libido, impotence, change in body image or structure

Social status
- *History:* conversational and interpersonal skills, size of social network, quality of relationships, degree of

trust in others, ability to function in social and occupational roles
- *Signs and symptoms:* withdrawal, lack of eye contact, inappropriate responses, aggressiveness, social isolation
- *Diagnostic test:* Social Adjustment Scale

Spiritual status
- *Medical history:* illnesses or trauma that caused a change in body image, chronic or terminal illness, disabilities, deformities
- *History:* religious affiliation, perception of faith and religious practices, support network (family, clergy, friends)
- *Signs and symptoms:* crying, despair, denial, withdrawal, social isolation, fanaticism
- *Diagnostic test:* Spiritual Well-Being Scale

DEFINING CHARACTERISTICS

- Actual change in body structure or function
- Avoidance of eye contact and social interaction
- Denial of loss
- Inability to look at or touch the affected part
- Intentional or unintentional hiding of the affected body part
- Missing body part
- Refusal or reluctance to learn care measures
- Social isolation
- Verbal response to perceived or actual change in structure, function, or appearance
- Withdrawal

ASSOCIATED DISORDERS

Alopecia; bone or skin cancer; burns; cerebrovascular accident; conditions requiring such surgeries as laryngectomy, limb amputation, mastectomy, tracheotomy; depression; dermatological conditions; facial tumors or trauma; missing digits; rheumatoid arthritis

EXPECTED OUTCOMES

Initial outcomes

- Patient acknowledges change in body image.
- Patient participates in aspects of care.
- Patient participates in decisions about care.
- Patient communicates feelings regarding change in body image.

Interim outcomes

- Patient talks with someone who has experienced a similar loss.
- Patient participates in rehabilitation program.
- Patient participates in counseling.

Discharge outcomes

- Patient expresses positive feelings about himself.
- Patient identifies limitations and develops strategies to compensate for loss.
- Patient engages in social interactions.
- Patient demonstrates ability to use new coping mechanisms.
- Patient can discuss deficit if confronted in a social setting.

INTERVENTIONS AND RATIONALES

Initial interventions

- Accept the patient's perception of himself and provide assurance that he can overcome this crisis *to validate his feelings.*
- While assisting the patient with self-care, talk to him and assess his coping patterns and level of self-esteem *to obtain a baseline against which to measure his psychological progress throughout hospitalization.*
- Encourage him to perform self-care *to foster a sense of independence and control over his situation.*
- Assess his willingness and readiness for decision making about care; then involve him in decisions when appropriate. *Involvement provides a sense of control over the present situation and fosters self-esteem.*
- Encourage the patient to express grief about his loss. *Grieving must precede acceptance of loss.*
- Provide continuity of care throughout hospitalization *to foster trust and establish a therapeutic relationship.*

Interim interventions

- Give the patient frequent opportunities to express his feelings about his altered body image and hospitalization *to allow him to express concerns and to correct misconceptions.*
- Help the patient identify positive aspects of his appearance *to foster a positive self-image.*
- Provide positive feedback and reinforce the patient's efforts to adapt to the change in his body image *to support continued adaptation and progress.*

- Encourage the patient to keep a journal during hospitalization to record feelings, goals, concerns, and progress. *A written record will help show him the progress he's made during hospitalization.*
- Discuss the patient's progress and point out where his condition has improved or stabilized *to foster a positive attitude.*
- Introduce the patient to someone who has coped with a similar situation. *Through discussion with someone who understands his concerns, the patient may learn new techniques for coping and adapting.*
- Encourage the patient's participation in a support group *to help him gain support and understanding.*
- If the patient is adapting poorly, refer him to a psychiatric liaison nurse or other mental health professional *for additional counseling.*

Discharge interventions
- Encourage the patient to describe the progress he's made throughout hospitalization *to foster a sense of self-esteem and help him recognize how he's adapted to body-image changes.*
- Teach and encourage healthy coping strategies *to help the patient overcome unproductive behavior.*
- Ask the patient which coping strategies have been most helpful *to assess his ability to adapt and to encourage appropriate coping patterns.*
- Refer the patient to such support services as the Candlelighters Childhood Cancer Foundation, Look Good Feel Better, and the American Cancer Society *to provide additional opportunities to improve body image.*

- Encourage family members to voice concerns. Refer them to family counseling *to help them adapt to the patient's altered body image and to enhance their abilities to provide support.*
- Encourage the patient to participate in activities and hobbies that he enjoyed before hospitalization, when possible, *to promote normalcy. Renewed interest in activities may help the patient reenter his social environment and gain independence and self-esteem.*

EVALUATION STATEMENTS

Patient:
- expresses feelings regarding change in body image.
- participates in care and decision making.
- expresses positive feelings about self.
- successfully uses coping strategies and problem-solving skills that he has learned.
- participates in rehabilitation program.
- participates in counseling.
- engages in activities and hobbies he enjoyed before entering hospital.
- identifies limitations and uses problem-solving strategies to overcome limitations.

  Family members:
- successfully provide needed emotional, physical, and social support.
- participate in counseling.

DOCUMENTATION

- Words patient uses to describe self, limitations, condition, and adaptive equipment
- Observations of patient's reaction to affected body part

- Observations of changes in structure and function of affected body part
- Patient's self-care abilities
- Health education, rehabilitation, and counseling services provided
- Nursing interventions and patient's response
- Observed interactions of patient and family members
- Evaluation statements.

Caregiver role strain

related to caring for a chronically ill relative

DEFINITION

Difficulty providing care because of increased and prolonged patient demands on family caregivers

ASSESSMENT

Cultural status
- *Family demographics:* age, sex, level of education, and occupation of members; nationality, race, ethnic group
- *History:* beliefs, attitudes, and values about health and illness; health practices, customs, rituals
- *Diagnostic test:* Cultural Assessment Guide

Family status
- *History:* marital status; roles in family; family rules; communication patterns; developmental stage; family alliances; goals, values, and aspirations; socioeconomic status; coping patterns; physical and mental health; social interactions; ability of family to meet physical and emotional needs of members
- *Diagnostic tests:* Family Environment Scale, Family Adjustment Device, Family Genogram, Dyadic Adjustment Scale, Family Awareness Scale, Index of Family Relations

Spiritual status
- *History:* religion, church affiliation, practices, support network
- *Diagnostic tests:* Spiritual and Religious Concerns Questionnaire, Spiritual Well-Being Scale

DEFINING CHARACTERISTICS

- Abusive or addictive behavior
- Ambivalence
- Anger
- Anxiety
- Denial
- Disruption of family life
- Emotional and social withdrawal
- Excessive involvement with chronically ill family member
- Frequent hospitalization of chronically ill family member
- Guilt
- Helplessness, hopelessness, powerlessness
- Ineffective problem solving
- Marital problems
- Poor communication
- Recent major life event
- Resentment
- Stress-related illnesses or symptoms
- Sudden, severe illness
- Unequal role responsibilities
- Unmet needs

ASSOCIATED DISORDERS

Anxiety disorder, depressive disorder, psychoactive substance use, somatoform disorder

EXPECTED OUTCOMES

Initial outcomes

- Family members discuss how illness has altered established roles and rules.
- Family members discuss inequities in care responsibilities for the chronically ill patient.
- Family members revise caregiving and household responsibilities to correct inequities.
- Family members don't resort to ineffective or dangerous coping methods, such as substance abuse, mistreatment of loved ones, absence from work or school, or withdrawal from or excessive involvement with the chronically ill family member.
- Family members involve support systems, such as extended family, community resources, and religious organizations, in care and emotional support of the patient.

Interim outcomes

- Family members discuss past experiences with crises and illnesses.
- Family members discuss perceived impact of illness on family function, such as interrupted goals, changes in social function, and living with the unpredictable course of a chronic illness.
- Family members establish limits on the patient's behavior and uphold them.
- Family members' emotional and physical needs are met.

Discharge outcomes

- Family communicates openly and honestly.
- Family members set realistic goals, such as learning stress-management strategies.
- Family outlook is supportive and positive.
- Family members recognize need for professional assistance.

INTERVENTIONS AND RATIONALES

Initial interventions

- Encourage family to discuss role changes that have occurred as a result of sudden illness, recurrent hospitalizations, or other major life events *to improve communication.*
- Facilitate negotiation among family members about responsibilities for household chores and caring for ill relative *to increase feelings of control, competency, and cooperation.*
- Encourage family members to discuss how they cope with relative's illness *to help them adjust to changes in roles and responsibilities.*
- Encourage family members to seek assistance such as stress-management training from outside resources *to decrease strain and to facilitate coping.*

Interim interventions

- Encourage discussion of the family's past experiences with crises and illnesses and invite comparison with the current situation. *Heightening family awareness that its members have weathered tough times before will increase self-confidence. Discussion will also facilitate resolution of past events and help the family decide which coping*

strategies used in the past may be relevant to the current crisis.
- Encourage family members to uphold established role behaviors and rules. *Maintaining routines and knowing which behaviors will and will not be accepted will help reduce anxiety among family members. It will also enhance feelings of manageability, closeness, and stability.*
- Assist family members to clarify needs and to develop plans to fulfill them. *If family life is centered around caring for a chronically ill relative, other members may feel deprived, mistreated, or unappreciated.*

Discharge interventions
- Facilitate open and honest communication *to decrease feelings of isolation, abandonment, and alienation.*
- Help family members set individual goals *to support independence and to increase sense of control, empowerment, and hope. Family members need help to avoid becoming stifled by the demands of caring for an ill relative.*
- Encourage involvement with religious and social networks *to enhance family well-being.*
- Refer the family to appropriate professional services such as stress management training *to ensure additional assistance as needed.*

EVALUATION STATEMENTS

Family members:
- share responsibilities equitably.
- adjust to changes in roles and rules brought on by current crisis.
- don't exhibit signs of stress.
- report diminished feelings of despair or of being overburdened.

- express optimism about their ability to manage crisis.
- report that communication is open and honest.
- plan short-term and future goals.
- support independent function of individual members.
- report improved relationships with each other and increased satisfaction as emotional needs are met.
- cope with the patient's ongoing changes and limitations.
- use community support resources, as necessary.
- seek additional professional help when necessary.

DOCUMENTATION

- Diagnostic test results
- Family's beliefs and attitudes about illness
- Role adjustment and flexibility of family members
- Coping patterns
- Stress-management strategies
- Attitudes about family life and future
- Expressions of feelings of empowerment, hope, and competence
- Indications of family members' abilities to recognize limitations and seek appropriate resources for help
- Immediate and future goals articulated by family members
- Evidence of increased involvement with activities unrelated to care of ill relative
- Use of support systems
- Referrals for additional professional help
- Evaluation statements.

Caregiver role strain

related to caring for chronically ill patients

DEFINITION

Staff member experiences difficulty caring for chronically ill patients

ASSESSMENT

Cultural status
- *History:* staff member's beliefs, attitudes, and values about health and illness; health practices

Hospital unit status
- *Roles:* clarity of staff member's role; responsibility to patient and family
- *Communication:* quality and frequency of communication with colleagues, patient, and family
- *Emotional needs:* resources for staff; support from supervisor and colleagues; resources for patient and family
- *Workplace factors:* staffing adequacy; caseload
- *Diagnostic test:* Work Environment Scale

Psychological status
- *History:* change in appetite, sleep pattern, energy level, motivation, involvement, self-esteem, mood, or physical health; alcohol or drug abuse
- *Diagnostic test:* Staff Burnout Scale for Health Professionals

Spiritual status
- *History:* attitudes about illness, death, and suffering; support network

DEFINING CHARACTERISTICS

- Absence from work
- Apathy, lack of concern for patient
- Attempt to fulfill role of patient's friend or family
- Beliefs and attitudes about health practices that conflict with patient's or family's values
- Excessive assignments
- Excessive feeling of responsibility for patient
- Excessive or inadequate involvement with patient or family
- Excessive patient dependency on staff
- Fatigue
- Impaired sleep
- Inadequate resources to meet patient's or family's emotional needs, inadequate staffing, lack of resources for staff support
- Irritability
- Multiple somatic complaints
- Poor communication with colleagues, patient, or family
- Poor appetite
- Refusal to accept assignments
- Substance abuse

ASSOCIATED DISORDERS

Mood disorder, substance abuse

EXPECTED OUTCOMES

Initial outcomes
- Staff member recognizes role strain.
- Staff member expresses understanding of the cause of role strain.

Interim outcomes
- Staff member decreases use of maladaptive coping methods.
- Staff member develops effective coping methods.

Concluding outcomes
- Increased support resources are made available to staff member.
- Staff member seeks support or assistance when needed.

INTERVENTIONS AND RATIONALES

Initial interventions
- Teach the staff member about the signs of role strain and contributing factors *to promote self-awareness.* Point out signs of role strain you've observed in the staff member.
- Help the staff member develop realistic expectations for herself and for patients *to decrease feelings of frustration and helplessness.*

Interim interventions
- Encourage the staff to express thoughts and feelings associated with working with the chronically ill *to alleviate strain and to reduce the risk of frustrations being acted out through substance abuse, work absences, or other nonproductive behaviors.*
- Teach adaptive coping strategies, such as exercise and meditation, *to replace maladaptive methods.*
- Provide additional training in working with the chronically ill through in-service sessions, conferences, and literature review *to increase staff self-confidence and to reduce role strain.*

Concluding interventions
- Provide information about support resources, such as employee assistance programs, staff support groups, community psychotherapists, and stress management workshops, *to increase the likelihood of use.*
- Facilitate supportive relationships among staff and between supervisor and staff (for example, by conducting a staff support group) *to increase social support among nurses.*

EVALUATION STATEMENTS

Staff member:
- expresses insight into role strain, its manifestations, and its causes.
- reduces use of maladaptive coping methods.
- participates in exercise program.
- attends conferences on care of chronically ill patients.
- receives a directory of staff support resources.
- expresses that work environment is supportive.

Coping, defensive

related to a vulnerable self-image brought on by a psychiatric disturbance

DEFINITION

Inability to acknowledge problems or the need for personal improvement because of perceived threats to self-esteem

ASSESSMENT

Cultural status
- *Demographics:* age, sex, level of education, occupation, nationality, race, ethnic group
- *History:* beliefs, attitudes, and values about health and illness; health customs, practices, and rituals

Family status
- *History:* marital status; household composition; family values and goals; communication patterns; conflict resolution methods; enmeshment or estrangement; ability of family to meet physical and emotional needs of its members; discipline pattern; history of alcoholism, sexual abuse, psychiatric disorders, or neurologic disorders
- *Economic status:* employment histories and related attitudes
- *Diagnostic tests:* Family Genogram, Holmes and Rahe Social Readjustment Rating Scale, Family Environment Scale

Neurologic status
- *History:* past medical disorders; head injury; drug or alcohol abuse, especially cocaine
- *Mental status:* appearance and attitude, level of consciousness, motor activity, thought and speech, mood and affect, perceptions, orientation, memory, general information processing, calculations, capacity to read and write, visual-spatial ability, attention span, abstraction, judgment and insight
- *Signs and symptoms:* irritability, mood swings, seizures, violent outbursts

- *Laboratory tests:* drug toxicology; plasma levels of lithium, carbamazepine, valproic acid, clonazepam; thyroid function
- *Diagnostic tests:* computed tomography scan, magnetic resonance imaging, positron emission tomography, electroencephalography

Psychological status
- *Substance abuse:* type of substance, effects on mood and behavior, signs of abuse or withdrawal, impact on functioning
- *Life changes:* developmental milestones, losses through separation or death, job loss, recent divorce, medical illness, legal difficulties
- *Psychiatric history:* age at onset of illness, symptoms and severity, impact on functioning, response to and compliance with treatment
- *Childhood development:* personality traits, adaptive behaviors, maladaptive behaviors, earliest memories, academic performance, relationships with peers, religious and social group involvement, recreational activities, sexual or physical abuse, signs of antisocial behavior
- *Adolescent development:* reaction to puberty and sexuality; relationships with peers, sexual partners, and authority figures; scholastic performance; occupational choices; extracurricular activities; delinquency; situational crises
- *Adult development:* military, education, and occupation histories; dating and marital history; hobbies and recreational activities; spirituality; reactions to illness and disability; coping methods; problem-solving strategies

- *Medications:* neuroleptics, antidepressants, anti-anxiety agents
- *Signs and symptoms:* changes in appetite, energy level, self-esteem, sleep pattern, sex drive, or competence
- *Diagnostic tests:* Minnesota Multiphasic Personality Inventory, Wechsler Adult Intelligence Survey, Brief Psychiatric Rating Scale, Narcissistic Traits Scale, revised version, Strauss-Carpenter Employment and Social Scales, Global Assessment Scale, Young Mania Rating Scale

Social status
- *History:* conversational and interpersonal skills, social network, quality of relationships, degree of trust in others, self-esteem, social and occupational role functioning
- *Signs and symptoms:* withdrawal, lack of eye contact, intrusiveness, inappropriate responses, aggressive behavior
- *Diagnostic test:* Social Adjustment Scale

DEFINING CHARACTERISTICS

- Denial of obvious problems or weaknesses
- Desire for instant gratification
- Difficulty establishing and maintaining relationships
- Discomfort in social situations
- Grandiosity or inaccurate perception of reality
- Hypersensitivity to criticism
- Intolerance of being alone
- Lack of genuine concern for others or superior attitude toward others
- Noncompliance with treatment or therapy
- Projection of blame or responsibility or rationalization of failures
- Strong desire to be center of attention
- Tendency to split and manipulate members of the treatment team.

ASSOCIATED DISORDERS

Alcohol-related disorders, amphetamine-related disorders, antisocial personality disorder, bipolar disorder, borderline personality disorder, brain tumor, chronic pain, cocaine-related disorder, histrionic personality disorder, mood disorder, narcissistic personality disorder, permanent disability or disfigurement, schizophrenia, temporal lobe epilepsy

EXPECTED OUTCOMES

Initial outcomes
- Patient expresses understanding of goals of hospitalization and treatment.
- Patient discusses family history and current crisis.
- Patient acknowledges personal responsibility for difficulties with relationships.
- Patient receives information about group therapy.

Interim outcomes
- Patient attains therapeutic plasma levels of medications.
- Patient undergoes individual therapy to stabilize mood swings and reduce defensive behavior.
- Patient participates in group, family, or marital therapy.

- Patient demonstrates increased ability to understand own behaviors and feelings.

Discharge outcomes

- Patient acknowledges need for medication, long-term therapy, and follow-up treatment after discharge.
- Patient meets goals of hospitalization and sets goals for outpatient therapy.
- Patient demonstrates ability to interact with others without becoming defensive, rationalizing behaviors, or expressing grandiose ideas.
- Patient evaluates group therapy experience and states commitment to additional group therapy as an outpatient.
- Patient identifies fears, feelings, and moods that precipitate exploitative or manipulative behaviors.

INTERVENTIONS AND RATIONALES

Initial interventions

- Tell the patient you understand that acknowledging problems may be difficult. *Grandiosity or immaturity may make it difficult for the patient to acknowledge weaknesses.* Encourage realistic appraisal of problems and efforts to set goals. *A supportive approach will help motivate the patient without threatening his self-esteem.*
- Assess the patient for mood swings, poor impulse control, inability to delay gratification, self-destructive tendencies, or potential to harm others. If necessary, place patient on special precautions, for example, keeping him within view at all times, *to assure the*

safety of the patient and those around him while he stabilizes.

- Have the patient perform self-care to the extent possible *to foster a sense of control.*
- Establish a structured daily routine *to provide the patient with alternatives to self-absorption.*
- Provide immediate, matter-of-fact, non-threatening feedback for inappropriate behavior *to make the patient aware of how other people perceive his behavior and to reduce inappropriate behavior.*
- Provide immediate, positive feedback for appropriate, responsible behavior *to increase the patient's confidence in his ability to cope.*
- Observe how the patient interacts with others *to assess his interpersonal skills.*
- Assess the patient's familial and marital relationships, noting behaviors that adversely affect relationships. *Assessment will help determine the patient's motivation to change and family members' willingness to maintain their relationship with him.*
- Evaluate the patient's eligibility for group therapy. *If the patient is highly symptomatic and his behavior is disruptive, he may need time to stabilize. Holding out the possibility of later selection for treatment may motivate the patient to comply with therapy.*

Interim interventions

- Allow sufficient time for medications to reach therapeutic levels *to increase the patient's sense of security and stability so that he can acknowledge vulnerability and pain.*

▪ Help the patient identify positive and negative traits *to encourage honest self-evaluation.*

▪ Help the patient identify situations that provoke defensive reactions. Use role playing to help him practice appropriate responses *to enhance his confidence and increase his ability to cope with difficult situations.*

▪ Provide information about the patient's diagnosis, causes of disorder, medications, and treatment *to enhance his ability to make informed decisions and to encourage him to participate in care. Therapy may include medications, electroconvulsive therapy, and individual, milieu, group, and family counseling.*

▪ Encourage the patient to participate in group therapy sessions *to increase his interpersonal problem-solving skills and help him understand the impact of his behavior on other people.*

▪ Encourage the patient and his family members to participate in family or marital therapy sessions *to decrease negative interactions and to educate family members about the patient's diagnosis and treatment.*

Discharge interventions

▪ Praise the patient for evidence of emotional growth such as increased expression of empathy *to promote his efforts to improve relationships with others,* and praise appropriate behavior *to strengthen his ability to monitor his behavior after discharge.*

▪ Encourage the patient to continue group therapy following discharge to practice discussing painful feelings and experiences; interacting with peers without grandiose, hostile, or intrusive behaviors; and speaking in front of others despite timidity. *This*

will help increase his positive feelings about self and further develop his interpersonal skills.

▪ Discuss the importance of follow-up treatment *to enhance the patient's decision-making ability and to increase his willingness to assume responsibility for his behavior.*

▪ Emphasize the importance of continuing family or marital therapy after discharge *to increase treatment benefits to all family members and to decrease the likelihood of relapse.*

EVALUATION STATEMENTS

Patient:

▪ expresses understanding of goals of hospitalization.

▪ reports fewer or less severe symptoms.

▪ initiates and completes at least two self-care activities daily.

▪ makes at least one decision daily about activities, self-care, or treatment.

▪ acknowledges responsibility for behavior and impact on others.

▪ socializes with others each day.

▪ acknowledges positive change in feelings and behavior through group therapy.

▪ discusses effective and ineffective behavior.

▪ discusses how behavior is influenced by feelings.

▪ discusses issues related to exploitative and manipulative behavior.

▪ expresses knowledge of diagnosis, medications, and discharge plan.

▪ demonstrates ability to follow through on decisions.

▪ participates in family therapy.

DOCUMENTATION

- Diagnostic test results and laboratory findings
- Goals established by patient
- Patient's statements indicating self-perception
- Social interaction patterns
- Use of defense mechanisms
- Knowledge of illness and treatment
- Nursing interventions and patient's responses to them
- Patient's response to therapeutic milieu and group and family therapy
- Evaluation statements.

Coping, family: Potential for growth

related to blending two existing families

DEFINITION

Potential for improved family functioning after marriage, when one or both partners already have children

ASSESSMENT

Family status
- *Family composition:* parents and stepparents; parentage of children in the home; number of grown, independent children
- *Children:* ages and developmental stages, educational levels, previous or current developmental problems, previous or current problems in school
- *Parents:* ages, educational levels, usual coping mechanisms, methods of discipline, knowledge of children's

common developmental issues, experience with child rearing, use of support systems
- *Original families:* conditions surrounding family break-ups, family alliances
- *Family alliances:* emotional triangles, stability, flexibility of family boundaries, difficulties of joining or leaving the family
- *Family roles:* perceptions of each member's responsibilities, financial responsibilities, discipline of children, nurturing
- *Family rules:* origin, equity, methods of enforcement
- *Communication patterns:* among family members, with members of extended families, with people outside the family
- *Family coping patterns:* major events preceding new marriage; methods of conflict resolution; methods for resolving crises of loss, separation, or trauma
- *Evidence of abuse:* physical, sexual, or emotional abuse experienced or inflicted by any family member
- *Family health history:* long-term or short-term disability or illness; substance or alcohol abuse and its treatments and treatment effectiveness
- *Physical security:* methods and resources used to meet needs, competition among family members to have needs met
- *Emotional security:* methods for meeting emotional needs, competition for support
- *Values:* efforts to establish cohesiveness, religious affiliation, adherence to religious values
- *Family customs:* beliefs, customs, attitudes, rituals, and behaviors

- *Diagnostic test:* Family Genogram

Psychological status
- *Family history:* losses or separations that preceded current marriage; episodic or long-term mental illness; emotional abuse; schizophrenia, depressive disorder, personality disorder, bipolar disorder, or other mental illness; past and current psychological treatment or psychotherapy; response to treatment
- *Medication history:* use by any family member of neuroleptic or anxiolytic drug, antidepressant, or lithium; effectiveness of drug treatment
- *Individual assessment:* anxiety level, self-esteem, body image, cognitive or perceptual difficulties, coping methods, support systems, past and present stressors
- *Diagnostic tests:* Piers-Harris Self-Esteem Scale, State-Trait Anxiety Inventory

Socioeconomic status
- *Demographics:* nationality and race; affiliations with racial, ethnic, and cultural groups
- *Economic factors:* adequacy of financial resources, including income, alimony, and child support; parents' employment histories and attitudes
- *Diagnostic test:* Cultural Assessment Guide

DEFINING CHARACTERISTICS

- Biological children favored over stepchildren
- Competition among stepchildren and one spouse for attention of other spouse
- Lack of contact between children and biological parents
- Parental demand for equal loyalties from all children
- Stepmother's expectation to be primary nurturer for all children
- Unreasonably strict family boundaries

ASSOCIATED DISORDERS

Attention-deficit disorder, conduct disorder, depressive disorder, separation anxiety disorder

EXPECTED OUTCOMES

Initial outcomes
- Children learn appropriate ways to express feelings of loss.
- Children are allowed to visit biological parents.
- Parents express understanding of children's developmental stages.

Interim outcomes
- Biological parents use appropriate discipline methods.
- Family members contact sources of support, such as teachers, clergy, or counselors.
- Family members report increased satisfaction with the way their emotional needs are met.

Discharge outcomes
- Family members report improved self-esteem.
- Family members demonstrate appropriate ways to express thoughts and emotions.
- Partners cooperate in performing parental responsibilities.

INTERVENTIONS AND RATIONALES

Initial interventions

- Complete Family Genogram with both spouses *to identify characteristics of family relationships, such as close relationships, poor relationships, and severed relationships.*
- Teach the children appropriate ways to express feelings *to help them cope with loss.*
- Encourage the parents to allow visits between biological parents and children *to decrease anxiety and discourage dysfunctional behavior patterns.*
- Help family members develop realistic expectations about forming new family bonds *to decrease frustration and disappointment.*
- Inform the parents about the children's stages of development *to increase their competence as nurturers.*

Interim interventions

- Allow family members to express feelings regarding strained loyalties *to help prevent development of dysfunctional behavior patterns.*
- Inform the biological parents about appropriate ways to discipline the children *to prevent abusive patterns of behavior.*
- Provide information about sources of support *to increase family members' confidence in outside intervention.*
- Help family members develop appropriate ways to express their emotional needs *to increase their abilities to have needs meet.*
- Facilitate discussion among family members about difficult issues, such as custody, visitation, and holidays, *to decrease anxiety levels, promote cooper-ation, and maintain original family relationships.*

Discharge interventions

- Instruct family members to seek additional counseling as needed to improve functioning and prevent a potential family crisis.

EVALUATION STATEMENTS

Family members:
- demonstrate appropriate ways to resolve conflicts among siblings, stepparents, parents, and stepchildren; and between biological parents and their children.
- report increased cohesiveness in blended family.

Children:
- report that visits to biological parents don't lead to conflict in new family.
- report absence of physical, emotional, and sexual abuse.
- indicate absence of substance abuse by any family member.
- function at appropriate developmental levels in school and in social relationships.

Parent and stepparent:
- function as co-parents and partners.

DOCUMENTATION

- Results of diagnostic tests
- Records of family sessions or therapy
- Reports of progress toward goals
- Reports and observations of emotional or physical abuse in the family
- Evaluation statements.

Coping, family: Potential for growth

related to marital conflict

DEFINITION

Family member seeks assistance in resolving marital conflict as a means to improve family functioning

ASSESSMENT

Cultural status
- *Demographics:* age, sex, level of education, occupation, nationality, race, ethnic group
- *History:* beliefs, values, and attitudes about marital contract and about health and illness; health customs, practices, and rituals
- *Diagnostic test:* Cultural Assessment Guide

Family status
- *Family roles:* formal and informal roles and performance
- *Family communication:* styles and quality of communication, methods of conflict resolution
- *Developmental stage of family:* lengths of relationships in family, how family adapts to change
- *Family subsystems:* conflict between family members, alliances between family members, effects of alliances on family stability and functioning
- *Physical and emotional needs:* ability of family to meet family member's emotional or physical needs, disparities between individual needs and family's willingness or ability to meet them

- *Family health history:* bipolar disorder, depressive disorder, suicide, schizophrenia, mental retardation, substance abuse, stress-related illness, medical illness
- *Diagnostic test:* Family Genogram

Psychological status
- *Current illness:* signs and symptoms (affective states, such as depression, mania, anxiety, calm)
- *Diagnostic tests:* Hamilton Rating Scale for Depression, Zung Self-Rating Depression Scale

Sexuality status
- *Signs and symptoms:* level of libido, sexual desire, or sexual responsiveness in parents; history of sexually transmitted diseases
- *Diagnostic tests:* tests for sexually transmitted diseases

DEFINING CHARACTERISTICS

- Descriptions of conflict or estrangement between parental pair
- Disruption in family communication patterns or in role performance
- Expressions of blame regarding children's behavioral or health problems
- History of depression in any family member
- History of stress-related medical illness
- Loss of libido or sexual responsiveness in either parent
- Problems in children's behavior or school performance
- Recent estrangement from extended family
- Recent history of sexually transmitted disease

ASSOCIATED DISORDERS

This diagnosis may coincide with any psychiatric diagnosis, depending on the patient and the circumstances of treatment.

EXPECTED OUTCOMES

Initial outcome
- Couple agrees to focus on making concrete steps to deal with crisis that brought them into treatment.

Interim outcomes
- Couple practices effective communication techniques.
- Couple reports that current crisis (medical or behavioral disturbance in one or more family members) has stabilized.

Discharge outcomes
- Couple agrees on a plan to develop their relationship.
- Couple finds health care practitioners to assist them in developing relationship.

INTERVENTIONS AND RATIONALES

Initial interventions
- Develop a Family Genogram with the couple *to help them understand family patterns and role expectations.*
- Arrange a family meeting to assess communication patterns, affective states of all members, and presence and nature of family secrets *to help them gain a better understanding of the current crisis.*

- If the couple is able to discuss conflict, encourage them to do so in an open and nonjudgmental way *to foster effective communication.*
- Restate comments made by the couple regarding the current crisis in a manner that separates fact from feeling. *Clarification is an essential therapeutic technique in crisis intervention.*

Interim interventions
- Work with the couple on effective communication and negotiation skills. *Open communication is necessary if the couple is to understand each other's perception of the crisis.*
- Model effective communication skills; for example, by using "I" statements and separating fact from feeling, *to help the couple distinguish between appropriate and inappropriate methods of communication.*
- Encourage the expression of feelings by communicating unconditional positive acceptance of the couple. *Positive reinforcement helps lower the anxiety level.*
- Coordinate the treatment team to plan further interventions for other members of the family; for example, provide additional counseling for a child with behavioral problems. *A consistent, cohesive approach limits the opportunity for conflict between the team members and the family.*

Discharge interventions
- Once the crisis is stabilized, help the couple focus on underlying problems in the marital relationship. *If handled appropriately, a family crisis can become the spark for developing healthier coping patterns.*

- Encourage the couple to view the recent crisis in the context of the history of their marital relationship *to help them gain better perspective.*
- If the couple asks for suggestions for further therapy, offer information and referrals only after consulting with other members of the treatment team. *Long-term support may be needed to maintain coping and stability.*

EVALUATION STATEMENTS

Family members:
- report that crisis is moving toward solution.

Couple:
- acknowledges that conflict between them has been a factor in family crisis.

Couple (or one partner):
- describes a plan to work on marital conflict.
- explores options for ongoing treatment.

DOCUMENTATION

- Results of diagnostic tests
- Family's current understanding of crisis or of member's illness
- Affective state of couple
- Level and style of communication between family members
- Plan developed to work on marital conflict
- Evaluation statements.

Coping, ineffective family

related to codependence

DEFINITION

Dysfunctional interaction in which the emotional lives of family members become enmeshed with the needs of a single family member, commonly a relative with a chemical dependency or personality or impulse control disorder

ASSESSMENT

Cultural status
- *Demographics:* ages, levels of education, and occupations of parents; age, sexes, and developmental stages of children
- *History:* nationality, race, religion, ethnic group, socialization pattern, customs, values, beliefs, attitudes toward role of women in family, safety of the community

Family status
- *History:* marital status, previous marriages (either partner), financial status, communication patterns, methods of conflict resolution, interaction with people and institutions outside the family (extended family, friends, schools, health care system), alliances between family members, triangles within the family, major life events and their meaning to family members
- *Developmental stage of the family:* addition of new members (birth, adoption, blended families), adolescent children, children living on their

own, dependent parents or grandparents, losses from death or separation
- *Coping patterns:* usual coping mechanisms, roles of family members (for example, decision maker, peace keeper, scapegoat, model child), flexibility or rigidity of boundaries, perception of the effectiveness of coping patterns
- *Family rules:* origin, enforcement, and rigidity of rules
- *Medical history:* episodic or chronic physical or mental illness or substance abuse, treatment, and patient's response
- *Signs and symptoms:* evidence of physical, emotional, or sexual abuse or neglect; denial of abuse; inability to recognize abusive behavior; development of strategies for hiding abuse; inability to meet developmental needs of children; inability to meet physical and emotional needs of any family member; conflict between the values and goals established for the family and those of individual family members; maladaptive rules, such as keeping family secrets or harsh parental discipline
- *Diagnostic test:* Family Genogram

Psychological status
- *History:* presence of chronically ill or handicapped family member, losses of family members through separation or death, family crises and their resolutions, childhood history of abuse or neglect by either parent, history of mental or physical illness (any family member) and reaction to treatment
- *Current illness:* evidence of drug or alcohol abuse, withdrawal, anxiety, depressive or impulsive behavior; failure

to comply with a medication regimen; stress-related medical illnesses
- *Laboratory tests:* blood and urine drug toxicology, human immunodeficiency virus testing
- *Diagnostic tests:* Piers-Harris Self-Esteem Scale, State-Trait Anxiety Inventory, Beck Depression Inventory, Brief Psychiatric Rating Scale

DEFINING CHARACTERISTICS

- Anxiety, compulsive behavior, depression, or hypervigilance (exhibited by family members)
- Evidence of physical, emotional, or sexual abuse
- Inability of family members to recognize personal needs of others
- Needs of one family member placed ahead of needs of all other members
- Presence of an abusive family member who is chemically dependent or who has a personality or impulse control disorder
- Rigid or weak individual and family boundaries

ASSOCIATED DISORDERS

Alcohol-related disorder, depressive disorder, stress-related disorders, substance-related disorder

EXPECTED OUTCOMES

Initial outcomes
- Family members agree to rules for safe, healthy interaction.
- Family exhibits a reduction in abusive behavior.
- Family members express desire for appropriate treatment; for example,

treatment for substance abuse, psychiatric disorders, or codependence.

Interim outcomes
- Family members gradually overcome their denial of family problems.
- Family members engage in family or individual therapy, as appropriate.
- Family members with drug or alcohol problems undergo treatment.
- Family members express personal feelings without fear of reprisal.
- Family members seek and use sources of support within the community.

Discharge outcomes
- Family members express satisfaction with the manner in which their individual needs are addressed.
- Family members exhibit improved self-esteem.
- Family members recognize and accept each other's goals.
- Family members report a reduction in the level of depression and anxiety within the family.
- Family members express commitment to maintaining a pattern of communication that encourages open expression of feelings.

INTERVENTIONS AND RATIONALES

Initial interventions
- Complete a Family Genogram to identify family patterns of substance abuse, violence, victimization, and isolation *to accurately define problem areas.*
- Talk with all family members about establishing rules for family interaction, such as prohibiting violence, requiring treatment for substance abuse (if indicated), holding regular family discussions, and identifying specific learning goals for each member to improve family interaction. *By agreeing to basic rules, the family members begin the therapeutic process of building a productive family unit.*

Interim interventions
- Encourage each family member to express his or her feelings and provide a safe environment in which they can do so. *When family members feel safe, they are more likely to disclose true feelings and overcome dysfunctional patterns of communication. This helps each member build self-esteem.*
- Encourage individual therapy or a support group for codependent members of the family, as indicated *to help codependent family members identify and express their own personal needs.*
- Introduce family members to the concept of codependency. Encourage them to explore ways in which they act as enablers to an abusive or chemically dependent relative. Emphasize the need for them to pay attention to their own needs and goals even in times of crisis. *Family members may need assistance in becoming aware of codependent behavior patterns.*
- Provide family members with information about community resources, such as schools, social services, churches, and youth organizations, *to reduce anxiety by disclosing the range of support services available to each member.*

Discharge intervention
- Encourage family members to seek counseling if new or reemerging issues

threaten the stability of the family *to prevent regression into dysfunctional patterns of family interaction.*

EVALUATION STATEMENTS

Family members:
- no longer tolerate abusive behavior.
- seek and continue appropriate ongoing treatment for chemical dependencies or psychological disorders.
- express understanding of the concept of codependency.
- express personal feelings and needs.
- exhibit diminished signs and symptoms of anxiety or depression.
- seek and use support services and systems in the community.

DOCUMENTATION

- Reports and observations of emotional or physical abuse
- Records of individual and family therapy sessions
- Progress of each family member toward personal goals
- Evaluation statements.

Coping, ineffective family

related to inability to support and care for patient with AIDS

DEFINITION

Behavior of family members or companion that indicates difficulty in adapting to the patient's diagnosis of acquired immunodeficiency syndrome (AIDS)

ASSESSMENT

Cultural status
- *Demographics:* age, sex, level of education, occupation, nationality, race, ethnic group
- *History:* family members' and patient's beliefs, values, and attitudes about health and illness; health customs, practices, and rituals; lifestyles

Family status
- *Relationship status:* patient's perception of significant relationships
- *Family roles:* formal and informal roles, role performance, degree of agreement on roles, interrelationships of roles
- *Family communication:* style and quality of communication, methods of conflict resolution
- *Developmental stage:* length and extent of patient's contact with family members; length of patient's relationship with companion; family members' abilities to adapt to change, shifts in role responsibility, problem-solving skills
- *Family subsystems:* effects of family alliances on individual members and family unit
- *Physical and emotional needs:* ability of family members and companion to meet patient's physical and emotional needs; disparities between patient's needs and willingness or ability of family and companion to meet them
- *Coping patterns:* major life events and their meanings to each family member and companion, usual coping patterns, perceived effectiveness of coping patterns

- *Health history (family members and companion):* bipolar disorder, depressive disorder, suicide, schizophrenia, mental retardation, substance abuse, stress-related illness, medical illness
- *Family goals and values:* extent of family members' understanding and articulation of mutual goals and values; family's acceptance of patient's goals and values; patient's and companion's perception of family goals and values
- *Diagnostic tests:* Family Environment Scale, Family Adjustment Device, Family Genogram

Sexuality status
- *History:* change in patient's body image, structure, or function
- *Attitudes:* family members' attitudes towards patient's sexuality; family members' and companion's knowledge of human immunodeficiency virus (HIV) and AIDS

Spiritual status
- *Patient's history:* religious affiliation; current perception of faith and religious practices; perceptions about life, death, and suffering; available support network (family, clergy, friends)
- *Diagnostic tests:* Spiritual and Religious Concerns Questionnaire, Spiritual Well-Being Scale

DEFINING CHARACTERISTICS

- Family members' behavior that suggests difficulty with patient's diagnosis, physical limitations, and psychological responses
- Family members' objections to companion participating in patient's care

- Family members' or companions' gradual withdrawal from participation in patient's care
- Patient's feelings of abandonment, agitation, or depression
- Patient's declining quality of relationships with family members
- Patient's disappointment in declining quality of relationship with companion

ASSOCIATED DISORDERS

AIDS, HIV encephalopathy, HIV infection, Kaposi's sarcoma, *Pneumocystis carinii* pneumonia

EXPECTED OUTCOMES

Initial outcome
- Family members and companion discuss their feelings about patient's illness and impact it has on their capacity to support him.

Interim outcome
- Family members and companion discuss ability to participate in patient's care.

Discharge outcomes
- Patient expresses greater understanding of demands on and limitations of family and companion.
- Patient reports feeling less dependent on companion and family members and seeks other sources of support when needed.

INTERVENTIONS AND RATIONALES

Initial interventions

- Work with patient to complete a Family Genogram *to determine key family patterns.*
- Arrange a time to allow family members and companion to verbalize their feelings *to allow them to realistically adjust to the patient's needs.*
- Encourage family members to express their feelings about the patient's companion and the extent to which he participates in care. Encourage the companion to express his feelings about family members' attitudes toward him and the patient. *All people close to the patient will need an opportunity to express feelings of frustration, anger, and grief. Disagreements about responsibility for the patient may inevitably lead to conflict.*

Interim interventions

- Assess family relationships *to identify realistic opportunities for reconciliation.* When appropriate, act as patient advocate to family members. Tell them he needs their support, not judgment. Remember, though, the patient and family members may not have time, motivation, or resources to resolve long-standing conflicts. *Because time is limited, you will need to establish priorities for family intervention.*
- Hold patient and family conferences to determine aspects of patient's care in which family members or his companion are still willing to participate. *Family members may find a group problem-solving approach helpful in conflict situations.*

- Encourage use of respite or other outside resources *to relieve family members or companion when they no longer have the energy to provide care.*

Discharge interventions

- Encourage the patient to join a support group *to find the emotional backing his family members and companion are unable to provide. Outside sources can make up for shortcomings in the family members' and companion's abilities to provide care.*
- Listen openly to the patient's expressions of pain over unresolved conflicts with family members or his companion and their inability to fully meet his needs. *Therapeutic listening may help the patient better understand himself, his family, and his companion and focus on new coping strategies.*
- Help the patient cope with loss by emphasizing the positive aspects of his relationship with family members. Help him understand that human weakness may prevent family members from doing what is right. *Beyond alienation, there is almost always love and caring among family members and regret for what ideally should have been.*

EVALUATION STATEMENTS

Family members and companion:
- demonstrate greater willingness to discuss feelings.
- support patient to extent that they are capable.
   Patient:
- takes steps to meet his own care needs.
- verbalizes an increased understanding of family members and companion and their limitations.

DOCUMENTATION

- Family members' and companion's stated responses to patient's illness and limitations
- Observation of interactions between family members and companion
- Patient's expressions of grief over family conflict
- Patient's expressions of grief over conflict with companion
- Evaluation statements.

Coping, ineffective individual

related to postpartum mood changes

DEFINITION

Decreased ability to meet demands of parenting, related to depression following childbirth

ASSESSMENT

Cultural status
- *Demographics:* age, marital status, level of education, occupation, nationality
- *History:* beliefs, values, and attitudes about health and illness; health customs, practices, and rituals
- *Diagnostic test:* Cultural Assessment Guide

Family status
- *Family roles:* formal and informal roles, role performance, degree of family agreement on roles, interrelationships of roles

- *Family rules:* rules that foster stability, rules that hinder adaptation, process for modifying rules
- *Family goals and values:* extent of members' understanding and articulation of family goals and values, extent of family's acceptance of individual goals and values
- *Family communication:* styles and quality of communication, methods of conflict resolution
- *Developmental stage of family:* relationships between members, adaptation to change, shifts in role responsibility, changes in problem-solving skills
- *Physical and emotional needs:* family's ability and willingness to meet patient's emotional needs
- *Socioeconomic factors:* economic status of family; sense of adequacy and self-worth; employment status; attitudes toward work; identification with racial, cultural, or ethnic group; influence of religious beliefs on values and practices
- *Coping patterns:* major life events and their meanings to each family member; family members' perception of effectiveness of coping patterns
- *Evidence of abuse:* physical and behavioral indicators
- *Family health history:* bipolar disorder, depressive disorder, suicide, schizophrenia, mental retardation, substance abuse, stress-related illness, medical illness

Neurologic status
- *Mental status:* appearance and attitude, level of consciousness, motor activity, thought and speech, mood and affect perceptions, orientation, memory, general knowledge, calcula-

tions, reading and writing ability, visual-spatial ability, attention span, abstraction, judgment and insight
- *Medications:* all prescribed and illicit drugs
- *Diagnostic test:* Folstein Mini-Mental Health Status Examination

Gynecological status
- *History:* pregnancy, labor, and delivery; previous pregnancies; pain history; symptoms of fatigue or sleep deprivation
- *Physical examination:* hormone levels (cortisol, estrogen, progesterone, prolactin, complete blood count, thyroid, and serotonin)

Nutritional status
- *History:* breast-feeding status, nutritional deficiency, use of nutritional supplements, exercise pattern, weight gain or loss, eating habits, diet
- *Laboratory tests:* hemoglobin level, hematocrit, serum iron levels

Psychological status
- *Developmental history:* birth order, number of siblings, occupation and plans after birth of child, hobbies and recreational activities
- *Health history:* illnesses that cause changes in body image
- *Signs and symptoms:* depression, anxiety, cognitive disturbances, sleep pattern disturbances, sexual drive, withdrawal
- *Diagnostic tests:* Minnesota Multiphasic Personality Inventory, Hamilton Rating Scale for Depression, Beck Depression Inventory

Self-care status
- *Ability to care for self and baby*

Spiritual status
- *Personal habits:* religious affiliation, current practices, support network (family, clergy, friends)

DEFINING CHARACTERISTICS

- Fatigue
- Lack of support from family or friends
- Major life stressors
- Mental illness in family
- Physical pain
- Poor prenatal treatment and education
- Traumatic birthing experience

ASSOCIATED DISORDERS

Depressive disorder, eating disorders, hormonal changes, mania

EXPECTED OUTCOMES

Initial outcomes
- Patient inflicts no self-injury or self-harm.
- Patient is free from fatigue.
- Patient uses appropriate methods for dealing with pain.
- Patient understands possible causes for her mood changes.
- Patient talks about the birth experience.
- Patient asks her health care provider questions related to her care.

Interim outcomes
- Patient understands dietary requirements and other health care measures.
- Patient reports decreased feelings of depression, anxiety, and anger.

Discharge outcomes
- Patient is able to ask for help with caring for baby and other responsibilities.
- Patient obtains referrals for support services.
- Patient establishes realistic goals for herself and her family.

INTERVENTIONS AND RATIONALES

Initial interventions
- Assess the patient's potential for suicide and remove harmful objects *to protect her. This is the top priority of care.*
- Assess the patient's level of pain and fatigue. *Pain and fatigue are major contributors to postpartum depression.*
- Allow the patient to express feelings of anger, guilt, and disappointment related to the birth experience *to help her achieve a better perspective on her experience.*
- Discuss the birth experience with the patient, including possible trauma. *To get past a traumatic experience, the patient must first acknowledge it.*
- Support the patient's efforts to talk to her health care provider *to bolster her confidence in her ability to get needed information.*

Interim interventions
- Teach the patient about nutrition and exercise *to help improve her general health and provide activities that will enhance her sense of control.*
- Teach relaxation skills *to facilitate pain management.*
- Help the patient improve her coping skills *to increase confidence and decrease powerlessness.*

- Explain the causes and contributing factors of postpartum depression to the patient and her family. *Understanding mood changes can help reduce anxiety and feelings of helplessness.*

Discharge interventions
- Tell the patient it's acceptable to ask others for help. *The patient may feel she needs permission to ask for help. An active support system can prevent the patient from feeling overwhelmed.*
- Ensure the father that his help is needed and give him the opportunity to express his feelings *to reduce his stress, make him feel valued, and encourage his involvement.*
- Help the patient make effective use of referrals *to ensure ongoing care.*
- Help the patient set realistic goals for herself and her family. *Achieving goals will promote feelings of self-worth.*

EVALUATION STATEMENTS

Patient:
- is able to talk about pregnancy, delivery, and child care in a calm and rational way.
- is aware of appropriate ways of taking care of herself.
- demonstrates ability to care for the baby.
- reports feeling less depressed and anxious.
- reports satisfaction with support systems.
- calls her health care provider as needed.

The baby's father:
- becomes more involved in child care.

DOCUMENTATION

- Evidence of depression or anxiety
- Evidence of denial of problems
- Patient's reported difficulty making decisions
- Nutrition and health teaching to patient and family and their responses
- Patient's goals for discharge
- Patient's reaction to medication and other treatments
- Observations of family's involvement in helping patient
- Referrals for ongoing care
- Statements patient makes about her baby
- Statements made by baby's father regarding his role in family
- Patient's ability to care for herself and baby
- Evaluation statements.

Coping, ineffective individual

related to psychiatric disturbance

DEFINITION

Lack of effective adaptive behaviors to cope with difficult life situations

ASSESSMENT

Cultural status

- *Demographics:* age, sex, level of education, occupation, nationality, race, ethnic group
- *History:* beliefs, values, and attitudes about health and illness; health customs, practices, and rituals

Family status

- *History:* household composition, developmental stage, family alliances, individual roles and role performances, changes in family roles and responsibilities over time, ability of family to fulfill physical and emotional needs of its members
- *Coping patterns:* adaptations to changes over time, support systems, usual coping methods and their effectiveness, conflict resolution methods
- *Family health history:* mood disorder, schizophrenia, suicide, mental retardation, substance abuse, stress-related illness, or medical illness
- *Socioeconomic factors:* financial status, employment histories and attitudes toward work
- *Diagnostic tests:* Family Genogram, Holmes and Rahe Social Readjustment Rating Scale, Family Environment Scale, Family Adjustment Device

Neurologic status

- *Medications:* neuroleptics, anxiolytic agents, anticonvulsants, antidepressants, antimanic agents, pain medications
- *Mental status:* appearance, attitude, level of consciousness, motor activity, thought and speech patterns, mood and affect, perceptions, orientation, memory, general information processing, calculations, reading and writing capacity, visual-spatial ability, attention span, ability to understand abstractions, and judgment and insight
- *Sensory status:* cortical function
- *Laboratory tests:* complete blood count, urinalysis, blood urea nitrogen and electrolyte levels, drug screening, toxicology, medication serum levels, serum glucose level, allergy tests

- *Diagnostic tests:* electroencephalography, computed tomography scan or magnetic resonance imaging

Psychological status
- *Drug history:* illicit drugs or alcohol, over-the-counter or prescribed drugs
- *Past psychiatric illness:* symptoms and severity, age at onset, impact on functioning, treatment and response, compliance with psychotropic drug regimen
- *Current illness:* patient's perception of condition, signs and symptoms, impact on function, coping methods
- *Childhood development:* developmental milestones, responses of others to child, adaptive and maladaptive behaviors, peer relationships, academic motivation and achievement, recreational and leisure activities, religious education, relationships with siblings, parents, and extended family
- *Adolescent development:* maturity level; participation in social, school, or religious activities; dating history; ability to achieve autonomy within family; delinquency; experimentation with drugs or alcohol
- *Adult development:* dating and marital history; military, academic, or work history; level of independence in work, finances, housing, social events, and daily living activities; health care; self-esteem
- *Diagnostic tests:* Minnesota Multiphasic Personality Inventory, Wechsler Adult Intelligence Survey, Cognitive Capacity Screening Examination, Merinda Leisure Finder, Hamilton Rating Scale for Depression, State-Trait Anxiety Inventory

Social status
- *Social interactions:* conversation skills, interpersonal skills, social network, quality of relationships, social and occupational role functioning, degree of trust in others
- *Signs and symptoms:* withdrawal, lack of eye contact, inappropriate responses
- *Diagnostic test:* Social Adjustment Scale

DEFINING CHARACTERISTICS
- Chronic fatigue and worry
- Compulsive behavior or obsessive thoughts
- Denial of change in health status
- Denial or anger regarding psychiatric illness
- Difficulty asking for help
- Frequent complaints of physical symptoms not confirmed by medical assessment
- Inability to meet basic needs and lack of independence
- Need for immediate gratification
- Poor coping and problem-solving skills

ASSOCIATED DISORDERS

Adjustment disorder, affective disorder, attention-deficit disorder, conversion disorder, head injury, hypochondriasis, mood disorder, personality disorder, schizophrenia, seizures, somatization disorder, somatoform disorder, substance abuse

EXPECTED OUTCOMES

Initial outcomes
- Patient participates in planning care.

- Patient expresses understanding of relationship between symptoms, emotional state, and behavior.
- Patient reduces use of manipulative behavior to gratify needs.

Interim outcomes
- Patient acknowledges responsibility for behavior.
- Patient identifies effective and ineffective coping methods.
- Patient participates in group therapy.

Discharge outcomes
- Patient expresses understanding of psychiatric illness, medications, and importance of continued treatment.
- Patient makes use of available support systems following discharge.

INTERVENTIONS AND RATIONALES

Initial interventions
- If possible, assign a primary nurse to the patient *to provide continuity of care and to promote development of a therapeutic relationship.*
- Spend consistent, uninterrupted periods of time with the patient and encourage open expression of feelings and emotions *to help the patient develop insight into himself and his circumstances.*
- As the patient expresses feelings more openly, discuss the relationship between feelings and behavior *to help the patient understand the connection between emotions and behavior.*
- Assist the patient only when necessary and provide positive reinforcement for independent behavior *to discourage dependent behavior and enhance self-esteem.*

- Encourage the patient to make decisions about care *to reduce his feelings of helplessness.*
- Recognize and set limits on the patient's manipulative behavior. *The patient may manipulate others to reduce his sense of insecurity and increase his feelings of power.*
- Describe consequences of unacceptable behavior and present clear expectations for appropriate behavior *to provide the patient with consistent guidelines and reduce inappropriate behavior.*

Interim interventions
- Provide information about the cause, diagnosis, and treatment of psychiatric disorders *to enable the patient to make reasonable, informed decisions and to encourage him to participate in his care.*
- Discourage the patient from blaming others for his mistakes. Help him accept responsibility for his actions *to foster positive change.*
- Encourage the patient to identify positive personal qualities and accomplishments *to increase his self-esteem and to reduce his perceived need to manipulate others.*
- Help the patient analyze the current situation and evaluate the effectiveness of coping strategies *to foster an objective outlook.*
- Praise the patient for identifying and implementing effective coping techniques *to reinforce appropriate behavior.*
- Teach alternatives to ineffective behaviors and discuss methods for adopting new behaviors *to encourage the patient's participation in care and to promote change.*

- Encourage the patient's attendance in group therapy sessions. Reassure him that he will not be forced to continue if group therapy causes discomfort *to increase the likelihood of his attendance and to reduce his fear of speaking before a group.*
- Role-play social situations with the patient *to allow him to practice interpersonal skills and improve the quality of peer interactions.*

Discharge interventions
- Provide referrals to outpatient group therapy programs *to ensure support as the patient rejoins the community and to encourage use of improved social and coping skills.*
- Encourage the patient to use support systems, such as a psychotherapist, his family, and his friends, *to ensure availability of long-term support and to help him maintain effective coping skills.*
- Emphasize the importance of seeking follow-up treatment *to help the patient make treatment-related decisions and to encourage his sense of responsibility for behavior.*

EVALUATION STATEMENTS

Patient:
- discusses emotions triggered by illness and usual coping behaviors.
- participates in developing plan of care.
- describes successful use of direct communication to have needs met.
- describes one difficult interpersonal situation that was solved by identifying the problem, choosing alternative ways to communicate, and taking action.

- describes at least two ineffective coping behaviors and appropriate alternative behaviors.
- enlists support and assistance from family and friends.
- expresses understanding of diagnosis, medication purpose and regimen, discharge plan, and need for continued care.
- accepts referral to group therapy.

DOCUMENTATION

- Diagnostic test results and laboratory findings
- Patient's stated perception of condition
- Symptoms of illness including patient's emotions and behaviors
- Nursing interventions and patient's response
- Response to group therapy
- Discharge plan
- Evaluation statements.

Coping, ineffective individual

related to a situational crisis

DEFINITION

Inability to use adaptive behaviors in response to difficult life situations, such as loss of health, a loved one, or a job

ASSESSMENT

Cultural status
- *Demographics:* age, sex, level of education, occupation, nationality, race, ethnic group

- *History:* beliefs, values, and attitudes about health and illness; health customs, practices, and rituals
- *Diagnostic test:* Cultural Assessment Guide

Family status
- *History:* patient's marital status, role in family, evidence of abuse, support systems, family history, family's ability to meet patient's physical and emotional needs, family communication patterns

Psychological status
- *History:* presence of mental illness, usual problem-solving techniques
- *Laboratory tests:* urinalysis, hemoglobin level, blood glucose level, liver function test, human immunodeficiency virus testing
- *Diagnostic tests:* Hamilton Rating Scale for Depression, Minnesota Multiphasic Personality Inventory

Self-care status
- *History:* ability to perform activities of daily living, willingness to perform self-care activities, use of problem-solving techniques

Social status
- *History:* ability to function in social and occupational roles

DEFINING CHARACTERISTICS

- Change in communication patterns
- Chronic fatigue and worry
- Denial of problems
- Dependent personality
- Difficulty asking for help
- Evidence of compulsive behavior
- Excessive consumption of alcohol
- Inability to meet role expectations or basic needs or to solve problems
- Inappropriate use of defense mechanisms
- Ineffective problem-solving skills
- Insomnia
- Irritability, impulsiveness
- Irritable bowel syndrome
- Lack of insight and judgment
- Low self-esteem, perceived self-victimization
- Muscular tension
- Overeating or lack of appetite
- Poor resources and support systems
- Psychosocial stressors
- Verbal manipulation
- Verification of situational crisis

ASSOCIATED DISORDERS

Acute myocardial infarction, alcoholism, anxiety disorders, brief psychotic disorder, cancer, depressive disorders, dissociative disorders, end-stage disease (renal, pulmonary, or cardiac), panic disorders, personality disorders, phobias, somatoform disorders, substance-related disorders or withdrawal

EXPECTED OUTCOMES

Initial outcomes
- Patient performs activities of daily living.
- Patient communicates feelings about present situation.

Interim outcomes
- Patient participates in planning own care.
- Patient identifies two or more adaptive coping techniques.
- Patient implements learned coping techniques.

Discharge outcomes

- Patient uses support systems, such as family and friends, to aid coping.
- Patient expresses feeling of increased control over present situation.
- Patient identifies personal strengths.
- Patient recognizes the need for ongoing outpatient treatment.

INTERVENTIONS AND RATIONALES

Initial interventions

- Help the patient perform daily activities *to increase his self-esteem and promote health and safety.*
- Encourage the patient to talk about his feelings with people he trusts *to help him come to terms with the current crisis.*

Interim interventions

- Encourage the patient to make decisions about his care *to increase his sense of self-worth and mastery over his current situation.*
- Help the patient identify underlying sources of his feelings *to help him grasp the situation and cope more effectively.*
- Teach the patient cognitive and behavioral techniques, such as replacing irrational beliefs, deep breathing, and relaxation, *to improve his coping skills.*
- Encourage the patient to try coping behaviors. *A patient in crisis may be more willing to try new coping behaviors.*
- Discuss with the patient which coping behaviors seem to work *to determine those that are best suited to his needs.*

Discharge interventions

- Teach the patient assertive behaviors *to help him manage anger and reduce feelings of helplessness.*
- Help the patient and family develop objectivity in thinking about the current crisis *to foster a realistic view of events.*
- Identify and praise the patient's successes in coping with the current crisis *to foster self-esteem.*
- Help the patient identify people, such as family and friends, whom he can turn to for support *to prevent isolation.*
- Refer the patient and family to psychological counseling and community support groups *to provide ongoing support.*

EVALUATION STATEMENTS

Patient:

- performs activities of daily living.
- expresses thoughts and feelings related to current crisis.
- exhibits adaptive techniques for managing physical and emotional reactions to crisis.
- develops realistic goals with his family.
- is aware of appropriate outpatient therapeutic options.

DOCUMENTATION

- Evidence of ability to perform activities of daily living
- Patient's verbal and behavioral expression of thoughts and feelings
- Description of patient's emotional status
- Patient teaching, including coping techniques and established goals

- Response of patient and family to teaching
- Referrals for outpatient therapy
- Evaluation statements.

Coping, ineffective individual

related to substance abuse

DEFINITION

Lack of adaptive and appropriate behaviors characterized by the use of alcohol or illicit drugs to cope with the stress of life's demands and roles

ASSESSMENT

Cultural status
- *Demographics:* age, sex, level of education, occupation, nationality, race, ethnic group
- *History:* beliefs, values, and attitudes about health and illness; health customs, practices, and rituals
- *Diagnostic test:* Cultural Assessment Guide

Patient status
- *History:* marital status, family and social roles, support systems, previous substance abuse, perception of present health problems
- *Laboratory tests:* drug toxicology, thyroid function test, serotonin levels, electrolyte levels, urinalysis, hemoglobin level, blood glucose level, liver function test, human immunodeficiency virus testing

Family status
- *History:* family roles, coping patterns, family's ability to meet patient's physical and emotional needs, history of substance abuse in family members
- *Diagnostic test:* Family Genogram

Psychological status
- *History:* self-esteem and self-image, functional ability, current independence level, problem-solving and coping skills, decision-making skills, anxiety level, history of mental illness
- *Social interaction:* interpersonal skills, social network, ability to function in occupation, level of trust in others, ability to seek assistance, aggressive behaviors
- *Diagnostic tests:* Hamilton Rating Scale for Depression, Minnesota Multiphasic Personality Inventory

Neurologic status
- *History:* use of prescribed and over-the-counter medications
- *Diagnostic tests:* electroencephalography, Folstein Mini-Mental Health Status Examination

Self-care status
- *Observation:* functional ability (muscle tone, size, and strength; range of motion; coordination), daily activities (dressing, grooming, bathing, toileting, and hygiene)

DEFINING CHARACTERISTICS

- Active withdrawal anxiety as evidenced by tremulousness, somatic complaints, impaired cognitive functioning, or cravings for alcohol or drugs
- Avoidance behaviors

- Denial
- Grandiosity to mask low self-esteem
- Impulsiveness
- Manipulative behavior

ASSOCIATED DISORDERS

Alcoholism, alcohol withdrawal, bipolar disorder, depressive disorder, personality disorder, schizophrenia, substance-related disorders

EXPECTED OUTCOMES

Initial outcomes
- Patient stops using abused substances.
- Patient doesn't experience injury during withdrawal.

Interim outcomes
- Patient admits that substance abuse is making his life unmanageable.
- Patient identifies resources to help him recover from addiction.
- Family members identify resources to help them cope with the patient's addiction.
- Patient uses available sources of support, such as Alcoholics Anonymous, Narcotics Anonymous, group therapy, educational programs, and individual counseling.
- Staff members coordinate care activities to prevent manipulation by patient.

Discharge outcome
- Patient expresses commitment to attend appropriate support groups and to participate in outpatient follow-up.

INTERVENTIONS AND RATIONALES

Initial interventions
- Remove products containing alcohol — such as mouthwashes and perfumes — from the patient's room and monitor visitors *to prevent substance abuse and to establish the expectation of abstinence. The patient needs to understand that abstinence is necessary for recovery.*
- Assess vital signs and neurologic status *to monitor for convulsions or dangerous increases in blood pressure caused by alcohol withdrawal.*
- Administer fluids and prescribed medications *to help stabilize blood pressure and neurologic status.*
- Spend time talking with the patient, especially when his craving for alcohol or drugs is intense. *This encourages him to talk about, rather than act on, impulses.*

Interim interventions
- Work with the patient to identify ways his impulsive acts harm him *to enhance his awareness of the harmful effects of addiction. Talking about his behavior can help the patient identify underlying feelings.*
- Encourage family members to discuss, in a compassionate way, the way the patient's drinking or drug use has affected their lives and relationships. Encourage family members' involvement in Al-Anon *to promote family healing. Ultimately, motivation to change must come from the patient; however, family members can influence the patient's choices.*
- Teach the patient about substance abuse and provide referrals for further

education about addiction as a disease and about alternate coping skills. Suggest problem-solving techniques that emphasize rational nonemotional responses to problems. *When the patient is no longer cognitively impaired by the effects of withdrawal, he may be more receptive to teaching.*
- Involve the entire treatment staff in discussions about the patient's progress. *During withdrawal, the patient may attempt to manipulate staff members by pitting one against another.*

Discharge interventions
- Provide referrals to Alcoholics Anonymous, Narcotics Anonymous, and educational or therapeutic programs that focus on addiction as a disease, awareness of feelings, coping skills, and problem-solving methods *to take advantage of teaching opportunities once cognitive impairment from the effects of withdrawal decrease.*
- Provide opportunities for staff to resolve conflicts involving the patient's care *to foster staff unity in managing the patient's denial and attempts to manipulate staff.*

EVALUATION STATEMENTS

Patient:
- does not use abused substances while in the hospital.
- does not experience life-threatening effects of withdrawal.
- acknowledges addiction.
- attends and participates in educational, treatment, and self-help programs related to his addiction.
- states his intention to attend community-based addiction treatment programs.

DOCUMENTATION

- Patient statements regarding addictive behavior
- Observations of patient's physical, nutritional, neurologic, and psychological status
- Nursing interventions
- Patient responses to nursing interventions
- Evaluation statements.

Coping, ineffective staff

related to the special patient

DEFINITION

Lack of adaptive and appropriate behaviors on part of staff in response to patient needs

ASSESSMENT

Patient status
- *History:* medical diagnosis, prognosis, perception of present health problems, coping behaviors, problem-solving methods, support systems, family behaviors, family's involvement with patient, family's role and functions

Staff status
- *History:* communication styles and methods of staff members; group cohesiveness; conflict resolution methods; professional goals, values, and beliefs of staff members; professional and personal boundaries

Organizational status
- *History:* methods for handling special patients, communication methods and patterns, nurse-physician communication patterns, use of interdisciplinary case review, specialized personnel and resources

DEFINING CHARACTERISTICS

- Development of exclusive relationships between staff members
- Divisions among or between nursing and medical staff
- Frequent patient complaints
- Inconsistency in nursing interventions and implementation of plan of care
- Lack of objectivity among staff
- Patient history of substance abuse or personality disorder
- Patient hospitalization longer than normal length of stay
- Patient failure to adhere to treatment

ASSOCIATED DISORDERS

Anxiety disorder, bowel disorder, chronic pain, conversion disorder, hypochondriasis, mood disorder, Munchausen syndrome, personality disorder, psychosis, schizophrenia, somatization disorder, substance-related disorder

EXPECTED OUTCOMES

Initial outcome
- Staff members identify problem with care delivery.

Interim outcomes
- Staff members state feelings about providing care for special patient.

- Staff members accept responsibility for their behavior.
- Staff members communicate clearly with each other.

Concluding outcomes
- Staff develops consistent plan of care for special patient.

INTERVENTIONS AND RATIONALES

Initial intervention
- Interview the staff (and the patient, if appropriate) and assess problems *to clarify treatment goals.*

Interim interventions
- Provide a forum for the staff to discuss feelings related to providing care for the special patient *to foster understanding of relationship between emotions and behavior and to allow the staff to assess interpersonal attitudes and behaviors.*
- Provide education on reality testing, limit setting, and establishing appropriate boundaries *to provide the staff with tools and knowledge to facilitate change.*
- Attend or facilitate a patient care conference *to improve staff communication regarding the special patient.*
- Encourage the staff to include the patient or family in the development of a plan of care *to decrease the patient's sense of powerlessness and foster a positive therapeutic relationship.*

Concluding interventions
- Help the staff develop a clear, consistent plan of care for the special patient *to promote development of therapeutic*

interventions and to ensure continued care.
- Periodically monitor staff members' relationships with the special patient *to assess the staff's ability to handle special patients.* Emphasize that staff members need to maintain flexibility in their approach to special patients.

EVALUATION STATEMENTS

Staff members:
- identify problems in treating special patient.
- communicate effectively with each other and with patient.
- develop and implement consistent plan of care.

DOCUMENTATION

- Initial consultations with staff
- Patient and family interviews
- Patient care conferences or forums to discuss patient cases
- Educational activities related to behavior management
- Nursing plan of care for the special patient
- Follow-up report on staff's ability to handle special patients
- Evaluation statements.

Decisional conflict

related to difficulty making health care choices

DEFINITION

State of uncertainty about health-related course of action when choice involves risk, loss, or challenge to personal life values

ASSESSMENT

Cultural status
- *Demographics:* age, sex, level of education, occupation, nationality, race, ethnic group
- *History:* beliefs, values, and attitudes about health and illness; health customs, practices, and rituals
- *Diagnostic test:* Cultural Assessment Guide

Family status
- *History:* roles, communication and coping patterns, developmental stage, socioeconomic factors

Neurologic status
- *Mental status:* appearance, attitude, level of consciousness, judgment, insight, orientation, memory, abstraction and calculation, mood and affect, thought and speech
- *Physical examination:* cerebellar function, cranial nerve function

Psychological status
- *History:* current illness, signs and symptoms, impact of illness on behavior and level of functioning, psychiatric and developmental history
- *Diagnostic tests:* Brief Psychiatric Rating Scale, Wechsler Adult Intelligence Survey

Social status
- *History:* interpersonal skills, quality of relationships, degree of trust in self and others

DEFINING CHARACTERISTICS

- Delayed decision making
- Expressions of concern about other people's role in decision-making
- Expressions of doubt concerning personal beliefs and values
- Expressions of mistrust in other people's opinions about health-related concerns
- Physical and psychological signs of distress

ASSOCIATED DISORDERS

This nursing diagnosis may accompany any condition that presents the patient with difficult decisions concerning his health care; for example, acquired immunodeficiency syndrome, brain death, cancer, end-stage renal disease, or total body failure.

EXPECTED OUTCOMES

Initial outcome

- Patient expresses concern about the potential for conflict between his needs and the wishes of other people involved in his care.

Interim outcomes

- Patient identifies decisions that he can make independently and those that require assistance.
- Patient identifies desirable and undesirable consequences of available options.
- Patient practices progressive muscle relaxation to decrease tension created by decisional conflict.

Discharge outcomes

- Patient reports feeling comfortable with his ability to make specific decisions.
- Patient accepts help from others when necessary without interpreting their help as interference.

INTERVENTIONS AND RATIONALES

Initial intervention

- Listen to the patient's concerns about making a decision *to demonstrate unconditional acceptance.*

Interim interventions

- Help the patient identify available options and their consequences *to encourage rational decision making.*
- Encourage the patient to make decisions about daily activities *to enhance his feelings of autonomy.*
- Teach progressive muscle relaxation techniques *to decrease physical and psychological signs of tension.*

Discharge intervention

- Help the patient identify decision-making areas that require assistance from others and provide appropriate referrals. *Providing referrals will ensure ongoing support. Putting the patient in touch with appropriate community resources will help him gain trust that others are genuinely interested in his well-being.*

EVALUATION STATEMENTS

Patient:
- expresses concerns about family, friends, or health team members interfering with decision making.

- distinguishes between decisions he can make independently and those that require assistance.
- expresses increased comfort accepting help.
- no longer interprets help as interference.
- uses progressive relaxation techniques to alleviate stress.

DOCUMENTATION

- Assessment factors including health status, cognitive functioning, psychological status, and available support systems
- Nursing interventions to help resolve decisional conflict
- Patient's responses to nursing interventions
- Evaluation statements.

Decisional conflict

related to family's choices regarding organ donation

DEFINITION

Inability of family members to address organ donation after the death of a loved one

ASSESSMENT

Cultural status
- *Demographics:* age, sex, level of education, occupation, nationality, race, ethnic group
- *History:* beliefs, values, and attitudes about health and illness; health customs, practices, and rituals

- *Diagnostic test:* Cultural Assessment Guide

Family status
- *Communication:* style and quality of communication, methods of conflict resolution, coping patterns
- *Developmental stage:* ages of family members
- *Alliances:* conflicts between members, support systems, effect of alliances on family stability
- *Physical and emotional needs:* family's ability to meet the needs of its members
- *Religion:* affiliation, values, ethics, customs, practices

DEFINING CHARACTERISTICS

- Anxiety, ambivalence, grief, helplessness, or powerlessness about loss of patient
- Conflict over organ donation
- Need for help in decision making

ASSOCIATED DISORDERS AND TREATMENTS

Brain death; coma; transplantation of lung, heart, liver, kidney; vegetative state

EXPECTED OUTCOMES

Initial outcome
- Family expresses feelings about loss of loved one.

Interim outcomes
- Family acknowledges that nothing more can be done for the patient medically.

- Family expresses feelings about organ donation.
- Family requests medical information about brain death.

Discharge outcome

- Family makes informed decision that is sensitive to feelings of each member.

INTERVENTIONS AND RATIONALES

Initial interventions

- Assess the family's comprehension of patient's medical condition *to determine possible need for crisis intervention.*
- Set aside time to listen to family members and encourage them to express their feelings *to convey understanding and support.*
- Discuss the patient's medical condition clearly and concisely *to promote understanding and to reduce distorted thinking.*
- Help family members understand the difference between coma, vegetative state, and brain death *to ensure the family's right to make fully informed decisions about organ donation.*
- Encourage family members to consult with clergy or another support person *to provide positive reinforcement and help them clarify beliefs and feelings.*

Interim interventions

- Identify the patient as potential organ donor *to fulfill professional responsibility.*
- Assist family members to begin grief process *to promote adjustment to loss.*

- Discuss donor option after the family has had time to assimilate clinical information and adjust to the finality of the patient's medical condition *to make family members aware of the donor option and reinforce their right to make an informed decision. Family members cannot be expected to initiate the idea of organ donation during a time of emotional stress.*
- Encourage questions *to promote understanding and to increase the family's ability to make an informed decision.*

Discharge interventions

- Once family members have made an informed decision, support their choice *to promote their sense of control during the crisis.*
- Help family members understand the grieving process by discussing the universal and self-limiting nature of the grieving process *to offer hope for relief and to provide comfort.*
- Provide information about sources of support *to aid adjustment to the grieving process.*

EVALUATION STATEMENTS

Family members:
- express feelings about loss of loved one.
- verbalize understanding of brain death, coma, and vegetative state.
- acknowledge the patient's medical status.
- are equipped to make informed decision about donor option.
- express feelings about decision whether to grant permission to donate organs.
- begin to move through the grieving process.

DOCUMENTATION

- Family's perceptions and feelings about organ donation
- Family members' behaviors
- Nursing interventions to aid coping
- Information given to family about patient's medical status
- Presentation of donation option
- Evaluation statements.

Decisional conflict

related to staff members' disagreement regarding end-of-life treatment decisions

DEFINITION

Feelings of uncertainty about how a staff member can best ensure that end-of-life treatment decisions respect a patient's right to self-determination, support the patient's interests, and adhere to ethical standards

ASSESSMENT

Cultural status

- *History (staff members and patient):* beliefs, attitudes, and values about health and illness, death, and dying, moral obligations of health care professionals, and patient and caregiver autonomy; health practices, customs, and rituals
- *Knowledge (staff members):* medical and social facts giving rise to the need for treatment decisions, accepted moral norms governing the withholding and withdrawing of life-sustaining treatment, professional moral respon-

sibilities, pertinent federal and state legislation, precedent-setting case law and legal implications of decisions, pertinent hospital policies

- *Hospital environment:* degree to which individual staff members are willing to get involved to prevent or resolve ethical conflict, existence of ethics consultation service and ethics committee
- *Professional responsibilities and skills:* authority for decision making, patient advocacy responsibilities, interpersonal skills and communication patterns, methods of conflict resolution, values and goals, coping patterns

Spiritual status

- *Personal beliefs (staff members and patient):* religious affiliation; religious meanings associated with life, suffering, illness, and death; importance of religious injunctions regarding treatment options

DEFINING CHARACTERISTICS

- Differences of opinion regarding staff members' legal responsibilities and potential liabilities
- Disagreement about when end-of-life treatment decisions should be made
- Uncertainty or lack of consensus about the moral norms that ought to govern decision making and of different members of the health care team
- Uncertainty or lack of consensus about the patient's identity, decision-making history, moral and religious values, and interests
- Uncertainty or lack of consensus about patient's underlying medical condition and its affect on his ability to function and achieve life goals

- Uncertainty or lack of consensus about who should serve as patient advocates when making end-of-life treatment decisions

ASSOCIATED DISORDERS

Acquired immunodeficiency syndrome; coma with brain death; end-stage cardiogenic shock; end-stage renal, pulmonary, or cardiac disease; metastatic cancer in the terminal stages

EXPECTED OUTCOMES

Initial outcome

- Staff members agree to identify areas of conflict and initiate strategies to resolve conflict.

Interim outcomes

- Staff members reach consensus about pertinent medical and social facts, which treatment decisions need to be made, and advocacy responsibilities of individual caregivers.
- Staff members evaluate existing treatment options, assessing potential benefits and risks.
- Staff members seek appropriate resources (for example, an ethics consultant) to resolve conflict.
- Staff members identify feelings, beliefs, and prejudices that contribute to the ethical dilemma.
- Staff members recommend a course (or competing courses) of action supported by ethical reasoning.
- Staff members show respect for the opinions and choices of colleagues who may be unable to accept the plan of care.
- Staff members assist with discharge or transfer of the patient if his preferences are incompatible with the hospital's stated philosophy.

Concluding outcome

- Staff members develop mechanisms to prevent ethical conflict in the future or to facilitate its early resolution.

INTERVENTIONS AND RATIONALES

Initial intervention

- Seek the assistance of an outside facilitator, if necessary, to assemble the involved parties and help them discuss the ethical dilemma. *Staff members must acknowledge the need for and agree to conflict resolution before the process can begin.*

Interim interventions

- Help staff members reach consensus about the pertinent medical and social facts, the required treatment decisions, and the advocacy responsibilities of individual caregivers. *Without a common understanding of these variables, discussion will be fruitless.*
- Encourage staff members to discuss existing treatment options, assessing potential benefits and harms. *Allowing caregivers to argue strongly for one option versus another may reveal underlying sources of conflict.*
- Encourage staff members to discuss ethical norms and legal considerations *to resolve the ethical dilemma.*
- If discussion reveals profound differences concerning the ethical norms that ought to guide decision making or the weight to be given to liability considerations, help staff members seek assistance *to resolve the ethical dilemma.*

- Invite an ethics consultant to participate in staff discussions *to help resolve differences.*
- Help staff members respect the options and ethical choices of colleagues unable to accept the plan of care *to ensure respect for the moral autonomy of health care professionals.*
- Encourage staff members to express willingness to discharge or transfer the patient if his treatment preferences are incompatible with the hospital's stated philosophy. Staff members need to acknowledge the limits placed on them by the principle of patient autonomy.

Concluding intervention
- Encourage staff members to discuss the development of mechanisms to prevent similar future ethical conflicts or to facilitate early resolution of conflict *to foster development of preventive ethics.*

EVALUATION STATEMENTS

Staff members:
- acknowledge need to identify areas of conflict and initiate strategies for achieving resolution.
- reach consensus about pertinent medical and social facts, required treatment decisions, and advocacy responsibilities of individual caregivers.
- evaluate existing treatment options, assessing potential benefits and risks.
- seek appropriate resources to resolve conflict, such as an ethics consultant.
- identify and discuss feelings, beliefs, and prejudices that contribute to the conflict.
- recommend a course (or competing courses) of action supported by ethical reasoning.

- respect conscience rights of caregivers who may be unable to accept the plan of care.
- agree to discharge or transfer patient if his stated preferences are incompatible with hospital's stated philosophy.
- develop mechanisms to prevent ethical conflict in the future or to facilitate early resolution of conflict.

DOCUMENTATION

- Nature of conflict
- Details of meeting to resolve conflict (date, time, place, participants, summary, recommendations)
- Use of outside resources, for example, ethics consultant or ethics committee
- Changes in plan of care
- Evaluation statements.

Denial, ineffective

related to fear or anxiety

DEFINITION

Conscious or unconscious attempt to disavow the knowledge or meaning of an event to reduce anxiety or fear to the detriment of health

ASSESSMENT

Cultural status
- *Demographics:* age, sex, level of education, occupation, nationality, race, ethnic group
- *History:* beliefs, values, and attitudes about health and illness; health customs, practices, and rituals

- *Diagnostic test:* Cultural Assessment Guide

Family status
- *History:* marital status, family role, family history, family's ability to meet patient's physical and emotional needs, evidence of abuse, support systems

Neurologic status
- *History:* general appearance, affect, mood, memory, orientation, communication, judgment, abstract thinking, insight
- *Diagnostic test:* Mini–Mental Status Examination

Psychological status
- *History:* body image, self-esteem, problem-solving ability, coping behaviors, awareness of diagnosis, effect of illness on lifestyle

DEFINING CHARACTERISTICS

- Attribution of symptoms to causes other than his illness
- Delay in seeking medical attention to detriment of health
- Displacement of fear of condition's impact
- Inability to admit impact of disease on life pattern
- Inappropriate affect
- Refusal to admit fear of death or invalidism
- Refusal to perceive personal relevance or danger of symptoms
- Refusal to seek medical attention
- Tendency to minimize symptoms
- Use of self-treatment to relieve symptoms

ASSOCIATED DISORDERS

Acquired immunodeficiency syndrome, acute myocardial infarction, alcoholism, anorexia nervosa, anxiety, bipolar disease (manic or depressive phase), cancer, bulimia nervosa, depressive disorder, end-stage disease (renal, pulmonary, or cardiac), substance-related disorder

EXPECTED OUTCOMES

Initial outcomes
- Patient expresses his knowledge and perception of present health problem.
- Patient describes his lifestyle and reports any recent changes.

Interim outcomes
- Patient describes the stages of grief.
- Patient demonstrates appropriate level of grieving.
- Patient discusses present health problem with doctor, nurses, family, and friends.

Discharge outcome
- Patient exhibits an increased awareness of reality.

INTERVENTIONS AND RATIONALES

Initial interventions
- Plan to spend uninterrupted non-care-related time with the patient each day. Use this time to talk to the patient *to build trust and encourage him to share his knowledge and feelings.*
- Encourage the patient to express his feelings about his present problem, its severity, and its impact on his life. *Ex-*

pressing feelings will help the patient confront and begin to resolve his fears.
- Communicate with the doctor frequently to assess the patient's knowledge about his illness *to foster a consistent, collaborative approach to patient care.*

Interim interventions
- Visit more frequently as the patient's denial lessens *to alleviate fears and foster accurate reality testing.*
- Listen to the patient and provide nonjudgmental feedback *to demonstrate positive regard for the patient's point of view.*

Discharge interventions
- Explain the stages of anticipatory grieving *to improve the patient's understanding of his emotions and ability to cope with them.*
- Encourage the patient to communicate with others and to ask any questions that will help resolve his concerns. *Patients fixated in denial may isolate themselves from others.*

EVALUATION STATEMENTS

Patient:
- describes present health problem.
- describes lifestyle patterns and reports any recent changes.
- communicates an understanding of the stages of grief.
- demonstrates behavior appropriate to his present phase in the grieving process.
- discusses health problem with doctor, nurses, family, and friends.
- displays increasing awareness of reality, either verbally or through behavior.

DOCUMENTATION
- Patient's perception of health problem
- Mental status (baseline and ongoing)
- Patient's knowledge of grief process
- Patient's behavioral responses to illness
- Nursing interventions
- Patient's response to nursing interventions
- Evaluation statements.

Diversional activity deficit

related to long-term hospitalization or frequent, lengthy treatments

DEFINITION

Restriction or decrease in patient's ability to use unoccupied time to his advantage or satisfaction

ASSESSMENT

Cultural status
- *Demographics:* age, sex, level of education, occupation, nationality, race, ethnic group
- *History:* beliefs, values, and attitudes about health and illness; health customs, practices, and rituals
- *Diagnostic test:* Cultural Assessment Guide

Self-care status
- *Observation:* functional ability (muscle tone, size, and strength; range of motion; coordination), daily activities (dressing, grooming, bathing, toileting, and hygiene)

Neurologic status
- *Mental status:* appearance and attitude, level of consciousness, thought and speech, mood and affect, perceptions, orientation, memory, general information

Musculoskeletal status
- *History:* neuromuscular disorders, accidents or trauma, degenerative joint diseases, extreme pathologies, exercise patterns
- *Signs and symptoms:* pain, joint swelling, stiffness, limited movement, muscle weakness
- *Laboratory tests:* serum uric acid level, rheumatoid factor level, erythrocyte sedimentation rate
- *Diagnostic tests:* Functional Mobility Scale, Muscle Strength Scale

Psychological status
- *Current illness:* effects of illness on energy level, motivation, personal hygiene, self-image, self-esteem, sleep pattern, daily functioning
- *History:* presence of psychological disorder, age of onset, type and severity of symptoms, impact on functioning, type of treatment, patient's response to treatment
- *Psychosocial status:* relationships with family or friends; hobbies and interests; favorite music, TV, or reading matter; changes or adaptations needed to carry out activities

DEFINING CHARACTERISTICS

- Expression of boredom or of wishing for something to do
- Hospital stay required past acute stage of illness
- Physical limitations that affect participation in usual activities
- Treatments performed more than once a day
- Treatments that require significant amounts of time

ASSOCIATED DISORDERS AND TREATMENTS

Burns, isolation for contagious diseases, multiple fractures, peripheral vascular ulcers, plastic surgery involving extensive skin grafting, pressure ulcers, spinal cord injury

EXPECTED OUTCOMES

Initial outcome
- Patient expresses interest in using leisure time meaningfully.

Interim outcomes
- Patient participates in chosen activity.
- Patient expresses interest in available activities.
- Patient states satisfaction with use of leisure time.
- Patient makes decisions about timing and spacing of treatments.
- Patient expresses satisfaction with established schedule of treatment routines.

Discharge outcome
- Patient makes adaptations that enable him to pursue interests and activities.

INTERVENTIONS AND RATIONALES

Initial interventions

- Encourage the patient to discuss past hobbies, interests, or skills. *Listening conveys a sense of caring and may help the patient to think of new activities to pursue.*
- Provide a radio or TV at the patient's request *to help relieve boredom and increase enjoyment of leisure time.*
- Engage the patient in conversation while carrying out procedures, if he desires. Discuss favorite topics. *Conversation during treatments reduces discomfort by diverting attention; it also increases the patient's sense of self-worth.*
- Encourage the family or significant other to bring in familiar objects for the patient's room. Provide space for favorite plants, cards, reading material, and hobby supplies. For bedridden patients, use ceiling for posters and other objects. *Providing objects with personal meaning to the patient relieves boredom and stimulates interest.*

Interim interventions

- Schedule time daily for the patient to pursue leisure activities; for example, have him sit at a desk in a wheelchair daily to use a paint-by-number kit. *Diversional activities improve the patient's quality of life. Scheduling activities helps to emphasize their value.*
- Encourage visitors to involve the patient in favorite activities, for example, discussion, reading, or attendance at programs available at the health care facility, if appropriate, *to reduce boredom.*

- Discuss current events with the patient; encourage him to read newspapers or books and watch TV or listen to the radio. *Keeping the patient informed of current events helps reduce the isolation of long-term hospitalization.*
- Schedule treatments to allow adequate rest periods and pursuit of favored activity; for example, restrict treatments between _____ and _____ (time) to allow the patient time for watching a favorite TV show. *This gives him increased control over his environment.*
- Streamline treatments as much as possible. Have all equipment ready before starting; thoroughly instruct new personnel in the routine and plan the schedule for minimal interruptions. *Efficiency conveys respect for the value of the patient's time.*

Discharge intervention

- Work with the patient and the family to find ways to carry out desired activities. Use imagination and creativity; for example, a former carpenter may adapt to carving small objects rather than building large ones. *Creative strategies may enable the patient to pursue previous activities within new limits.*

EVALUATION STATEMENTS

Patient:

- expresses desire to participate in activity during leisure hours.
- engages in chosen activity.
- reports decrease in feelings of boredom.
- makes decisions about timing and spacing of treatments.

- expresses a positive attitude about the treatment schedule.

DOCUMENTATION

- Patient's expressions of boredom, desire to carry out leisure activity, and frustration at being restricted
- Patient's interests, skills, and abilities to carry out activity
- Observations of patient's skill level and extent of participation in activity
- Patient's expression of satisfaction with use of non-treatment-related time
- Evaluation statements.

Family process alteration

related to dysfunctional behavior

DEFINITION

Ineffective family functioning causing psychological, emotional, and social impairment of its members

ASSESSMENT

Cultural status
- *Demographics:* age, sex, level of education, occupation, nationality, race, ethnic group
- *History:* beliefs, values, and attitudes about health and illness; health customs, practices, and rituals
- *Diagnostic test:* Cultural Assessment Guide

Family status
- *History:* marital status; developmental stage of family; family roles; family rules; communication patterns; family alliances; family goals, values, and aspirations; socioeconomic status; evidence of abuse; family health history; ability of family to meet physical and emotional needs of its members
- *Diagnostic tests:* Family Environmental Scale, Family Genogram, Primary Communication Inventory, Index of Family Relations

Parental status
- *Diagnostic tests:* Child Attitude Toward Father and Mother Scales, Index of Parental Attitudes

DEFINING CHARACTERISTICS

- Alcohol or substance abuse
- Frequent family crises
- Imbalance in family members' roles and responsibilities
- Inability of family to meet physical and needs emotional needs of its members
- Inability to resolve family conflicts
- Inflexible, inconsistent, or inappropriate rules
- Intolerance of individual differences and autonomy of family members
- Low self-esteem among family members
- Minimal or absent social networks
- Overbonding and overdependence on family by members
- Poor communication between family members
- Poor problem solving
- Recurrent hospitalizations for psychiatric or medical illnesses
- Rigid or contradictory roles
- Unhealthy or harmful beliefs and customs
- Unrealistic expectations for children

- Verbal, physical, emotional, or sexual abuse

ASSOCIATED DISORDERS

Attention-deficit disorder; anxiety disorders; conduct disorder; delirium, dementia, and amnestic and other cognitive disorders; dissociative disorders; eating disorders; factitious disorder; personality disorders; sexual disorders; schizophrenia; somatoform disorder; substance-related disorders

EXPECTED OUTCOMES

Initial outcomes
- Adults will establish clear lines of authority with children.
- Family members do not abuse alcohol or other substances.
- Family members do not experience verbal, physical, emotional, or sexual abuse.

Interim outcomes
- Family members communicate clearly, honestly, consistently, and directly.
- Family members establish clearly defined roles and responsibilities that are age-appropriate and equitable.
- Family members express understanding of rules and expectations.
- Family members report that methods of solving problems and resolving conflicts have improved.
- Family members report a decrease in the numbers and intensity of family crises.

Discharge outcomes
- Family members describe role expectations that are realistic and promote

individual growth and improved self-esteem.
- Family members report that family rules have changed to adapt to the changing needs of individual members.
- Family members report increased feelings of competence and autonomy.
- Family members report increased social contacts.
- Family members seek ongoing treatment.

INTERVENTIONS AND RATIONALES

Initial interventions
- Meet with adult family members alone *to establish levels of authority and responsibility within the family.*
- In counseling sessions, arrange seating so the adults present a unified front *to reinforce their function as a decision-making unit. In dysfunctional families, one adult may align himself with certain children, while his spouse or partner is aligned with other children.*
- Hold adults accountable for their alcohol or substance abuse and have them sign "Use Contracts" *to decrease denial, increase trust, and promote change. The contract states that the adult will not abuse substances or will seek help for substance abuse.*
- Assist family members to set limits on abusive behaviors and have them sign "Abuse Contracts" *to foster feelings of safety and trust, promote individual accountability and control, and protect individuals from further injury. The contract states that the adults will not abuse or beat each other or that they will seek help for controlling abusive tendencies.*

• Encourage the adults to support each other in setting limits on children's behavior and enforcing rules *to foster adult authority and a consistent approach to discipline.*

Interim interventions

• Teach family members how to communicate clearly and directly *to increase their abilities to express thoughts and feelings and create a climate that fosters honest communication.*
• Guide family members in discussion of roles and responsibilities *to encourage flexibility, promote age-appropriate behavior, and ensure balanced responsibilities.*
• Help the adults establish rules that are appropriate, consistent, and realistic *to help them establish consistent and supportive family discipline.*
• Help family members identify, discuss, and work out problems *to help them develop confidence in their abilities to resolve conflicts and to help them view the family as a safe place to express feelings.*

Discharge interventions

• Encourage family members to recognize improvement in their abilities to communicate with one another *to reinforce the benefits of developing communication skills.*
• Instruct family members to evaluate roles and rules periodically *to ensure flexibility to allow for individual growth and needs fulfillment.*
• Encourage family members to expand their social network *to foster emotional development and build support.*
• Discuss situations or problems that may require further treatment and provide appropriate referrals *to ensure continued professional support.*

EVALUATION STATEMENTS

Adults:
• listen to children and respect their thoughts and feelings, while retaining authority and enforce family rules.
  Family members:
• demonstrate understanding of family roles and rules.
• describe roles and rules that are consistent, realistic, and age-appropriate.
• do not abuse alcohol or other substances.
• do not experience verbal, physical, emotional, or sexual abuse.
• report that family communication is open, spontaneous, honest, and direct.
• report that differences of opinion are respected.
• identify problems and work together to solve them.
• report increased success in resolving conflicts.
• report fewer crisis situations.
• expand their social networks.
• report improved self-esteem.
• recognize need for further treatment.

DOCUMENTATION

• Problems and conflicts described by family members
• Behavioral contracts signed by family members
• Family alliances and changes in alliances over the course of treatment
• Changes in family roles and rules and how these changes were negotiated
• Evidence of changes in family communication patterns

- Nursing interventions and family members' responses
- Unresolved conflicts and problems
- Patient concerns regarding termination of treatment and resources for additional help
- Referrals provided for further treatment
- Evaluation statements.

Family process alteration

related to organ transplantation (awaiting procedure)

DEFINITION

Altered family structure and function during wait for donor organ or tissue

ASSESSMENT

Cultural status
- *Demographics:* age, sex, level of education, occupation, nationality, race, ethnic group
- *History:* beliefs, values, and attitudes about health and illness; health customs, practices, and rituals
- *Diagnostic test:* Cultural Assessment Guide

Family status
- *Roles:* formal and informal roles, role performance, interrelationship between family roles
- *Communication:* style and quality of communication, methods of conflict resolution
- *Developmental stage:* ages of family members

- *Alliances:* conflicts between members, support systems, effect of alliances on family stability
- *Physical and emotional needs:* family's ability to meet needs of its members
- *Socioeconomic factors:* financial status, cultural identity, ethnic identity
- *Religion:* affiliation, values, mores, and practices
- *Diagnostic tests:* Family Environment Scale, Family Adjustment Scale

DEFINING CHARACTERISTICS

- Anticipatory grieving prior to transplantation
- Difficulty with role performance while waiting for transplantation to occur
- Fear and anxiety related to lack of knowledge about transplantation and need to wait for an available donor organ
- Fear of death of loved one while awaiting donor organs
- Feelings of powerlessness while waiting for transplantation to occur

ASSOCIATED DISORDERS AND TREATMENTS

Amyloidosis; cirrhosis of the liver; chronic obstructive pulmonary disease; congenital anomalies of the heart, kidney, or liver; end-stage cardiac disease; hepatitis; renal failure; transplantation of heart, kidney, or liver

EXPECTED OUTCOMES

Initial outcome
- Family members use coping skills during period prior to relative's surgery.

Interim outcome
- Family expresses understanding of purpose, method, and potential complications of transplantation.

Discharge outcome
- Family continues to provide support as patient enters surgery.

INTERVENTIONS AND RATIONALES

Initial interventions
- Assess family members' fear and anxiety *to determine their ability to cope with the impending surgery.*
- Establish a therapeutic relationship with family members *to encourage them to share their feelings. Validation of feelings is necessary to foster hope.*

Interim interventions
- Provide clear, accurate information to family members regularly *to reduce anxiety and to increase their sense of control.*
- Assess psychological effect of patient's prognosis on family members *to determine their needs and plan interventions to prevent maladaptive responses.*
- Encourage participation in a support group for transplant patients and families *to provide an opportunity for family members to share their feelings and to learn more about transplantation.*

Discharge intervention
- Encourage family members to remain supportive of the patient and use coping skills throughout transplantation and recovery periods *to foster effective family functioning.*

EVALUATION STATEMENTS

Family members:
- discuss fears and concerns regarding anticipated transplantation.
- express anxiety while waiting for a donor organ to become available.
- express hope regarding anticipated transplantation.
- identify and use effective coping mechanisms.
- strengthen their ability to support each other.

DOCUMENTATION

- Diagnostic test results
- Family members' statements reflecting their feelings about anticipated organ transplantation
- Family members' statements indicating their understanding of the purpose of transplantation, the procedure, and the associated risks
- Nursing interventions
- Family members' responses to nursing interventions
- Evaluation statements.

Family process alteration

related to organ transplantation (following procedure)

DEFINITION

Disruption in structure and function of family system following organ transplantation

ASSESSMENT

Cultural status
- *Demographics:* age, sex, level of education, occupation, nationality, race, ethnic group
- *History:* beliefs, values, and attitudes about health and illness; health customs, practices, and rituals
- *Diagnostic test:* Cultural Assessment Guide

Family status
- *Roles:* formal and informal roles, role performance, interrelationship between roles
- *Communication:* style and quality of communication, methods of conflict resolution
- *Alliances:* conflicts between members, support systems, effect of alliances on family stability
- *Physical and emotional needs:* family's ability to meet needs of its members
- *Religion:* affiliation, values, mores, and practices
- *Coping:* usual patterns, perception of effectiveness of coping patterns
- *Diagnostic tests:* Family Environment Scale, Family Adjustment Device

DEFINING CHARACTERISTICS

- Anxiety and powerlessness expressed over relative's condition following organ transplantation
- Decreased coping energy following organ transplantation
- Fear that relative will develop complications after organ transplantation
- Role uncertainty following relative's organ transplantation

ASSOCIATED DISORDERS AND TREATMENTS

Amyloidosis; chronic obstructive pulmonary disease; cirrhosis of the liver; congenital anomalies of the heart, kidney, or liver; end-stage cardiac disease; hepatitis, transplantation of heart, kidney, or liver; renal failure

EXPECTED OUTCOMES

Initial outcomes
- Family members communicate physical and emotional needs.
- Family members report that basic physical and emotional needs are met.

Interim outcome
- Family copes successfully with stress related to risk of rejection or infection and other complications of organ transplantation.

Discharge outcomes
- Effective family function is restored.
- Family resumes their former roles or roles are modified as needed.

INTERVENTIONS AND RATIONALES

Initial interventions

- Assess factors interfering with family members' ability to communicate needs and concerns *to prioritize interventions.*
- Encourage the family to express feelings and concerns by listening actively and expressing empathy *to help them cope with unpredictable outcomes of transplantation.*

Interim interventions

- Educate the family about what to expect following transplantation. Explain the risks of rejection and infection *to empower family members through increased awareness and knowledge.*
- Mediate between family members and members of the transplant team *to ensure consistency of treatment and continuity of care.*
- Identify effects of role changes on family function *to determine appropriate interventions.*

Discharge interventions

- Teach each family member how to recognize signs of infection and rejection and adverse effects of immuno-suppressive medications *to foster responsibility, provide direction, and reduce feelings of helplessness.* Emphasize the importance of follow-up care.
- Provide referrals to support groups or community resources *to reduce emotional stress during the transition from hospital to home and community.*
- Emphasize the importance of maintaining communication with the transplant team after discharge *to assure the family of ongoing support and to increase their feelings of control.*

EVALUATION STATEMENTS

Family members:
- openly share feelings and concerns.
- express understanding of immuno-suppressant drug therapy and other measures to prevent transplant rejection.
- list signs and symptoms of transplant rejection, infection, and adverse effects of drug therapy.
- understand behaviors that may promote effective family functioning and factors that may interfere with effective functioning.
- express readiness to contact transplant team as needed.
- discuss potential effects of prolonged recovery on family functioning.
- report that they have resources necessary to follow prescribed treatment regimen.

DOCUMENTATION

- Statements by family members indicating their feelings and concerns regarding organ transplantation and recovery
- Names and phone numbers of contact people at transplant center
- Discharge instructions
- Family members' statements indicating their ability and willingness to assist patient as needed
- Family's adaptation to patient's return home after discharge
- Referrals to community resources
- Evaluation statements.

Fatigue

related to adverse effects of medications

DEFINITION

An overwhelming, sustained sense of exhaustion and decreased capacity for physical and mental work following ingestion of prescribed medication

ASSESSMENT

Cultural status
- *Demographics:* age, sex, level of education, occupation, nationality, race, ethnic group
- *History:* beliefs, values, and attitudes about health and illness; health customs, practices, and rituals
- *Diagnostic test:* Cultural Assessment Guide

Neurologic status
- *Mental status:* appearance, attitude, thought and speech patterns, mood, affect, perceptions, orientation, attention span, abstraction, judgment and insight
- *Physical examination:* motor and sensory function, reflexes
- *Laboratory tests:* serotonin levels, drug toxicology, electrolyte levels, thyroid function, liver function, urinalysis, blood glucose levels
- *Diagnostic tests:* electroencephalography (EEG), sleep-deprived EEG

Psychological status
- *Effects of current illness:* motivation, changes in appetite, energy level
- *Life changes:* recent divorce, illness, job loss, loss of loved one
- *Psychiatric history:* presence of psychiatric illness, type of treatment, patient's response to treatment, medication history
- *Alcohol or drug abuse:* type of substances, evidence of abuse or withdrawal
- *Diagnostic tests:* Hamilton Rating Scale for Depression, Beck Depression Inventory

Self-care status
- *History:* presence of neurologic, sensory, or psychological impairment, exercise, nutrition
- *Observation:* functional ability (muscle tone, size, and strength; range of motion; coordination), daily activities (dressing, grooming, bathing, toileting, and hygiene)

Sleep-pattern status
- *Prior medical conditions:* sleep disorders
- *History:* usual hours of sleep, circadian pattern, energy level after sleep, rest and relaxation patterns
- *Medications:* sleep aids, caffeine, alcohol, amphetamines, benzodiazepines
- *Signs and symptoms:* difficulty falling asleep, nocturnal awakening, early morning awakening, hypersomnia, insomnia, sleep pattern reversal

DEFINING CHARACTERISTICS

- Abnormal EEG findings
- Addiction to sleep aids
- Depression
- Disorganized sleep schedule

- High level of caffeine consumption
- History of drug or alcohol abuse
- Insufficient help while adjusting to medication changes or adverse effects
- Lack of exercise

ASSOCIATED DISORDERS

Adverse effects of neuroleptics, anxiolytics, and sedatives of the barbiturate class; extrapyramidal adverse reactions; mood disorders; organic mental syndromes; substance abuse

EXPECTED OUTCOMES

Initial outcomes
- Patient acknowledges that medication use or illness contributes to fatigue.
- Patient describes sleep schedule.
- Patient describes times of day when fatigue is at its worst.

Interim outcomes
- Patient stays in bed at night.
- Patient remains out of bed during daytime, except for designated rest periods.
- Patient participates in activities.
- Patient performs self-care measures.

Discharge outcomes
- Patient maintains a standard sleep schedule.
- Patient maintains an exercise and nutrition program.

INTERVENTIONS AND RATIONALES

Initial interventions
- Observe and document the patient's level of fatigue *to determine realistic activity goals.*
- Teach the patient about the possible correlation between medication use, mental health, and fatigue *to increase his understanding of his condition.*
- Ask the patient to describe his sleep patterns *to understand the relationship between sleep patterns and fatigue.*

Interim interventions
- Encourage the patient to identify times and situations when fatigue is increased *to plan a strategy for reducing fatigue.*
- Provide designated times of rest *to foster sleep at night.*
- Discuss the patient's activity and self-care schedule with him. Encourage him to get out of bed at appropriate times *so that he can maintain activities.*
- Teach the patient relaxation techniques. *Relaxation induces sleepiness.*

Discharge interventions
- Discuss with the family ways to modify the patient's home environment *to reduce overexertion, minimize feelings of being overwhelmed, and increase his ability to participate in activities and perform self-care.*
- Help the patient plan his sleep and rest schedule and a balanced nutrition and exercise program while he is taking the prescribed medication *to encourage an appropriate sleep schedule and decrease the risk of fatigue.*

- Encourage the patient to notify his doctor of any severe adverse reactions to the medication *to encourage him to get help with serious medication problems.* Teach him ways to deal with uncomfortable but nonthreatening adverse reactions.

EVALUATION STATEMENTS

Patient:
- attends group and mealtime activities.
- sleeps _____ hours per night.
- performs self-care measures without undue fatigue.
- eats three well-balanced meals a day.
- maintains nutrition, exercise, activities, and sleep schedule after discharge.
- describes helpful changes in his home.

DOCUMENTATION

- Group meetings and mealtimes attended by patient
- Number of hours patient sleeps at night and during daytime rest periods
- Degree of fatigue reported by patient
- Medication taken by patient
- Patient and family teaching regarding medication
- Patient's discharge schedule
- Evaluation statements.

Fatigue

related to mood disturbance

DEFINITION

Generalized, persistent fatigue (lasting 6 months or more), accompanied by muscle pain and emotional and cognitive changes that severely impair daily functioning

ASSESSMENT

Cultural status
- *Demographics:* age, sex, level of education, occupation, nationality, race, ethnic group
- *Personal habits:* beliefs, values, and attitudes about health and illness; health customs, practices, and rituals
- *Diagnostic test:* Cultural Assessment Guide

Musculoskeletal status
- *Effects of current illness*
- *Signs and symptoms:* persistent fatigue that interferes with daily activities, muscle pain following activity, reduced physical fitness resulting from inactivity, dizziness resulting from the effects of extreme inactivity on autonomic function

Sleep pattern status
- *Personal habits:* usual hours of sleep, circadian pattern, energy level after sleep, rest and relaxation patterns
- *Signs and symptoms:* sleep pattern disturbances, daytime fatigue resulting from poor or unrefreshing sleep

- *Diagnostic test:* Sleep electroencephalography

Psychological status
- *History:* current illness; recent stressful events; ability to function in occupation; attitudes, beliefs, and behaviors; activity level
- *Family history:* presence of psychological disturbances
- *Signs and symptoms:* irritability, poor concentration, loss of interest in activities or surroundings, depression, fatigue, headache, forgetfulness, irritability, confusion, tearfulness (especially when tired)

DEFINING CHARACTERISTICS

- Attitudes, beliefs, and behaviors that tend to perpetuate symptoms and exacerbate fatigue
- Avoidance of activity
- Family history of depressive disorder
- Helplessness
- Inability to function in occupation
- Myalgia
- Persistent fatigue that interferes with daily activities
- Poor cognition
- Prior episodes of depressive illness
- Recent episode of viral illness
- Recent loss or stressful event
- Seasonal episodes of mood disorder
- Sleep disorder

ASSOCIATED DISORDERS

Alcoholism, anxiety disorders, chronic fatigue syndrome, chronic mononucleosis, chronic postviral syndrome, dyssomnia, Epstein-Barr virus syndrome, immunologic defects, mood disorders, myalgic encephalomyelitis, parasomnia, somatization disorder, sleep apnea, substance-related disorders

EXPECTED OUTCOMES

Initial outcomes
- Patient is not injured.
- Patient uses prescribed medication.
- Patient adheres to scheduled sleep and rest periods.
- Patient reports reduced myalgia with use of medication.
- Patient identifies own baseline level of activity tolerance.

Interim outcomes
- Patient gradually increases activity level above the established baseline.
- Patient participates in appropriate individual, group, couples, or family therapy.

Discharge outcomes
- Patient identifies maladaptive thinking patterns and behaviors.
- Patient demonstrates an understanding of the relationship between symptoms and psychological factors or psychiatric disorder.
- Patient identifies feelings of regaining control over his own life through a continued gradual increase in activity.
- Patient participates in defining goals for continuing treatment.

INTERVENTIONS AND RATIONALES

Initial interventions
- Develop an activity and rest schedule based on the patient's tolerance. Discuss the importance of regular

sleep and rest periods *to prevent excessive fatigue, which may lead to injury.*
- Teach the patient about the purpose of medication and administer medication as prescribed *to decrease daytime fatigue.*
- Encourage the patient to identify symptoms that follow activity *to help him understand activity intolerance.*
- Help the patient follow scheduled sleep and rest periods *to promote effective sleep patterns.*
- Arrange for a medical evaluation of the patient's physical deconditioning *in order to establish a baseline activity and rest level.*

Interim interventions
- Help the patient establish an appropriate activity schedule with graded increases in activity level. Establish rest periods between activities *to improve function, mood, and feelings of well-being.*
- Help the patient plan a schedule that is conducive to attending therapy appointments and completing homework assignments between appointments. *Homework assignments can help the patient identify unproductive thinking patterns and behavior.*

Discharge interventions
- Help the patient identify his own symptoms and behaviors *to encourage him to change unproductive thinking patterns and behaviors.*
- Collaborate with the patient in setting precise and realistic treatment goals for improving his functioning *to motivate him to continue treatment.*
- Encourage and support the patient and family members to continue a graded increase in patient activity (fol-

lowed by rest periods), even when symptoms occur. *Participation in activity helps the patient reestablish a feeling of control over his life.*

EVALUATION STATEMENTS

Patient:
- does not experience injury.
- develops improved sleep and rest patterns.
- demonstrates increased energy and activity level and improved function, mood, and feeling of well-being.
- offers alternatives to maladaptive or depressive thinking patterns and demonstrates changes in behavior.
- agrees to continuing treatment and rehabilitation.
- verbalizes realistic goals for functioning rather than expecting a cure.

DOCUMENTATION

- Nursing interventions performed to decrease daytime fatigue
- Nursing interventions performed to improve function, mood, and feeling of well-being
- Patient's response to nursing interventions
- Referrals for specialized evaluations and treatments
- Evaluation statements.

Fatigue

related to postpartum status

DEFINITION

An overwhelming, sustained sense of exhaustion experienced by a new mother during the first 3 months after delivery

ASSESSMENT

Cultural status

- *Demographics:* age, level of education, employment during or after pregnancy, marital status
- *History:* beliefs, attitudes, and values about health, illness, and child rearing

Cardiovascular status

- *History:* use of tobacco and caffeine, nutrition and exercise patterns before, during, and after pregnancy
- *Physical examination:* mobility, activity tolerance, skin color, vital signs, including temperature, pulse, respirations, blood pressure
- *Prior medical conditions:* postpartum hemorrhage, primary or pregnancy-induced hypertension, diabetes mellitus (gestational or other), heart disease, thyroid disease
- *Laboratory tests:* hemoglobin and hematocrit levels, blood glucose level, thyroid function tests

Family status

- *Family roles:* formal and informal roles, role performance, commitment by family members to traditional roles

in child rearing, role changes after addition of a child to family unit
- *Family communication:* quality of communication
- *Developmental stage of family:* changes in roles over time, problems adapting to change
- *Family subsystems:* family alliances, conflict between family subsystems, supportive relationships within family, family's ability to help with new baby, disparities between individual's needs and family's willingness or ability to meet them
- *Socioeconomic factors:* employment status, attitudes toward work
- *Coping patterns:* usual coping patterns, reaction to childbirth, reaction to other major life events
- *Diagnostic tests:* Family Environment Scale, Family Adjustment Device, Primary Communication Inventory, Index of Family Relations

Nutritional status

- *History:* usual exercise pattern, typical daily food intake, type of infant feeding
- *Physical examination:* height, weight, basal energy expenditure, anthropometric measurements
- *Signs and symptoms:* weight change during or since pregnancy, nutritional deficiencies, nausea and vomiting, fainting, pallor, irritability, cravings
- *Medications:* use of iron and other minerals, multivitamins, vitamin B_{12}, other nutritional supplements; use of laxatives and prescription and over-the-counter drugs
- *Laboratory tests:* hemoglobin and hematocrit levels, serum iron, total protein, serum transferrin levels

- *Diagnostic tests:* Eating Attitudes Test, Concern Over Weight and Dieting Scale

Psychological status
- *Reactions to birth:* changes in energy level, motivation, sleep, sexual drive; reaction to new body image and temporary limitations; significance attached to birth
- *History:* self-esteem, psychiatric history, hobbies and recreational activities, primary depression, postpartum depression, substance abuse before or during pregnancy, stress related to pregnancy or other factors
- *Medications:* narcotics, psychotropic drugs
- *Laboratory tests:* blood and urine drug toxicology
- *Diagnostic tests:* Center for Epidemiological Study-Depressive Symptomatology Scale, Spielberger State-Trait Anxiety Inventory, Impact of Event Scale, The Problem Solving Inventory, Self-Efficacy Scale

Sleep pattern status
- *History:* usual hours of sleep, circadian pattern, energy level after sleep, rest and relaxation patterns, changes in sleep patterns since birth, infant sleep patterns
- *Medications:* sleeping aids, caffeine, alcohol, amphetamines
- *Signs and symptoms:* sleep pattern disturbances, depression, sleep apnea, nocturnal or early awakening, hypersomnia and insomnia

DEFINING CHARACTERISTICS

- Breast-feeding
- Decreased self-esteem, difficulty with problem solving, discomfort with body image
- Difficulty adapting to demands of parenting
- Difficulty introducing baby to siblings
- Early return to work after delivery
- Extremes in parity
- Greater than average blood loss
- History of high-risk pregnancy, labor, or delivery
- Inability to rest and relax or limited opportunities for recreation
- Irritable infant who sleeps poorly
- Lack of support from family members
- Low hemoglobin and hematocrit levels
- Multiple roles in family and in community
- Poor nutrition and hydration
- Postpartum depression, lethargy, listlessness
- Prolonged use of narcotics for postpartum pain or other substance use
- Socioeconomic stresses
- Teenage or late-life pregnancy
- Underlying medical conditions

ASSOCIATED DISORDERS

Anemia, cesarean deliveries, heart disease, hypertensive disorders, muscle atrophy (following prolonged bed rest during pregnancy), postpartum depression, thyroid disease

EXPECTED OUTCOMES

Initial outcome
- Mother has significant stretches of time (specify) to rest within 48 hours after delivery.

Interim outcomes
- By the 3rd day after delivery, mother lists ways to ameliorate fatigue.
- By the 2nd week after delivery, mother identifies resources to help lessen her expenditure of energy.

Discharge outcomes
- By the end of the 6th week after delivery, mother incorporates measures to modify fatigue into her daily routine.
- At 3 months postpartum, mother has more energy and can describe a plan for ongoing fatigue management.

INTERVENTIONS AND RATIONALES

Initial intervention
- During the first 48 hours of the postpartum period, reduce unnecessary stimulation. Organize nursing procedures and education within compressed time periods and encourage rest *to conserve the mother's energy and avoid exhaustion.*

Interim intervention
- At 3 days postpartum, teach strategies to increase comfort and rest, such as using a sidelying position for breastfeeding, paying attention to nutrition, resting frequently, and performing light exercises. *These strategies can help the mother decrease fatigue.*
- From 3 days through 2 weeks postpartum, encourage the mother to obtain needed help. Encourage her to use spouse or partner, family, friends, church members, or neighborhood teenagers *to help her conserve her energy.*

Discharge intervention
- Review with the mother plans for integrating fatigue management into her life. *Fatigue is an ongoing issue with parenthood.*

EVALUATION STATEMENTS

Mother:
- by 48 hours postpartum feels more rested than immediately after delivery.
- by 3 days postpartum can describe three strategies to decrease fatigue.
- by 2 weeks postpartum obtains needed help.
- at 3 months postpartum reports increased energy levels.

DOCUMENTATION

- Amount mother rests following delivery
- Mother's description of strategies for obtaining help and rest
- Evidence of assistance by family members and other sources of support
- Mother's plan for ongoing management of fatigue
- Evaluation statements.

Fluid volume excess

related to excess fluid intake (water intoxication)

DEFINITION

A self-induced fluid imbalance due to excessive water intake (psychogenic polydipsia) and inability to excrete excess fluid, resulting in dangerously low sodium levels leading to behavior changes and seizures

ASSESSMENT

Cultural status
- *Demographics:* age, sex, level of education, occupation, nationality, race, ethnic group
- *History:* beliefs, values, and attitudes about health and illness; health customs, practices, and rituals
- *Diagnostic test:* Cultural Assessment Guide

Renal status
- *Prior medical conditions:* history of conditions that impair renal function
- *History:* drinking pattern; water, coffee, tea, and alcohol intake; smoking
- *Physical examination:* general observations, skin color and turgor, urine output, presence of edema, vital signs, weight changes throughout day
- *Signs and symptoms:* decreased or excessive urine output, edema (periorbital swelling, distended abdomen), hypothermia, thirst, weight gain, bedwetting, elevated blood pressure, hypothermia, sudden dramatic weight gain during the day, varied patterns of excessive urine excretion at night
- *Laboratory tests:* serum sodium and plasma sodium levels, midday urine specific gravity

Neurologic status
- *Mental status:* appearance and attitude, level of consciousness, motor activity, thought and speech, mood and affect, perceptions, orientation, memory, general information, calculations, capacity to read and write, visual-spatial ability, attention span, abstraction, judgment and insight
- *Prior medical conditions*
- *Medications:* neuroleptic drugs, anticonvulsants, antipsychotic agents, antidepressants, alcohol, illicit drugs
- *Signs and symptoms:* sudden onset seizure, altered gait, increased irritability, slurred speech, confusion, disorientation, agitation, delusions, poor concentration, drowsiness, apathy, restlessness, deteriorating level of alertness as the day progresses, neuroleptic-induced dry mouth

Psychological status
- *Prior psychiatric conditions*
- *Personal habits:* thoughts and behaviors associated with fluid intake and excretion
- *Signs and symptoms (thought content):* delusional reasons for drinking, such as need to purify the body or wash away evil spirits; self-medication to suppress auditory hallucinations or to get high; boredom; socially impoverished behavior
- *Signs and symptoms (behavioral):* frequent trips to the water fountain, compulsion to drink out of toilets and shower, taking drinks from other patients' meal trays, hoarding drink containers, drinking own urine, continuous drinking during waking hours, no nighttime drinking while excess fluid is voided, bed-wetting
- *Laboratory tests:* urinalysis, electrolyte levels

DEFINING CHARACTERISTICS

- Changes in mental status, including poor concentration, apathy, lethargy, confusion, agitation

- Chronic psychiatric illness
- Decreased level of alertness during the day
- Diurnal weight gain (weight may return to normal levels at night)
- Drinking that begins around breakfast time and continues until evening, no drinking during the night
- Endocrine dysfunction
- Episodes of bed-wetting
- History of water intoxication
- Impaired renal function
- Massive water ingestion (more than 20 to 25 liters per day) accompanied by hyponatremia
- Midday serum sodium level less than 130 mEq/liter or midday plasma sodium level less than 120 mmol/liter (may return to normal levels overnight)
- Midday urine specific gravity between 1.010 and 1.003 (may return to normal levels overnight)
- Sudden onset of seizures with no apparent cause
- Urinary incontinence during the night

ASSOCIATED DISORDERS AND TREATMENTS

Bipolar disorder, diabetes insipidus, major motor seizure, psychosis with auditory hallucinations, renal disease (chronic or acute), tardive dyskinesia, schizophrenia (chronic)

This diagnosis also may be associated with use of the following drugs: chlorpropamide or tolbutamide, opioids, barbiturates, vincristine, clofibrate and carbamazepine, thiazide diuretics, neuroleptic agents, and psychotropics.

EXPECTED OUTCOMES

Initial outcome
- Patient attains fluid balance within normal limits as evidenced by sodium serum level within normal range and maintenance of established weight.

Interim outcomes
- Patient maintains fluid balance within normal limits as evidenced by diurnal weight variation within targeted range and normal urine specific gravity.
- Patient participates in learning activities related to water intoxication.
- Patient identifies stressors that trigger excessive fluid intake.
- Patient uses learned relaxation techniques to reduce stress and anxiety.
- Patient describes signs and symptoms of water intoxication.
- Patient participates in activities aimed at controlling his water intake.
- Patient uses nontoxic oral rewards, such as sugar-free hard candy or gum.

Discharge outcomes
- Family members demonstrate an understanding of symptoms and treatment of water intoxication.
- Patient demonstrates evidence of controlling own fluid balance by maintaining weight within specified range.
- Patient express understanding that water intoxication is potentially lethal.

INTERVENTIONS AND RATIONALES

Initial interventions
- Monitor the patient and divert his attention from water intake. Strategies may include one-on-one supervision,

seclusion, controlling access to bathrooms, monitoring showers, restricting use of water fountains, taking away drinking cups, and limiting drinks. Use restraints as a last resort. *Initially, strict control is needed to control excessive water intake.*
- Monitor serum sodium levels at times of peak symptoms *to assess fluid balance.*

Interim interventions
- Teach the patient how to maintain a log to monitor his own diurnal weight and how to use his target weight as an indicator of excessive water intake. Discuss how to recognize signs and symptoms of water intoxication. *These measures will help the patient understand water intoxication.*
- Teach the patient how to identify triggers that produce anxiety and use relaxation techniques *to help him establish inner controls.*
- Collaborate with the patient in establishing a written contract to decrease water intake *to enhance patient participation in care and foster a sense of control.*
- Provide gum and sugar-free hard candies *as substitutes for the use of water.*
- Monitor the patient's serum sodium levels and diurnal weight *in order to maintain water balance.*

Discharge interventions
- Give the patient an opportunity to drink or refuse water at specified times of the day *to reinforce his control of water intake.*
- Offer rewards, such as passes to visit family or to participate in off-floor ac-

tivities, *to reinforce the patient's control of water intake.*
- Teach family members or friends the precise amount, frequency, and duration of oral fluids recommended for the patient *to help manage water intake at home.*

EVALUATION STATEMENTS

Patient:
- maintains targeted weight.
- sodium levels within normal range.
- identifies signs and symptoms of water intoxication.
- describes lethal effects of water intoxication.
- participates in the treatment plan.
- signs a behavioral contract.
- uses relaxation techniques in response to identified triggers.
- uses hard candy or gum as alternative, nontoxic means of achieving oral gratification.

Family members or friends:
- demonstrate the ability to manage the patient's fluid intake schedule and monitor his behaviors.

DOCUMENTATION

- Physiologic symptoms of excess fluid intake
- Alterations in symptoms in response to treatment
- Nursing interventions performed to limit fluid intake
- Patient teaching
- Patient's response to nursing interventions
- Patient's level of participation in treatment
- Patient's willingness to honor behavioral plan

- Patient's use of relaxation techniques at times of stress or anxiety
- Patient's use of alternative methods of oral gratification or rewards to substitute for water consumption
- Patient's response to fluid intake restriction (verbal and behavioral)
- Follow-up care, continuing treatment, and referrals
- Evaluation statements.

Grieving, anticipatory

related to anticipated divorce or separation

DEFINITION

Grief reaction to anticipated personal loss resulting from a divorce or separation

ASSESSMENT

Cultural status

- *Demographics:* age, sex, level of education, occupation, nationality, race, ethnic group
- *History:* beliefs, values, and attitudes about health and illness; health customs, practices, and rituals
- *Diagnostic test:* Cultural Assessment Guide

Family status

- *History:* marital status or live-in arrangement, duration of relationship, reasons for separation, initiator of separation, acceptance level of both parties, children's understanding of separation, previous relationships and reasons for cessation

- *Family composition:* number and ages of children, elderly relatives or other dependents in the home, pets
- *Family traits:* culture; ethnic background; religion; communication style; conflict resolution methods; physical, emotional, or sexual abuse; health status
- *Socioeconomic factors:* economic level, community status, social network, support from extended family and friends
- *Diagnostic tests:* Family Genogram, Holmes and Rahe Social Readjustment Rating Scale, Index of Family Relations, Index of Spouse Abuse

Neurologic status

- *Examination:* cognitive functioning
- *Mental status:* appearance and attitude, level of consciousness, motor activity, thought and speech, mood and affect, perceptions, orientation, memory, general information, calculations, capacity to read and write, visual-spatial ability, attention span, abstraction, judgment and insight
- *Laboratory tests:* complete blood count, urinalysis, human immunodeficiency virus test, endocrine functions
- *Diagnostic tests:* none unless specified for positive findings

Psychological status

- *History:* signs and symptoms; changes in self-esteem, concentration level, memory, appetite, weight, sleep pattern, sexual interest and fulfillment, parental ability, social interactions, occupational competence; change in relationships with extended family and friends; past psychiatric illness; previous treatment or hospitalization

- *Childhood development:* parental modeling of marriage and relationships; sibling birth order; relationships with peers, teachers, and authority figures; personality traits; overall health and history of childhood diseases; social involvement; academic performance; maladaptive behaviors
- *Adolescent development:* ability to individuate from family of origin, peer relationships, dating, sexual behavior, school involvement, work, leisure activities, relationships with parents and siblings
- *Adult development:* self-esteem and ability to achieve intimacy, ability to give emotionally and psychologically to others, job stability, military history, dating and marital history, parenting skills, children's development, financial responsibility, relationship with family of origin, coping strategies, social and leisure activities
- *Medication history:* antidepressants, antipsychotics, antimanic agents, anticonvulsants, analgesics, hormone replacement therapy, use of alcohol, illicit substance use
- *Diagnostic tests:* Minnesota Multiphasic Personality Inventory, Beck Depression Inventory, State-Trait Anxiety Inventory

DEFINING CHARACTERISTICS

- Conflict between partners regarding major issues, such as child rearing practices or life goals
- Discrepancy in developmental stages of partners
- Domestic violence
- Extramarital affair
- Financial conflict

- Marriage after less than 6-month relationship or after engagement longer than 3 years
- Marriage that follows significant loss
- Marriage used as a means to separate from family of origin
- Partners from divergent backgrounds
- Physical, emotional, or sexual abuse
- Physical or mental illness in family
- Poor communication skills
- Poor relationship with siblings or parents
- Substance abuse

ASSOCIATED DISORDERS

Endocrine dysfunction, impulse-control disorder, menopause or climacteric, mood disorder, organic mental disorder, personality disorder, physical disorder, posttraumatic stress disorder, relational problems, sexual dysfunction

EXPECTED OUTCOMES

Initial outcomes

- Patient seeks treatment for dysphoria, anxiety, or suicidal thoughts.
- Patient seeks treatment for changes in sleep pattern, appetite, or activity levels.
- Patient discusses behaviors and emotions related to expected loss.
- Patient expresses concerns about changes in lifestyle and relationships after separation or divorce.
- Patient discusses future association with former partner.
- Patient expresses concern regarding her ability to maintain future long-term relationships.

Interim outcomes

- Patient acknowledges effect of separation or divorce on emotional state.
- Patient expresses understanding of grieving process.
- Patient describes coping strategies used successfully in the past.
- Patient develops a time line of expected events and activities during separation or divorce.
- Patient describes plans for coping with expected changes.
- Patient agrees to work on strengthening personal relationships.

Discharge outcomes

- Patient presents plan for resolving legal issues, visitation schedule, alimony, housing, or other issues related to separation or divorce.
- Patient acknowledges that separation was a stimulus for emotional growth in other areas of her life.
- Patient demonstrates effective coping strategies.
- Patient describes actions to promote emotional growth.
- Patient participates in role-playing exercises to strengthen financial and occupational planning skills.
- Patient acknowledges stages and expected duration of grief reaction.
- Patient participates in group therapy.

INTERVENTIONS AND RATIONALES

Initial interventions

- Evaluate the patient's safety. If she is endangered by suicidal thoughts or thoughts of harming others, discuss the option of entering the hospital *to communicate to the patient that, while you can help evaluate her situation, ultimately she is responsible for her own behavior.*
- Encourage the patient to verbalize feelings about her current problem *to enable her to evaluate her current need.*
- Encourage realistic appraisal of the significance of the relationship's end *to help the patient understand that ending the relationship will bring changes to many aspects of her life.*
- Acknowledge that the patient's pain is real but assure her that it will abate as therapy and time progress *to sustain hope in the midst of depression.*
- Explain the purpose of prescribed antidepressant or antianxiety medications. *Drug therapy may be prescribed during the acute stage of crisis to enable the patient to work through the grieving process. Once the acute crisis is past, drugs may be discontinued.*
- Emphasize the need for short-term counseling *to help the patient realize she will return to her former state of health.*
- Encourage the patient to initiate plans to deal with impending changes related to separation or divorce *to help decrease uncertainty and pain and to help her come to terms with feelings of guilt or unrealistic expectations regarding reconciliation.*
- Encourage the patient to address her concerns and seek therapy as needed *to provide an opportunity for her to work on areas of her choosing, such as interpersonal relationships.*

Interim interventions

- Offer cognitive reframing of illogical ideas *to help break the all-or-nothing thought patterns that are common in depressed patients and to foster hope.*

Help the patient view reality from a healthier perspective.

- Discuss coping strategies that the patient has used successfully in the past *to encourage use of established effective behaviors and help the patient draw on her strengths.*
- Teach ways the patient can confront approaching changes instead of just responding passively to events *to foster positive action and to decrease anxiety.*
- Explain the stages of grieving to the patient. Tell her that her experiences may be similar to people who face other traumatic losses, such as the death of a loved one. She may experience denial, protest, despair, remorse, anger and guilt. *Teaching will increase the patient's understanding of the grieving process.*
- Help the patient develop a timetable describing events that she can anticipate during her separation or divorce and appropriate activities *to help her anticipate future events, encourage her to take action, and to promote assertive behavior.*
- Determine the patient's willingness and ability to take part in group therapy *to provide an opportunity to express feelings about loss and receive feedback from others who are enduring a similar experience. She may come to realize that others have similar hardships and learn to appreciate that change is an inherent part of human existence.*

Discharge interventions

- Reinforce positive, mature, goal-directed statements and behaviors *to increase positive behavior and to promote reality testing.*
- Encourage the patient to make concrete plans *to foster emotional growth.*

- Role-play anticipated discussions with children, parents, friends, and colleagues regarding the separation or divorce *to help the patient evaluate her situation, to reduce depression and anxiety, and to promote effective responses to anticipated changes. Children may experience depression or conflicting loyalties during a divorce. Relationships with relatives may need to be reevaluated, especially relationships with in-laws if there are children. Friendships may change when the patient is no longer part of a couple. Exploring these issues will help the patient understand that change is an inherent part of life.*
- Encourage the patient to discuss housing, finances, and the possible need to return to work. *For many women and children, financial resources are diminished after a separation or divorce. Increased awareness will foster realistic planning.*
- Note evidence of grief reaction stages in the patient's behavior and explain that working through these feelings may be an ongoing process *to affirm the patient's progress and give her permission to work on issues surrounding grief.*
- Monitor adherence to the timetable established by the patient for activities related to separation or divorce *to assist her efforts to assume greater responsibility and control. The patient may have ambivalent feelings about assuming control and need your support.*
- Acknowledge the patient's personal growth and increased self-esteem as individual and group therapy progresses *to encourage active participation in treatment.*

EVALUATION STATEMENTS

Patient:
- does not harm self or others.
- states intention to contact hospital, therapist, hot line, or other support system if suicidal or homicidal thoughts recur.
- verbalizes plan to use effective coping strategies.
- demonstrates ability to address children's concerns about separation or divorce and to effectively communicate with friends, family, and colleagues.
- discusses plans to cope with expected changes in status, finances, and employment.
- acknowledges that feelings and behaviors are part of the grieving process.
- expresses understanding of the benefits of group therapy.
- agrees to take personal control of the separation or divorce schedule.
- evaluates her progress and acknowledges her increased ability to deal with the separation or divorce and personal growth in other aspects of her life.

DOCUMENTATION

- Diagnostic test results
- Nursing interventions to help patient cope with immediate crisis
- Nursing interventions to link patient with sources of support
- Positive coping strategies used in the past, as described by the patient
- Nursing interventions to help the patient evaluate her finances, housing options, and employment options and referrals to outside agencies for help with these needs

- Evidence of patient's progress through the stages of grieving
- Patient's timetable describing the separation or divorce
- Referral to group therapy
- Evidence of patient's future plans
- Referrals to mediators, lawyers, or social services as needed
- Evaluation statements.

Grieving, anticipatory

related to potential loss of family member

DEFINITION

Family's distress in response to anticipated loss of one of its members

ASSESSMENT

Cultural status
- *Demographics:* age, sex, level of education, occupation, nationality, race, ethnic group
- *History:* beliefs, values, and attitudes about health and illness; health customs, practices, and rituals
- *Diagnostic test:* Cultural Assessment Guide

Family status
- *History:* marital status, developmental stage, roles, rules, communication, coping patterns, family members' goals and aspirations, family's ability to meet physical and emotional needs of its members, socioeconomic status, family's health history
- *Diagnostic tests:* Family Environment Scale, Family Adjustment De-

vice, Family Genogram, Dyadic Adjustment Scale, Family Awareness Scale, Index of Family Relations

Spiritual status
- *Medical conditions:* chronic or terminal illness
- *Personal data:* family's religious affiliation, current perception of faith and religious practices, support network
- *Diagnostic tests:* Spiritual and Religious Concerns Questionnaire, Spiritual Well-Being Scale

DEFINING CHARACTERISTICS

- Alteration in family's roles, rules, or lifestyle
- Blame, shame, and guilt
- Conflicting or erroneous beliefs and expectations regarding cause, course, and outcome of illness
- Emotional withdrawal
- Past loss or illness
- Potentially harmful folk beliefs
- Social withdrawal

ASSOCIATED DISORDERS

Acquired immunodeficiency syndrome, Alzheimer's disease, cancer, end-stage renal, cardiac, or pulmonary disease

EXPECTED OUTCOMES

Initial outcomes
- Family members discuss past experience with loss and illness, beliefs about anticipated loss, and the anticipated course of illness and expected outcome.

- Family members discuss pre-illness roles, rules, goals, and aspirations, and anticipated changes in roles, rules, goals, and aspirations.
- Family members express feelings openly.
- Family members participate in patient's care.
- Family members seek needed information about illness and treatment options, and obtain information about community resources.

Interim outcomes
- Family members continue to adapt roles and rules to changes brought about by illness.
- Family members discuss ongoing sources of distress.
- Family members participate in treatment decisions.
- Family members direct activities toward realistic and meaningful life goals and maintain social network and community involvement.

Discharge outcomes
- Family members work on resolving problems in their relationships with each other and with the patient.
- Family members obtain information and support needed to make necessary treatment decisions.
- Family members preserve cultural, ethnic, and religious practices.
- Family members resolve loss through grief and mourning.

INTERVENTIONS AND RATIONALES

Initial interventions
- Use a genogram to map family members' past losses and illnesses and eth-

nic and cultural health practices *to encourage communication between them, to review how crises were managed in the past, and to foster resolution of unresolved issues.*

- Facilitate family discussion about thoughts and expectations regarding the patient's illness *to encourage effective communication and appropriate expression of feelings and to clarify misconceptions.*
- Discuss usual family roles and rules and recent changes *to assess family reorganization during crisis.*
- Encourage family members to participate in the patient's care *to increase their sense of control and competence, to foster realistic expectations, and to decrease denial and fears of abandonment, isolation, and separation.*
- Provide current information and encourage family members to ask questions *to foster trust, to reduce fear and anxiety, and to increase feelings of control and empowerment. Providing information also reduces misconceptions and helps the family cope in their struggle with denial, despair, and hope.*
- Discuss community resources and religious affiliation *to foster a sense of community, to decrease isolation, and to reinforce effective cultural, ethnic, and religious practices.*

Interim interventions
- Facilitate family discussion about changing roles and rules *to encourage flexibility as family functions are reallocated.*
- Encourage family discussion about stressors, such as fatigue, financial strain, and alterations in family relationships and lifestyles, *to enable the caregivers to express feelings of guilt, an-*

ger, and resentment and to reduce conflict. Family members need to be told that their feelings are natural.
- Promote family members' continued participation in treatment and decision making *to reduce feelings of guilt, blame, and shame and to foster a sense of control.*
- Help family members establish and prioritize realistic goals *to enhance family stability.*
- Encourage the family's involvement with social networks, their religious community, and support groups *to increase their emotional support, to provide help with coping and caregiving tasks, and to decrease feelings of isolation.*

Termination interventions
- Allow family members to spend time alone with the patient *to help them accept his condition and to facilitate the process of letting go and saying good-bye.*
- Encourage discussion of feelings of loss, separation, and being left behind *to help family members acknowledge loss as the patient deteriorates.*
- Assure family members that the patient's comfort level will be maintained *to provide reassurance that the loved one is free of pain and suffering and to decrease their feelings of guilt and blame.*
- Support the family's treatment decisions *to decrease feelings of guilt if aggressive treatments are discontinued and to increase feelings of competence.*
- Refer family members to appropriate professional services *to ensure availability of additional help.*

EVALUATION STATEMENTS

Family members:
- discuss past experiences with loss and identify unresolved issues.
- identify helpful and harmful beliefs and expectations about the cause, course, and outcome of illness.
- identify current roles and rules and discuss changes that have occurred since the onset of illness.
- discuss thoughts and feelings about loss.
- participate in patient care and in making treatment decisions.
- do not report overwhelming feelings of guilt, shame, isolation, abandonment, and lack of control.
- face inevitable loss with a sense of empowerment.
- enlist the help of a social network or religious community.

DOCUMENTATION

- Cultural and religious beliefs described by family members
- Past experience with loss and unresolved issues described by family members
- Coping patterns family members report having used successfully in the past
- Beliefs and expectations regarding anticipated loss
- Family members' description of how illness has altered roles and rules
- Nursing interventions to increase family's knowledge and decision-making capability
- Family members' participation in care
- Family's support network
- Evaluation statements.

Grieving, anticipatory

related to potential loss of patient

DEFINITION

Grief among staff members in anticipation of a patient's death

ASSESSMENT

Hospital unit status
- *Staff communication:* methods, patterns, and quality of communication between staff members; communication with patient and family
- *Coping patterns:* frequency of patient deaths, effect of death on each staff member, effectiveness of usual coping patterns
- *Emotional and psychological factors:* job satisfaction, morale, unit atmosphere, ability to meet needs of dying patients and grieving families, staff self-awareness
- *Social and cultural factors:* alliances between staff members, quality of relationships, beliefs, and attitudes about death and dying

DEFINING CHARACTERISTICS

- Beliefs and attitudes of staff members that are incompatible with patient's and family's beliefs
- Denial of feelings among staff members
- Frequent sick calls
- High staff turnover rate
- Ineffective interventions with dying patients and grieving families

- Isolation from colleagues
- Job dissatisfaction
- Lack of empathy for patients and family
- Lack of staff self-awareness
- Low staff morale
- Multiple patient deaths
- Maladaptive staff coping
- Poor communication between staff and patient or family
- Poor communication between staff members
- Refusal of staff members to take breaks

ASSOCIATED DISORDERS

Acquired immunodeficiency syndrome, cancer, end-stage renal, cardiac, or respiratory disease

EXPECTED OUTCOMES

Initial outcomes
- Staff members examine their beliefs and attitudes about death and dying.
- Staff members discuss thoughts and feelings about dying patients and grieving families.

Interim outcomes
- Staff members share information about effective coping methods with each other.
- Staff members report increased self-awareness of their own grieving.
- Staff members seek support and assistance from each other as needed.

Concluding outcomes
- Family members report satisfaction with emotional care from staff.

- Staff members report increased job satisfaction and morale.

INTERVENTIONS AND RATIONALES

Initial interventions
- In consultation with the unit nurse manager, develop a staff support group *to enable discussion of beliefs, attitudes, thoughts, and feelings about death and dying.*
- Establish the frequency and length of sessions, goals, and ground rules of the support group *to increase participation, to decrease anxiety of members, and to foster trust.*
- Help staff members examine their beliefs and attitudes about death and dying. *Staff members' beliefs and attitudes have an important effect on the patient and family.*
- Help the staff identify and express thoughts and feelings related to working with dying patients and grieving families *to help them accept and work through painful feelings.*

Interim interventions
- Encourage the staff to share methods of coping with the patient death *to foster examination of maladaptive coping methods and to reinforce adaptive methods.*
- Provide information about the grieving process *to increase staff members' empathy for patients and families and increase their awareness of their own feelings.*
- Encourage staff members to share their experiences with patients and families on an ongoing basis *to encourage cooperation in problem solving and*

decrease dependence on the group facilitator.

Concluding interventions

- Encourage role playing of staff interactions with the dying patient and grieving family *to increase staff competence and to foster communication between staff members, patients, and families.*
- Encourage the staff to discuss examples of productive and satisfying interactions with patients and families *to increase job satisfaction and to improve staff morale.*

EVALUATION STATEMENTS

Staff members:
- express insight into beliefs and attitudes about death and dying.
- express thoughts and feelings regarding working with dying patients and their families.
- identify and use adaptive coping methods.
- report increased awareness of their own grief response.
- seek support from colleagues.
- demonstrate improved morale and express greater job satisfaction.
    Patient and family:
- report improved emotional support from staff members.

Grieving, dysfunctional

related to recent loss

DEFINITION

An individual's exaggerated, delayed, prolonged, or absent response to loss of a significant person, ideal, status, object, or body part

ASSESSMENT

Cultural status
- *Demographics:* age, sex, level of education, occupation, nationality, race, ethnic group
- *History:* beliefs, values, and attitudes about health and illness; health customs, practices, and rituals; religious identification; influence of religious beliefs on values and practices
- *Diagnostic test:* Cultural Assessment Guide

Family status
- *Composition:* marital status, ages of members, elderly relatives or others living with family
- *Family roles:* formal and informal roles, roles performance, degree of family agreement on roles, interrelationships of roles
- *Family communication:* style and quality of communication, methods of conflict resolution
- *Developmental stage of family:* lengths of patient's relationships with family members, family's adaptation to change and shifts in role responsibility, problem-solving methods

- *Family alliances:* effects on stability of family unit
- *Physical and emotional needs:* ability of family to meet patient's physical and emotional needs
- *Family goals, values, and aspirations:* understanding and articulation of goals and values, acceptance of individual goals and values
- *Socioeconomic factors:* economic status; sense of adequacy and self-worth of members; employment and attitudes toward work
- *Coping patterns:* major life events and their meanings to each member, usual coping patterns, family's perception of effectiveness of coping patterns
- *Family health history:* bipolar disorder, depressive disorder, suicide, schizophrenia, mental retardation, substance abuse, stress-related illness, medical illness

Psychological status

- *Signs and symptoms:* changes in appetite, energy level, motivation, personal hygiene, self-image, self-esteem, sleep pattern, or sexual drive
- *Alcohol or drug abuse:* type of substance, effects on mood and behavior, evidence of abuse or withdrawal
- *Psychiatric history:* presence of illness, age of onset, type and severity of symptoms, type of treatment and patient's response
- *Developmental history:* reactions to losses through separation or death, life events in childhood
- *Diagnostic tests:* Hamilton Rating Scale for Depression, Beck Depression Inventory

Sleep status

- *History:* presence of sleep pattern disturbances
- *Medications:* sleep aids, caffeine, alcohol, amphetamines, benzodiazepines

Social status

- *Personal habits:* size of social network, quality of relationships, trust in others, level of self-esteem, ability to function in social and occupational roles
- *Signs and symptoms:* withdrawal from social relationships

Spiritual status

- *Personal habits:* current perception of faith and religious practices, religious affiliation, perceptions about life and death, support network

DEFINING CHARACTERISTICS

- Absence of normal grieving
- Delayed emotional response to loss
- Denial of potential loss
- Expression of anger or sadness
- Expressions of guilt regarding loss
- Frequent crying
- Lack of friendships
- Poor social skills
- Poor support systems
- Preexisting psychiatric illnesses, personality disorders, or depressive disorders
- Previous losses

ASSOCIATED DISORDERS

Anxiety, depressive disorder, substance-related disorder

EXPECTED OUTCOMES

Initial outcomes
- Patient expresses feelings of grief.
- Patient verbalizes loss and its meaning.

Interim outcome
- Patient expresses reduced feelings of guilt and self-blame.

Discharge outcomes
- Patient increases involvement with others.
- Patient makes plans for the future.

INTERVENTIONS AND RATIONALES

Initial interventions
- Observe the patient for lack of grieving. *Absence of emotion may mean the work of grieving is delayed or blocked.*
- Encourage the patient to express feelings *to help him work through delayed emotional reactions.*
- Help the patient work through excessive, distorted, and delayed emotional reactions *to reduce depression.*

Interim interventions
- Support the patient. Explain that grieving is normal and painful. Suggest that he has the strength to experience these feelings without harm *to help him accept his need to experience sadness and suffering as part of the grieving process.*
- Discourage rumination about guilt feelings. Instead, encourage expression of other feelings, such as sadness, helplessness, and anger. *Rumination about guilt prevents the experience of deeper feelings that the patient may perceive as unacceptable and frightening.*

Discharge interventions
- Refer the patient and family to appropriate support groups *to provide group support from others who have similar experiences.*
- Help the patient make simple plans for the future *to give him a sense of control and renewed hope.*

EVALUATION STATEMENTS

Patient:
- discusses loss and associated feelings of anger, sorrow, and guilt.
- demonstrates less guilt and self-blame for loss.
- expresses willingness to attend a support group meeting.
- shares grief with others and expresses desire to see family and friends.

DOCUMENTATION

- Patient's statements and behavior indicating dysfunctional grieving
- Patient's feelings about the loss and of isolation
- Patient's statements of suicidal ideation, guilt, or hopelessness
- Statements indicating improved energy, decreased hopelessness, and willingness to use support systems
- Patient's participation in the decision-making process.
- Evaluation statements.

Health maintenance alteration

related to inability to self-regulate symptoms of mental illness

DEFINITION

Inability to maintain healthy state due to inadequate ability to manage symptoms of mental illness

ASSESSMENT

Cultural status
- *Demographics:* age, sex, level of education, occupation, nationality, race, ethnic group
- *History:* beliefs, values, and attitudes about health and illness; health customs, practices, and rituals
- *Diagnostic test:* Cultural Assessment Guide

Family status
- *History:* marital status, members of current household, roles and role performance, shifts in role responsibility, interrelationships of roles
- *Family communication:* style and quality of communication, methods of conflict resolution
- *Physical and emotional needs:* family's ability to meet physical and emotional needs
- *Socioeconomic factors:* economic, educational, and occupational status of family
- *Coping patterns:* major life events and their meanings to each family member, usual coping patterns, family's perception of effectiveness of coping patterns, support systems
- *Family health history:* history of psychiatric or medical illness, mental and physical health promotion practices, family's perception of and involvement in patient's illness, family's understanding of symptoms and the difference between symptoms and annoying behaviors
- *Diagnostic tests:* Family Genogram, Family Environment Scale, Family Adjustment Device

Neurologic status
- *History:* anxiety disorders, attention-deficit disorder, seizures, hypoxia, head injury, schizophrenia, mood disorders, substance-related disorders, chronic pain
- *Medications:* neuroleptic agents, anxiolytic agents, anticonvulsants, antidepressants, antimanic agents, pain medications
- *Mental status:* appearance and attitude, level of consciousness, thought and speech, mood and affect, perceptions, orientation, memory, general information, calculations, capacity to read and write, visual-spatial ability, attention span, abstraction, judgment and insight
- *Physical examination:* motor and sensory function, reflexes, presence of tardive dyskinesia or other adverse effects of medication
- *Laboratory tests:* complete blood count, urinalysis, electrolyte level, drug screening, toxicology, medication serum levels, blood urea nitrogen level, blood glucose level, allergy testing

- *Diagnostic tests:* electroencephalography, computed tomography, magnetic resonance imaging

Psychological status
- *History:* patient's perception of present health problem or crisis; symptom type, frequency, severity, changes, and impact on functioning; coping styles
- *Psychiatric history:* age of onset, type and severity of symptoms, impact on functioning, type of treatment, patient's response to treatment; use of illicit drugs and alcohol; use of over-the-counter drugs; adherence to mental and physical preventive health practices
- *Childhood development:* birth order, developmental milestones, intelligence quotient, personality traits, perception of mental illness, responses of others, maladaptive behaviors, school performance, relationships with siblings, parents, and extended family
- *Adolescent development:* involvement in church, synagogue, or clubs; recreational interests; relationship with parents, authority figures, or therapists; sexual activities; academic and social comfort and performance; experimentation with cigarettes, drugs, and alcohol
- *Adult development:* level of independence; social activities; sexual behavior; academic, military, and occupational history; dating and marital history; spirituality; reactions to mental illness; hobbies and recreational activities; support systems; health care and health promotion activities; perception of self-esteem
- *Signs and symptoms:* withdrawal, lack of eye contact, inappropriate responses or personal habits, poor interpersonal skills, inability to function in social and occupational roles
- *Diagnostic tests:* Wechsler Adult Intelligence Inventory, Cognitive Capacity Screening Examination, Brief Psychiatric Rating Scale, Hamilton Rating Scale for Depression, State-Trait Anxiety Inventory, Social Adjustment Scale

Self-care status
- *Observation:* functional ability (muscle tone, size, and strength; range of motion; coordination), daily activities (dressing, grooming, bathing, toileting, and hygiene), location of personal belongings, noise, privacy, and space
- *Knowledge:* understanding of psychiatric condition, understanding of medication regimen, readiness to learn
- *Diagnostic tests:* Functional Ability Scale, Self-Care Assessment Tool

DEFINING CHARACTERISTICS
- Impaired perceptual or cognitive functioning
- Impaired short-term or long-term memory
- Inability to concentrate or to follow instructions
- Lack of appropriate responses to thoughts, feelings, or behaviors
- Lack of understanding of symptoms or the type and pattern of psychiatric illness
- Lack of understanding of steps to maintain mental health

ASSOCIATED DISORDERS
Schizophrenia or other recurrent and chronic psychiatric illnesses

EXPECTED OUTCOMES

Initial outcomes

- Patient and family members express an understanding of the patient's illness.
- Patient and family members define their understanding of the term "target symptom."
- Patient lists symptoms that led to his current need for treatment.
- Patient monitors "target symptoms" and their frequency.
- Patient describes the physical, social, and personal setting in which symptoms usually occur.
- Patient describes one common situation that increases symptoms.
- Patient discusses the relationship between his environment and his symptoms.
- Patient describes techniques for self-monitoring of symptoms.

Interim outcomes

- Patient identifies the changes in his thoughts, feelings, and behavior that precede onset of a symptom.
- Patient identifies the most important indicators of symptom onset.
- Patient evaluates the difference between persistent and target symptoms.
- Patient demonstrates skill in evaluating which symptoms indicate recurrence or relapse.

Discharge outcomes

- Patient describes one method of controlling persistent symptoms or forestalling a relapse.
- Patient describes the response of companions to his self-control methods.

- Patient identifies people who can provide support when symptoms exist or become intolerable and difficult to self-control.

INTERVENTIONS AND RATIONALES

Initial interventions

- Assess the patient's and family members' understanding of and attitude toward schizophrenia *to determine both the learning needs and the level of involvement that can be expected from each person.*
- Help family members communicate with the patient and understand what his behaviors mean *to reduce the patient's feelings of helplessness and give him a sense of control.*
- Administer a symptom rating scale (Brief Psychiatric Rating Scale) *to determine the type, frequency, and severity of his current symptoms.*
- Review the past history of the illness, focusing on episodes of relapse or recurrence of symptoms *to assess the course and pattern of the patient's symptoms.*
- Educate the patient and family members about schizophrenia *to correct any misperceptions about the illness.* Explain that the patient's lack of energy and withdrawal are real symptoms, not laziness, and that family members can help most by encouraging the patient to gradually regain his former skills.
- Educate the patient and family members about target symptoms. These are recurring symptoms, such as hallucinations or delusions, that are triggered by stress or tension *to foster greater un-*

derstanding of symptoms of schizophrenia.

- Explain to the patient that self-regulation of symptoms is a form of health maintenance *to give him greater control over his mental health.*
- Teach him that he can self-monitor for symptoms *to tell whether medications are working, to recognize warnings of a relapse, and to cope with symptoms that persist despite medication.*
- Ask questions to foster self-monitoring skills, such as:
– How do you define a symptom? How is it not normal?
– Have symptoms increased since you first became ill?
– Which symptoms become worse every time you get sick?
– During the current crisis, did your medication or treatment change because of an increase in symptoms?
– Do you have methods to reduce symptoms?
– Which symptoms do you pay closest attention to?
– Are there daily situations that make you uncomfortable or give you distress? Are the situations exacerbate your symptoms?
These questions will help the patient understand situations that increase symptoms and determine his ability to monitor himself.
- Depending on their level of understanding, assign the patient and family members homework to enhance self-monitoring skills. Assignments may include listing symptoms that led to the present crisis; tracking the frequency of one symptom in an 8-hour period; or identifying the physical, social, and personal setting where a symptom usually occurs. *Homework assignments*

reinforce learning, focus patient and family members on concrete goals, help them develop a better understanding of self-monitoring, and help them better manage their mental health.

Interim interventions
- Provide feedback on homework *to assess learning and provide encouragement.*
- Review information presented during the initial interventions *to clarify any gaps in learning or misunderstanding.*
- Readminister the Brief Psychiatric Rating Scale *to determine changes in type, frequency, and severity of symptoms.*
- Educate the patient and family members in self-evaluation techniques, such as observing, describing, and analyzing cues to relapse and distinguishing between signs of relapse and persistent symptoms. *Such common cues as sleep difficulties, withdrawal, poor concentration, and other changes may warn of a relapse several days in advance. Using self-evaluation techniques, the relapsing patient may better judge the difference between fantasy and reality.*
- Ask the patient questions such as:
– Do specific changes in your thoughts, feelings, or behavior signal that you are getting sick?
– What is the most reliable indicator of a relapse?
– What is the difference between the symptoms you always have and the ones that indicate a relapse? What makes these cues significant and when do you recognize them?

– Who is most helpful in assisting you to evaluate thoughts, feelings, and behavior?

These questions may help the patient evaluate behaviors and thoughts that precede the onset of illness.

▪ Depending on their level of understanding, assign the patient and family members homework. Assignments may include comparing the patient's record and an observer's record of all changes in thoughts, feelings, and behavior that occurred just before the onset of the symptom *to reinforce self-evaluation techniques.*

Discharge interventions

▪ Provide feedback on completed homework assignments to assess learning and provide encouragement.

▪ Review information that was presented in the interim interventions *to clarify any gaps in learning or misunderstanding.*

▪ Educate the patient and his family about the self-reinforcement techniques *to control persisting symptoms or forestall a relapse.* Emphasize the difference between effective measures and ineffective measures, such as alcohol abuse or stopping medication, that may lead to feeling worse and a relapse.

▪ Ask the patient questions such as:

– Do you have any specific methods that reduce your symptoms and in what situations do they work?

– How did you learn these self-control measures?

– Who helps you the most to control your symptoms?

These questions will help evaluate the patient's ability to self-control symptoms.

▪ Assign homework, such as having the patient list two effective self-control responses to a symptom and having a family member list two examples of positive reinforcement given to the patient for his efforts. *Homework assignments reinforce learning, focus on concrete goals, and help develop a better understanding of self-reinforcement techniques.*

▪ Encourage the patient to continue self-regulation strategies and refer him to appropriate mental health professionals *to provide ongoing help.*

▪ Help the family and companions identify available community resources, such as the National Alliance of the Mentally Ill, *to help them gain social support and information.*

EVALUATION STATEMENTS

Patient:

▪ describes impact of illness on self and others.

▪ expresses understanding of the course and pattern of his symptoms.

▪ describes situations that increase symptoms.

▪ describes behavioral cues that signal the onset of symptoms.

▪ analyzes the difference between target and persistent symptoms.

▪ employs effective self-control measures to extent possible.

Patient and family members:

▪ complete homework assignments.

▪ identify and contact sources of support.

Family members:

▪ assist patient as needed.

DOCUMENTATION

- Patient's and family members' expression of concern about the patient's inability to maintain mental health
- Observations of the patient's impaired ability to self-regulate symptoms
- Patient's response to nursing interventions
- Patient's response to homework assignments
- Changes in patient's symptoms shown by scores on the Brief Psychiatric Rating Scale
- Information given to the patient and family members and their demonstrated skill in carrying out the teaching program
- Referrals
- Evaluation statements.

Health maintenance alteration

related to perceptual or cognitive impairment

DEFINITION

Inability to maintain a healthy state

ASSESSMENT

Cultural status
- *Demographics:* age, sex, level of education, occupation, nationality, race, ethnic group
- *History:* beliefs, values, and attitudes about health and illness; health customs, practices, and rituals

- *Diagnostic test:* Cultural Assessment Guide

Family status
- *History:* marital status, family role, family history, family's ability to meet patient's physical and emotional needs, evidence of abuse, support systems, family communication patterns

Neurologic status
- *History:* medical problems, neurologic symptoms, exposure to toxins, pain management, medications
- *Neurologic examination:* appearance; level of consciousness; thought patterns; motor activity; judgment, orientation, memory

DEFINING CHARACTERISTICS

- Difficulty adapting to changes in environment
- Impaired perceptual or cognitive functioning
- Impaired short-term or long-term memory
- Inability to concentrate or to follow instructions
- Inability to fulfill basic health needs
- Lack of interest in health maintenance
- Self-care deficits

ASSOCIATED DISORDERS

Alzheimer's disease, anoxic encephalopathy, autism, brain tumor, cerebrovascular accident, dementia, head injury, Huntington's disease, Laënnec's cirrhosis, mental retardation, mood disorders, schizophrenia, substance-related disorders

EXPECTED OUTCOMES

Initial outcomes
- Patient maintains current health status.
- Patient sustains no harm or injury.

Interim outcomes
- Patient, family member, or companion expresses feelings and concerns.
- Patient, family member, or companion explains health maintenance program.

Discharge outcomes
- Patient, family member, or companion demonstrates ability to perform steps of health maintenance program.
- Patient, family member, or companion identifies available health resources.
- Patient, family member, or companion demonstrates appropriate coping skills.

INTERVENTIONS AND RATIONALES

Initial interventions
- Determine the patient's self-care status, degree of support from family or companion, and motivation level *to obtain a baseline for evaluating future functional changes.*
- Collaborate with doctors by performing prescribed treatments, monitoring progress, and reporting responses *to enhance the patient's wellbeing and develop an appropriate plan of care.*
- Help the patient, family, or companion identify steps for maintaining the patient's health *to provide a basis for future interventions.*

- Help the family or companion communicate with the patient and understand his behavior *to reduce their feelings of helplessness and to increase their sense of control.*
- Reorient the patient as often as necessary. Display personal objects from the patient's home so that the environment appears familiar *to enhance his reality testing and mental status.*

Interim interventions
- Discuss current disabilities with the patient, family member, or companion and provide a structured care program in writing *to increase the patient's and family's feelings of security.*
- Try to arrange for one person to provide care on an ongoing basis *to increase stability.*
- Describe fully all aspects of care *to ensure the patient's understanding.*
- When discussing care, give short, simple explanations at the patient's level of understanding *to increase cooperation.*
- Prepare the patient for possible changes in his health care regimen *to minimize disruptions.*
- Provide ample time for the patient to perform health maintenance tasks *to reduce frustration and to foster success.*

Discharge interventions
- Teach health maintenance practices, such as bathing, feeding, and reality orientation, and ask the family member or companion to demonstrate them *to provide support to caregivers and reduce their anxiety about providing care.*
- Advise the family member or companion how to maintain a safe envi-

ronment *to reduce risk of injury to the patient.*

- Encourage the patient and caregivers to express concerns about health maintenance *to provide them an opportunity to ask questions, increase their level of understanding, and improve their health management skills.*
- Teach the family member or companion methods to improve coping skills *to reduce maladaptive coping strategies.*
- Inform caregivers about social and community resources such as support groups *to help them obtain social support, to provide an outlet for expressing feelings about the patient's disorder, and to make available additional sources for information.*
- Provide the family member or companion with referrals to a psychiatric liaison nurse, social services, or other appropriate resources *to help prevent caregiver burnout.*

EVALUATION STATEMENTS

Patient:
- maintains health status.
- shows no signs of injury.
- discusses impact of illness and health maintenance needs on others' lives.
- performs health maintenance practices as well as possible, with assistance from family member or companion as needed.
- copes with current situation without experiencing severe emotional upset.
    Family member or caregiver:
- describes three health maintenance strategies.
- identifies and contacts sources of support.

- discuss feelings about patient's illness.
- demonstrates effective coping skills.

DOCUMENTATION

- Expressions of concern by patient and family or companion regarding patient's health maintenance
- Observations of patient's ability to perform self-care activities
- Nursing interventions
- Patient's response to treatments and nursing interventions
- Instructions given to patient and family or companion
- Patient's and caregiver's levels of understanding
- Demonstrations of health maintenance skills by patient, family members, or companion
- Referrals for patient and family or companion
- Evaluation statements.

Health-seeking behaviors

related to perceived risk of mental illness

DEFINITION

An individual's pursuit of improved mental health through participation in group therapy

ASSESSMENT

Cultural status
- *Demographics:* age, sex, level of education, occupation, nationality, race, ethnic group

- *History:* beliefs, values, and attitudes about health and illness; health customs, practices, and rituals
- *Diagnostic test:* Cultural Assessment Guide

Family status
- *Family history:* marital status; composition of current household; relationships among family members; level of enmeshment or estrangement; communication patterns; conflict resolution; ability of family to meet social, spiritual, physical, and emotional needs of its members; family values, goals, and plans; family activities
- *Health history:* history of physical or mental disorders, hospitalization or therapy for mental illness
- *Diagnostic tests:* Family Genogram, Holmes and Rahe Social Readjustment Rating Scale, Family Environment Scale

Neurologic status
- *Physical examination:* sensory and motor status, reflexes, ability to process environmental cues, ability to perform daily living activities, cognitive skills
- *History:* cerebrovascular accident, head injury, or seizures
- *Laboratory tests:* complete blood count; urinalysis; glucose, blood urea nitrogen, and electrolyte levels; drug toxicology screening; medication serum levels; allergy tests
- *Diagnostic tests:* Folstein Mini-Mental Health Status Examination, electroencephalography, electrocardiography, magnetic resonance imaging, electromyography (if indicated), computed tomography

Psychological status
- *Current illness:* presenting problems; signs and symptoms; feelings about possible susceptibility to mental illness; changes in self-care ability, self-image, self-esteem, motivation, perception of having control, coping methods, appetite, sleep cycle, activity level, sexual activity patterns
- *Signs and symptoms:* pain, discomfort, anxiety, depression
- *Childhood development:* developmental milestones; personality traits; adaptive and maladaptive behaviors; relationships with parents, siblings, extended family, and peers; role models of how to cope; academic performance; recreational activities; religious education
- *Adolescent development:* sports and recreational activities; spiritual groups; dating history; academic accomplishments; relationships with peers, family members, and authority figures; sense of individuality; sexual behavior; delinquency
- *Adult development:* dating and marital history; leisure activities; educational achievements; military history; legal problems; relationships with parents, siblings, spouse, children, extended family, friends, and peers; employment stability and satisfaction with occupation; coping strategies; health care status; motivation to improve health status
- *Medication history:* analgesics, anti-anxiety agents, antidepressants, antimanic agents, antipsychotics, anticonvulsants, hormone replacement therapy, use of alcohol or illicit drugs
- *Diagnostic tests:* Minnesota Multiphasic Personality Inventory, Wechsler Adult Intelligence Survey, Cognitive

Capacity Screening Examination, Myers-Briggs Type Indicator, State-Trait Anxiety Inventory, Zung Self-Rating Depression Scale, Merinda Leisure Finder

RISK FACTORS

▪ Expressed or observed desire for increased control over mental health
▪ Expressed or observed desire to improve mental health status
▪ Expressed or observed lack of knowledge about mental health–promotion behaviors
▪ Expressed or observed unfamiliarity with community mental health resources
▪ Familial predisposition to mental disorder or disease
▪ Fear of susceptibility to mental illness

ASSOCIATED DISORDERS

Affective disorders, anxiety disorders, arthritis, cardiac disease, cancer, diabetes mellitus, endocrine disorders, mood disorders, neurologic impairment, personality disorders, posttraumatic stress disorder

EXPECTED OUTCOMES

Initial outcomes
▪ Patient identifies concerns regarding mental health and reasons for participating in group therapy.
▪ Patient discusses perceived susceptibility to mental illness.
▪ Patient seeks information about group therapy for mental health promotion and stress reduction.
▪ Patient participates in group therapy screening process.
▪ Therapist prepares learning exercises (didactic and experiential) for group members.

Interim outcomes
▪ Patient acknowledges behaviors that may adversely affect his mental health.
▪ Patient learns about factors that may increase his risk for mental illness.
▪ Patient learns about genetic factors associated with mental illness, especially as they relate to his family of origin.
▪ Patient obtains needed information about group therapy.
▪ Patient agrees to attend and participate in specified number of therapy sessions, arrive on time, try to be open with group members and therapists, complete homework, and maintain confidentiality of group members.
▪ Patient participates in learning exercises and discusses how they apply to his personal history.

Discharge outcomes
▪ Patient describes behaviors to promote mental health, including stress reduction activities.
▪ Patient acknowledges risk factors (genetic history, dietary habits, occupation, activity and rest patterns) that can affect his own mental health.
▪ Patient completes homework assigned in group therapy.
▪ Patient continues group therapy and agrees to practice exercises for a specified amount of time after sessions end.
▪ Patient shares his feelings with group members and offers feedback to others.

INTERVENTIONS AND RATIONALES

Initial interventions

- Help the patient identify specific concerns with regard to his health *to promote interest and compliance.*
- Help the patient focus on fears of susceptibility to mental illness *to expedite a change in behavior.*
- Assess the patient's history for risk factors of mental illness *to help determine appropriate interventions. Consider the patient's family background to determine if there may be genetic risk factors in addition to the patient's own behavioral history.*
- Screen participants *to avoid group members who are unable to participate in or benefit from group therapy or assigned exercises. For example, actively psychotic clients or severely depressed clients may not benefit from this type of care.*
- Prepare lessons for group members in such topics as health education, progressive relaxation, guided imagery, meditation, refuting irrational ideas, coping-skills training, exercise, assertiveness training, time management, thought stopping, nutrition, or other appropriate topics *to educate groups. Structured lessons may help group members feel more comfortable.*

Interim interventions

- Encourage the patient to identify steps for decreasing unhealthy behavior and steps for increasing stress-reducing behavior *to enforce his sense of responsibility and control.*
- Educate the patient about factors that may pose risks to his mental health *to encourage responsible decisions about changing behavior.*
- Help the patient apply what he has learned to his own history *to enable him to make meaningful decisions.*
- Discuss the group therapy contract *to promote a sense of responsibility and cooperation.*
- Direct the patient in experiential exercises (for example, progressive relaxation exercises) during therapy sessions *to allow practice, feedback among members, and positive role modeling.*
- Assign homework *to reinforce learning and increase skills.*

Discharge interventions

- Instruct the patient to maintain a diary or record of behavior changes *to reinforce and promote positive change.*
- Discuss the patient's specific risks and susceptibility to mental illness *to assess comprehension and increase motivation to change behavior.*
- Encourage the patient to discuss his personal history and mental health risks in group therapy *to allow him to verbalize thoughts, bond with group members, test new behaviors, and receive feedback.*
- Offer positive feedback about accomplishments in group therapy *to reinforce benefits and to encourage use of stress-reduction techniques after treatment.*

EVALUATION STATEMENTS

Patient:
- identifies risks to his mental health and possible susceptibility to mental illness.

- discusses his personal history and fears regarding mental illness with group members.
- signs group therapy contract.
- participates in group therapy sessions.
- completes homework assigned in group.
- identifies his comfort level with different stress-reduction techniques.
- selects two or three stress-reduction methods to practice and use regularly.
- describes what he has learned from group therapy.

DOCUMENTATION

- Diagnostic test results
- Laboratory test findings
- Nursing interventions and the patient's response
- Observed behavior changes in patient
- Signed group therapy contract
- Patient's attendance record
- Patient's statements about stress-reduction techniques
- Progress reports
- Patient's assessment of group therapy
- Follow-up surveys
- Evaluation statements.

Hopelessness

related to chronic illness

DEFINITION

Perceived lack of alternatives or personal choices causing inability to act on own behalf

ASSESSMENT

Cultural status
- *Demographics:* age, sex, level of education, occupation, nationality, race, ethnic group
- *History:* beliefs, values, and attitudes about health and illness; health customs, practices, and rituals
- *Diagnostic test:* Cultural Assessment Guide

Health status
- *History:* changes in appetite, energy level, motivation, personal hygiene, self-image, sleep pattern, sexual drive, or behavior; life changes; current illness; patient's response to treatment
- *Developmental history:* military history, occupation and job changes, dating and marital history, hobbies and recreational activities, spirituality, prior medical conditions, reactions to illness and disability

DEFINING CHARACTERISTICS

- Decreased affect, involvement in care, and verbalization
- Despondence
- Deteriorating condition
- Frequent sighing
- Increased sleep
- Lack of concentration, interpersonal contact, spontaneity, initiative, interest, or motivation
- Loss of faith and spiritual values
- Low self-esteem
- Minimal eye contact, shrugging in response to questions, turning away from speaker, or other nonverbal cues
- Poor personal grooming
- Verbal expressions of hopelessness

ASSOCIATED DISORDERS

Acquired immunodeficiency syndrome, Addison's disease, bipolar disorder, burns, cancer, cardiovascular disease, chronic respiratory disease, chronic renal disease, Cushing's disease, depressive disorder, diabetes mellitus, endocrine disorder, hepatitis, leukemia and related lymphomas, systemic lupus erythematosus, multiple sclerosis, organ transplant, pancreas and liver diseases, Parkinson's disease, schizophrenia

EXPECTED OUTCOMES

Initial outcomes

- Patient verbalizes feelings of hopelessness.
- Patient expresses increased acceptance of limitations caused by chronic illness.

Interim outcomes

- Patient demonstrates ability to experience stages of grief.
- Patient identifies and uses effective coping mechanisms.
- Patient expresses understanding of benefits of social interaction.
- Patient participates in self-care activities.
- Patient participates in developing plan of care.

Discharge outcomes

- Patient resumes and maintains as many former roles as possible.
- Patient reports increased self-esteem.
- Patient reports increased feelings of hope.

INTERVENTIONS AND RATIONALES

Initial interventions

- Assess for evidence of self-destructive behavior and suicide potential. *Maintaining patient safety is the first nursing care priority.*
- If possible, assign a primary nurse to the patient *to foster a therapeutic relationship.*
- Converse with the patient about non-care-related subjects for a specific amount of time each shift. Encourage verbal responses by using open-ended statements and questions. If the patient chooses not to talk, spend time in silence. *These measures will help establish rapport with a depressed patient.*
- Provide appropriate physical outlets for expression of feelings — such as a punching bag or a place to walk — *to help the patient release hostilities and decrease feelings of tension and anxiety.*

Interim interventions

- Encourage the patient to develop and use adaptive coping skills *to enhance self-esteem, to reduce feelings of dependence, and to show support for positive behavior.*
- Encourage the patient's expressions of depression, anger, guilt, and sadness, and acknowledge the legitimacy of his feelings *to help him cope with chronic illness.*
- Encourage the patient to identify and use his abilities and skills *to promote optimal functioning.*
- Encourage the patient's fullest possible participation in self-care *to reduce feelings of helplessness.*

- Help the patient participate in as many activities as strength, energy, and time permit *to foster self-esteem.*
- Encourage the patient to identify and participate in enjoyable diversions *to decrease negative thinking and to enhance self-esteem.*
- Encourage positive thinking and express confidence in the patient's ability to cope with illness *to promote an optimistic outlook.*
- Encourage the patient to establish a self-care schedule *to enhance his feelings of control.*
- Assist the patient with hygiene and grooming needs *to help enhance his self-esteem.*
- Offer the patient and his family a realistic appraisal of his health status and convey hope for the immediate future *to facilitate acceptance of illness, promote patient safety and security, and encourage planning for future health care needs.*
- Encourage the patient to identify spiritual needs and facilitate fulfillment of those needs *to help him come to terms with chronic illness and the limitations it imposes.*
- Involve the patient and his family or companion in the plan of care. Teach them how to manage illness, prevent complications, and control environmental factors that affect the patient's health *to enable family members to participate in his care.*

Discharge interventions
- Allow the patient to increase his level of involvement in care as his outlook improves. *Once cognitive disturbances due to anxiety or depression decrease, the patient should be encouraged to make choices.*

- Refer the patient and his family or companion to a dietitian, social worker, clergy, mental health clinical nurse specialist, or other caregivers, as appropriate, *to ensure continued care.*
- Refer the patient to an appropriate support group *to enable him to discuss his illness with others who are capable of empathizing with his condition.*

EVALUATION STATEMENTS

Patient:
- talks about negative feelings instead of acting on them.
- expresses understanding of lifestyle changes imposed by chronic illness.
- discusses impact of illness and expresses realistic view of future.
- demonstrates ability to solve problems and make decisions.
- acknowledges belief in self.
- demonstrates increased energy level and will to live.
- states that feelings of hopelessness occur less frequently.
- interacts with others and increases his involvement in life experiences.
- demonstrates involvement in own health care.
- expresses understanding that self-care is necessary to enable optimal functioning.

DOCUMENTATION

- Patient's perception of chronic illness
- Patient's responses to treatment regimen
- Patient's baseline and ongoing mental and emotional status
- Patient education and counseling

- Precautions taken to maintain or enhance patient's level of functioning
- Nursing interventions to help patient cope with daily stress
- Nursing interventions to protect patient from harming self
- Patient's responses to nursing interventions
- Evaluation statements.

Injury, high risk for

related to dysphagia

DEFINITION

Accentuated risk of self-harm caused by dysphagia

ASSESSMENT

Cultural status
- *Demographics:* age, sex, level of education, occupation, nationality, race, ethnic group
- *History:* beliefs, values, and attitudes about health and illness; health customs, practices, and rituals
- *Diagnostic test:* Cultural Assessment Guide

Neurologic status
- *Mental status:* level of consciousness, thought processes, speech, memory, attention span, judgment and insight
- *Motor system:* muscle tone, strength, and symmetry; motor activity; cranial nerve function
- *Medications:* neuroleptics, antimanic agents, barbiturates

- *Signs and symptoms:* aspiration, dyskinesia, dysphagia, lethargy, tremors, paresthesia, paresis, chorea, poor coordination, numbness, fasciculation, coughing, choking
- *Diagnostic tests:* Bedside Dysphagia Evaluation, Modified Barium Swallow Videoflouroscopic Evaluation

Nutrition status
- *History:* typical daily food intake, use of drugs or alcohol, nutrient deficiencies
- *Signs and symptoms:* weight loss

Respiratory status
- *Physical examination:* rate, depth, and pattern of respirations; effect of breathing difficulty on eating
- *History:* lung disease
- *Signs and symptoms:* coughing, shortness of breath
- *Diagnostic tests:* pulse oximetry, transcutaneous oxygen monitoring

Sensory status
- *Physical examination:* sense of taste and smell; appetite; weight; position awareness; sensitivity to touch, temperature, superficial pain, and deep pain
- *Medications:* neuroleptics
- *Signs and symptoms:* olfactory hallucinations; tactile hallucinations; paresthesia; change in senses of smell and taste, appetite, or weight

Psychological status
- *Current illness:* presence of psychiatric illness, effect on functioning, treatment

Self-care status

- *History:* use of adaptive equipment, devices, or supplies
- *Observation:* daily activities (dressing, grooming, bathing, toileting, and hygiene)
- *Signs and symptoms:* decreased ability to carry out activities
- *Diagnostic tests:* Functional Ability Scale, Self-Care Assessment Tool

RISK FACTORS

- Antipsychotic-drug-induced movement disorder that affects swallowing (tardive dyskinesia)
- Aspiration pneumonia, coughing, or choking
- Decreased self-care skills
- Diminished memory
- Dysphagia
- Neurologic injury causing sensory or motor problems of the head and neck
- Poor pulmonary function
- Weight loss

ASSOCIATED DISORDERS

Cerebrovascular accidents, dementia, head injury, malignant brain tumor, movement disorder, multiple sclerosis, neurologic disease or injury, Parkinson's disease, psychiatric disorder, tardive dyskinesia

EXPECTED OUTCOMES

Initial outcomes

- Patient receives nothing by mouth to protect against aspiration.
- Patient undergoes Bedside Dysphagia Evaluation or Modified Barium Swallow Videoflouroscopic Evaluation, as prescribed.

Interim outcomes

- Patient receives foods of recommended consistencies only.
- Patient practices aspiration precautions while eating.

Discharge outcomes

- Patient states which food consistencies he can swallow safely.
- Patient states intention to continue aspiration precautions.

INTERVENTIONS AND RATIONALES

Initial interventions

- Remove food that may be available to the patient *to help ensure safety.*
- Inform the patient he cannot have oral foods *to prevent accidental choking.*
- Explain dysphagia evaluation procedures *to encourage the patient to participate in evaluation.*

Interim interventions

- Help the patient identify and remember food consistencies that can be safely eaten (clear liquid, thick liquid, puree, soft solid, or solid) *to increase his knowledge and sense of responsibility for his safety.*
- Teach aspiration precautions, including proper body position and posture, appropriate bite size and position in mouth, and to completely swallow before taking a new bite. *These measures help ensure safety.*

Discharge interventions
- Reward appropriate eating behavior *to help reinforce safe eating habits.*
- Make a referral to an appropriate agency, if needed, *to ensure ongoing care and implementation of feeding regimen.*

EVALUATION STATEMENTS

Patient:
- expresses understanding of the need to have nothing by mouth.
- cooperates in dysphagia evaluations.
- lists food consistencies that can be eaten safely.
- demonstrates measures to prevent aspiration.
- agrees to receive ongoing rehabilitation to revise his diet over time.

DOCUMENTATION

- Results of Bedside Dysphagia Evaluation and Modified Barium Swallow Videoflouroscopic Evaluation
- Patient's understanding of problem
- Nursing interventions
- Patient's willingness and ability to follow treatment recommendations
- Referrals to specialists and outside agencies
- Evaluation statements.

Injury, high risk for

related to overdose or withdrawal

DEFINITION

Accentuated risk of physical harm to oneself, others, or the physical setting as a result of substance abuse, withdrawal, or overdose

ASSESSMENT

Cultural status
- *Demographics:* age, sex, level of education, occupation, nationality, race, ethnic group, religion
- *History:* beliefs, values, and attitudes about health and illness; health customs, practices, and rituals

Cardiac status
- *Physical examination:* vital signs (temperature, pulse, respirations, blood pressure), heart sounds, skin condition, level of consciousness
- *Signs and symptoms:* palpitations, tachycardia, hypertension, abnormal heart sounds, decreased level of consciousness, altered skin color and temperature
- *Laboratory tests:* blood enzymes, cholesterol, and triglyceride levels
- *Diagnostic test:* electrocardiography

Gastrointestinal status
- *Health history:* dietary habits, changes in appetite, history of peptic ulcer or esophageal varices
- *Physical examination:* swallowing or gag reflex, stool characteristics, abdominal inspection, palpation, and auscultation
- *Signs and symptoms:* abdominal pain, nausea and vomiting, food intolerance, diarrhea
- *Laboratory tests:* complete blood count, hematocrit, prothrombin time, folic acid, and ammonia levels
- *Diagnostic tests:* barium enema, esophageal swallowing

Integumentary status
- *Signs and symptoms:* pruritus, rash, ecchymosis, edema, petechiae, spider angiomas

Neurologic status
- *Health history:* head injury, malignant brain tumor, dementia, schizophrenia, drug and alcohol abuse (age at onset, severity of symptoms, prescribed treatment and patient's response)
- *Medication history:* anticonvulsants, neuroleptics, antidepressants, antimanic agents, barbiturates, analgesics, alcohol, illicit drugs
- *Mental status:* appearance and attitude, level of consciousness, motor activity, thought and speech, mood and affect, perceptions, orientation, memory, general information, visual-spatial ability, attention span, abstraction, judgment and insight
- *Motor system:* muscle tone, strength, and symmetry; gait, cerebellar function
- *Cranial nerve function*
- *Signs and symptoms:* lethargy, restlessness, headache, vertigo, seizures, syncope, tremors, paresthesia, impaired movement or coordination, numbness, tics
- *Diagnostic tests:* Glasgow Coma Scale, Folstein Mini-Mental Health Status Examination, Abnormal Involuntary Movement Scale

Nutritional status
- *History:* usual exercise pattern, typical daily intake of food (type and amount), use of dietary supplements
- *Health history:* malabsorption, nutritional deficiencies
- *Physical examination:* height, weight, basal energy expenditure, anthropomorphic measurements, abdominal examination
- *Signs and symptoms:* weight loss, cravings, loss of appetite

Family status
- *Family development:* ability of family to meet patient's physical and emotional needs, usual coping patterns, perceived effectiveness of coping patterns, style of interaction, evidence of codependence or dysfunctional behavior, history of incarceration (specify reason)
- *Family roles:* formal and informal roles and role performance, interrelationship of roles, conflict within family concerning roles,
- *Health history:* depressive or other psychiatric disorders, suicide, substance abuse
- *Diagnostic test:* Family Genogram

Psychological status
- *Child and adolescent development:* family size and dynamics, losses through death or separation, academic performance, peer relationships, socialization, recreational activities, antisocial or maladaptive behaviors, reaction to puberty and sexuality, authority relationships, delinquency, situational crises
- *Adult development:* military experience, higher education, job or occupation changes, dating and marital history, hobbies and recreational activities, spirituality
- *Signs and symptoms:* flushed face; slurred speech; loss of inhibitions; mood lability; changes in behavior, energy level, motivation, personal hy-

giene, self-image, self-esteem, sleep pattern, sexual drive or ability; inability to function; expressions of anger, anxiety, depression, excitation, grandiosity, pathologic jealousy, self-pity, suicidal ideation, suspicion, unreasonable resentment
■ *Signs of dependency:* withdrawal symptoms follow episodes of abuse, rationalization of irresponsible or self-destructive behavior, episodes of "swearing off" alcohol or drugs, irrational fears, panic attacks, social isolation
■ *Early signs of addiction:* loss of control over daily events, blackouts, denial of substance abuse problem, frequent outbursts of anger, lying to cover up alcohol or substance use, anger, guilt, paranoia, extravagant behavior, increase in physical injuries or disorders, problems in key relationships
■ *Late signs of addiction:* breakdown in value system, frequent physical injuries from substance abuse, weight loss, inadequate nutrition, tremors, breakdown in body systems, anxiety, hallucinations, paranoia, failure to uphold family responsibilities, severe financial, legal, and marital problems
■ *Laboratory tests:* urinalysis, electrolyte levels, liver function tests, human immunodeficiency virus testing, blood and urine drug screens
■ *Diagnostic tests:* Brief Psychiatric Rating Scale, Behavioral Checklist, Hamilton Rating Scale for Depression, Self-Rating Anxiety Scale, Impact of Event Scale

Sensory status
■ *Health history:* neurologic injuries, psychiatric disorders, use of tobacco, alcohol, drugs (prescribed, over-the-

counter, illicit), hazardous substances (such as inhaled glue fumes, aerosol propellants, lighter fuel gases)
■ *Signs and symptoms:* hallucinations (visual, auditory, olfactory, tactile), changes in taste or sense of smell, dental caries
■ *Diagnostic tests:* visual, auditory, olfactory, and tactile examinations

Sleep pattern status
■ *Health history:* usual hours of sleep, circadian pattern, energy level after sleep, rest and relaxation patterns, use of amphetamines, use of alcohol or medication to aid sleep
■ *Signs and symptoms:* difficulty falling asleep, nocturnal awakening, early morning awakening, hypersomnia or insomnia, sleep pattern reversal

Social status
■ *Social development:* interpersonal and social skills, social network, ability to trust others, ability to function in social and occupational roles
■ *Signs and symptoms:* emotional withdrawal, suspicion, lack of eye contact, intrusiveness, inappropriate responses, aggressive behavior
■ *Diagnostic test:* Social Adjustment Scale

RISK FACTORS

■ Behavior changes, such as restlessness, confusion, ataxia, anxiety, lethargy, altered sleeping patterns
■ Blackouts
■ Change in pattern of use of alcohol or drugs
■ Family history of dysfunctional behavior (substance abuse, role reversal,

ineffective coping methods, physical, emotional, or sexual abuse)
- Feeling overwhelmed or victimized by events
- Hiding reserves of alcohol or drugs at home, in car, at work
- Lying to cover up substance use or abuse
- Personal history of substance abuse
- Physical signs of substance abuse, overdose, or withdrawal including tachycardia, hypertension, increased temperature, hyperreflexia, tremors in extremities, dilated or pinpoint pupils, diaphoresis, skin changes (ecchymosis, angiomas), abdominal tenderness, hepatomegaly, splenomegaly, weight loss, frequent upper respiratory infections, elevated blood enzymes, prolonged clotting time
- Poor coping skills, low self-esteem, poor self-concept, fear of failure
- Social relationships and activities that focus on alcohol or drugs
- Trouble maintaining relationships with spouse, coworkers, children, peers
- Use of alcohol, drugs (prescribed, over-the-counter, illicit), or both as coping mechanisms

ASSOCIATED DISORDERS

Bipolar disorder, dyssomnia, mood disorders, parasomnia, substance dependence, substance intoxication, substance-related disorders

EXPECTED OUTCOMES

Initial outcome
- Patient develops no further or potentially lethal complications as a result of overdose.

- Patient goes through withdrawal or recovers from overdose without sustaining injury.
- Patient doesn't engage in self-destructive behavior while in hospital.

Interim outcomes
- Patient starts to explore circumstances surrounding substance abuse.
- Patient identifies signs of overdose or withdrawal.
- Patient exhibits less denial about substance abuse or dependency.
- Patient cooperates with psychiatric evaluation and attends teaching sessions, individual and family counseling, and appropriate support group.

Discharge outcomes
- Patient takes first step in exploring interpersonal problems related to substance use.
- Patient states his intention to continue treatment for substance abuse after discharge, for example, by attending counseling sessions and meetings of appropriate support groups.
- Patient demonstrates improved self-esteem and self-concept.

INTERVENTIONS AND RATIONALES

Initial interventions
- Ascertain the type, amount, and time of ingestion of substance, as well as any other medications taken, *to determine the appropriate treatment.*
- Follow the medical regimen to manage physical injuries, detoxification, or symptoms of overdose or withdrawal *to ensure the patient's safety and promote optimal recovery.*

- Administer sedatives as prescribed *to reduce agitation, prevent exhaustion, and promote sleep.*
- Monitor the patient frequently for signs of oversedation. *Oversedation may mask neurologic complications.*
- Monitor vital signs at half-hour intervals *to prevent potentially lethal complications, such as circulatory collapse, hyperthermia, respiratory arrest, seizures, subdural or epidural hematoma, subarachnoid hemorrhage, or massive infarction.*
- Monitor fluid and electrolyte levels and blood urea nitrogen to guide fluid maintenance therapy. *Up to 6 liters of fluid (including 1½ liters of 0.9% sodium chloride solution) may be needed to counter fluid loss through perspiration and agitation.*
- Place an unconscious patient on his side *to prevent aspiration.*
- As needed, use soft restraints *to calm the patient and prevent injury.*
- As prescribed, administer antiemetics *to control nausea and vomiting.*
- As prescribed, administer vitamins *to improve patient's nutritional status.*
- Assess the patient for social withdrawal or isolation, self-destructive thoughts or acts, or outbursts of anger or violence *to provide a basis for developing interventions.*
- If the patient has expressed suicidal thoughts, remove any potentially dangerous items from the room, such as belts, glass objects, ties, or razor blades *to protect the patient.*
- Provide the patient with a quiet, soothing environment. Monitor the patient's mood and behavior for signs of anxiety, fear, or paranoia. *Patients often experience anxiety, especially if the medical regimen includes detoxifica-*

tion. A safe, calm environment and quiet talks about his fears help calm the patient, build trust, and lessen the risk of further injury.

Interim interventions
- Schedule noncare-related time to talk privately with the patient about his thoughts and feelings *to promote trust and afford the patient an opportunity to safely explore circumstances surrounding his substance abuse.*
- Firmly, compassionately, and persistently confront the patient with evidence of his substance abuse. Assess his level of denial. *Denial, a hallmark of substance abuse and addiction, is the major impediment to recovery. Recovery can begin only after the patient admits that a problem exists and demonstrates his willingness to participate in treatment.*
- Encourage the patient to attend group teaching sessions on the psychological and physiological effects of substance abuse *to help him better understand the causes and outcomes of his behavior.*
- Teach the patient about substance abuse, including risk factors, disease course, and potential outcomes of specific substance related disorders. Based on his understanding of events leading up to his hospitalization, review with him the signs and symptoms of withdrawal and overdose *to educate him about the potentially fatal effects of his illness.*
- Talk to members of the patient's family about their feelings regarding the patient's substance abuse problem. Be alert for signs of codependence and assess their ability to assist the patient. *Substance abuse affects the entire fami-*

ly. *Encouraging family members to express their feelings helps you assess for denial, codependence, and other dysfunctional family dynamics. Denial by family members is common. Family members may need to address personal issues related to substance abuse before they can help in the patient's treatment.*
▪ Encourage the patient and family members to attend counseling sessions while the patient is in the hospital *to help them understand the disorder and its effects.*
▪ Encourage the patient to attend meetings of an appropriate support group (for example, Alcoholics Anonymous) during hospitalization *to foster peer support and further opportunities to explore substance abuse.*
▪ Talk to the patient about the importance of accepting help from others and conforming to reasonable limits on behavior. Provide positive feedback when he asks the staff for help and when he complies with limits on behavior appropriate for the hospital setting. *Positive feedback promotes self-esteem and feelings of competency, reinforces appropriate social behavior, and encourages independence in complying with the treatment regimen.*

Discharge interventions
▪ Encourage the patient to explore interpersonal relationships during therapy sessions, during meetings of support groups, or with family members or a close friend. Identifying, acknowledging, and understanding interpersonal and social difficulties help prepare the patient to modify behavior.
▪ Involve the patient, staff, and family members (when possible) in developing an effective outpatient plan for

treatment and support *to ensure continuity of care by establishing short- and long-term goals and to promote self-esteem and self-control.*

EVALUATION STATEMENTS

Patient:
▪ recovers from withdrawal or overdose without experiencing complications.
▪ expresses his feelings regarding reason for hospitalization and possible substance abuse problem.
▪ begins to acknowledge the relationship between troubled personal relationships and substance abuse.
▪ cooperates with drug abuse evaluation.
▪ participates in counseling sessions (individual, group, family) and support groups.
▪ identifies triggers for episodes of substance abuse.
▪ expresses less denial concerning substance abuse or dependency.
▪ discusses potential harmful effects of substance abuse, overdose, and withdrawal.
▪ develops an effective support network comprised of family members, friends, support groups, and appropriate counselors.
▪ states his intention to continue treatment after discharge.
▪ reports less anxiety and improved self-esteem.

DOCUMENTATION

▪ Diagnostic test results
▪ Patient's physical and emotional reactions to treatment, detoxification, or both

- Aggressive or violent comments or behaviors
- Nursing interventions to manage the physiologic effects of overdose and withdrawal
- Nursing interventions to confront patient with evidence and effects of his substance abuse
- Nursing interventions to teach patient about substance dependency and addiction
- Family's level of denial and codependence and their ability to assist in patient care
- Patient's and family's response to nursing interventions
- Participation in therapy sessions (individual, group, family)
- Plan for continued outpatient treatment
- Evaluation statements.

Injury, high risk for

related to use of restraints

DEFINITION

Accentuated risk of physical harm caused by patient's psychological status and the need for using restraints

ASSESSMENT

Neurologic status
- *Mental status:* appearance and attitude, level of consciousness, motor activity, thought and speech, mood and affect, perceptions, orientation, memory, abstraction, judgment and insight

- *Physical examination:* motor and sensory function, reflexes
- *History:* head injury, frontal lobe injury
- *Laboratory tests:* serotonin levels, drug toxicology screening
- *Diagnostic tests:* electroencephalography (EEG), magnetic resonance imaging (MRI)

Psychological status
- *History:* use of phencyclidine, alcohol, or other substances; past episodes of violence or family history of violence; incarceration
- *Signs and symptoms:* agitation, irritability, suspiciousness, sleep deprivation, anger, rage, hostility, cursing, verbal threats, obscene gestures, throwing objects, pacing

RISK FACTORS

- Abnormal EEG or MRI results, abnormal serotonin levels, or positive drug toxicology screen
- Aggressive behavior, such as shouting, threatening talk, shaking fists, display of weapons, chair swinging, pounding fists, slamming doors
- Family history of violence
- History of drug or alcohol abuse
- Mood changes, such as disorientation, agitation, manic excitement, anger, suspiciousness
- Personal history of violence
- Poor judgment and insight
- Presence of command hallucinations or persecutory delusions

ASSOCIATED DISORDERS

Alcohol- or amphetamine-related disorders, antisocial personality disorder, bipolar disorder, borderline personality disorder, brief psychotic disorder, cocaine- or inhalant-related disorders, delusional disorder, dementia, intermittent explosive disorder, obsessive-compulsive disorder, panic disorder, paranoid schizophrenia, phencyclidine-related disorders, posttraumatic stress disorder, temporal lobe epilepsy

EXPECTED OUTCOMES

Initial outcomes
- Patient does not injure others.
- Patient does not injure self while under restraints.

Interim outcomes
- Patient maintains adequate intake of food and fluid.
- Patient's hygienic and toileting needs are met during period of restraint.
- Patient tolerates environmental stimuli without aggressive behavior.
- Patient does no harm to self or others when restraints are removed.

Discharge outcomes
- Patient uses nondestructive means such as exercise to ventilate frustration.
- Patient seeks help when he begins to feel out of control.

INTERVENTIONS AND RATIONALES

Initial interventions
- Designate one nurse to communicate with the patient and to direct other staff members *to minimize opportunities for the patient to exhibit hostility and to build trust.*

- Keep sufficient staff nearby for a show of strength, if necessary, *to show your control of the situation and to protect staff members.*
- Present a calm attitude to the patient and give matter-of-fact responses to verbal hostility. *Anxiety is contagious, but a calm attitude conveys a sense of control and a feeling of security to the patient.*
- Maintain a low level of stimuli *to minimize the patient's anxiety, agitation, and suspiciousness.*
- Keep all sharp objects, glass or mirrored items, belts, ties, and smoking material out of the patient's environment *to maintain his safety.*
- Before restraining the patient, consider alternatives, such as walking with the patient or administering prescribed medications, *to provide the least restrictive alternative to restraints.*
- If the patient poses a serious and imminent threat to himself or others, immediately request that a doctor examine him and order restraints *to ensure the safety of the patient and people around him.* Keep the following points in mind:
– The written order for restraints should include results of the physical examination, a description of the patient's behavior, the type of restraints, the duration of use, and the schedule for removing restraints and checking the patient's vital signs *to protect the patient's rights and to avoid liability.*
– In an emergency, you may apply restraints without delay, but be sure to obtain a written order from the patient's doctor as soon as possible *to meet legal requirements.*
– If a patient who was voluntarily admitted decompensates to the point of

needing restraints, court intervention to determine competency and authorize involuntary commitment may be required *to preserve the patient's rights.*
- When applying restraints, use the following guidelines *to prevent allegations of battery and false imprisonment:*
– Do not use or threaten to use undue force.
– Use only legally permissible forms of restraint.
– Use restraints only to the extent necessary to prevent injury.
- Explain the purpose of restraints and the time period they will be needed to the patient in plain and nonpunitive terms *to help him understand that restraints are a therapeutic intervention, not a punishment.*
- Document carefully the decision-making process that led to the use of restraints and review their need on a continuing basis *to protect against liability and charges of false imprisonment.*

Interim interventions
- Observe the patient every 15 minutes and document your findings *to ensure that his needs for circulation, nutrition, hydration, and elimination are met and to protect against injury.*
- Feed the restricted patient in an upright position *to minimize his risk of choking and aspirating food.*
- Explain to the patient the behavior required of him before you remove restraints *to help him begin to regain control of his behavior.*
- Taking the proper precautions, partially release the patient in restraints every 2 hours *to evaluate the need for continued restraints and to maintain circulation.*

- When the patient's behavior improves, and based on a doctor's order, remove the restraints one at a time *to minimize risk of injury to the patient and staff.*

Discharge interventions
- Encourage the patient to enter into a contract whereby he agrees to maintain control of his behavior *to get the subject of violence out in the open and make the patient responsible for controlling his behavior.*
- Teach the patient methods for maintaining self-control, such as strenuous daily exercises or initiating discussion with others before his anger gets out of hand, *to help him develop internal control mechanisms.*
- Discuss with the patient and staff members the circumstances that led to the use of restraints and other concerns related to the use of restraining devices *to help the patient and staff members resolve any emotional or intellectual conflicts regarding the way the situation was handled.*
- Refer the patient to appropriate mental health professionals and agencies, as needed, *to ensure continuity of care.*

EVALUATION STATEMENTS

Patient:
- experiences no injury and does not harm others.
- controls impulses and demonstrates a reduction in aggressive behavior.
- identifies causes and effects of violent episodes.
- learns appropriate ways to vent frustration and channel angry impulses.

- expresses the need for ongoing treatment and agrees to seek help when he begins to feel out of control.

DOCUMENTATION

- Diagnostic test results
- Patient's behaviors that indicate need for restraints
- Nursing interventions to reduce or prevent violence
- Nursing interventions to ensure the safety of other patients and staff members
- Patient's vital signs, circulation, nutrition, hydration, mental status during use of restraints
- Patient's behavior that indicates increased ability to control aggression
- Patient's response to nursing interventions
- Referrals to mental health professionals and appropriate agencies
- Evaluation statements.

Knowledge deficit

related to drug therapy in cognitively impaired patients

DEFINITION

Inability to understand or perform skills for proper drug administration because of cognitive limitations

ASSESSMENT

Cultural status
- *Demographics:* age, sex, level of education, occupation, race, nationality, ethnic group

- *History:* beliefs, values, and attitudes about health and illness; health customs, practices, and rituals

Family status
- *History:* family's ability to meet physical and emotional needs of its members, family members' understanding of patient's illness, family's ability to assist patient with drug regimen

Neurologic status
- *Mental status:* appearance and attitude, level of consciousness, motor activity, thought and speech, mood and affect, perceptions, orientation, memory, general information, calculations, capacity to read and write, visual-spatial ability, attention span, abstraction, judgment and insight

Psychological status
- *History:* level of motivation, self-image, personal hygiene
- *Psychiatric history:* presence of psychiatric disorder, age at onset, type and severity of symptoms, impact on functioning, type of treatment, patient's response to treatment

Self-care status
- *Health maintenance:* neurologic, sensory, or psychological impairment; medication history; compliance with drug therapy; response to drug therapy

DEFINING CHARACTERISTICS

- History of noncompliance with drug regimens
- Inability of family to meet patient's physical and emotional needs

- Inability to perform personal hygiene
- Inability to read
- Lack of motivation
- Memory deficits
- Poor self-image

ASSOCIATED DISORDERS

Amnestic and other cognitive disorders, dementias, learning disorders, mental disorders due to general medical condition, mood disorders, schizophrenia

EXPECTED OUTCOMES

Initial outcome
- Patient participates in teaching sessions regarding medication regimen.

Interim outcomes
- Patient complies with drug regimen while in the hospital.
- Patient uses visual aids to promote compliance with drug regimen.

Discharge outcome
- Patient demonstrates proper self-medication techniques.

INTERVENTIONS AND RATIONALES

Initial interventions
- Assess the patient's ability to understand spoken and written communications *to establish a basis for planning effective teaching.*
- Encourage the patient to attend group teaching sessions about medications and provide incentives, when

possible, *to reinforce learning and promote compliance.*

Interim interventions
- Teach the patient about the purpose, schedule, dosage, type, and adverse effects of each drug *to reduce his anxiety and enhance compliance.*
- Provide the patient with tools that enhance his understanding, such as pictures, charts, calendars, or a pill box or envelopes for medications *to provide visual cues for adhering to the medication schedule.*
- Provide the patient with positive feedback when he follows the prescribed regimen *to enhance self-esteem and encourage compliance.*

Discharge interventions
- Assess the patient's ability to independently follow the medication regimen *to identify the need for further teaching.*
- Encourage the patient to continue to use proven visual aids *to help him maintain the prescribed medication schedule after returning home.*
- Consult with members of the patient's family and members of the health care team, such as a visiting nurse or outpatient therapist, about the patient's medication regimen *to enlist their assistance in encouraging and monitoring the patient's compliance.*

EVALUATION STATEMENTS

Patient:
- maintains eye contact during teaching sessions about medications.
- asks questions about his medication regimen.

- takes medication without argument or struggle.
- maintains a readily available chart or calendar of his medication schedule.
- identifies members of a support network who can assist with the medication regimen.

DOCUMENTATION

- Medication teaching topics presented to the patient and family members
- Verbal and behavioral responses to teaching sessions
- Incidence of hiding or hoarding medications
- Nursing interventions to help the patient understand the effect of each medication and its proper administration
- Name, route, dosage, and schedule for all prescribed medications
- Demonstrations of proper self-medication by the patient
- Discussions with family and other support network members regarding the patient's medication schedule
- Evaluation statements.

Knowledge deficit

related to informed consent

DEFINITION

Patient's inability to understand information communicated to him about a treatment or procedure

ASSESSMENT

Cultural status
- *Demographics:* age, sex, level of education, occupation, nationality, race, ethnic group
- *History:* beliefs, values, and attitudes about health and illness; health customs, practices, and rituals

Family status
- *History:* marital status, family roles, family communication, developmental stage of family, family health history

Neurologic status
- *Mental status:* appearance, attitude, level of consciousness, motor activity, thought and speech, mood and affect, orientation, memory, capacity to read and write, judgment and insight

Legal status
- *History:* patient's authority to give his own consent, presence of legal guardian, nature of treatment (invasive, risky, experimental), presence of signed consent form

DEFINING CHARACTERISTICS

- Inability to repeat or explain important information about condition or treatments
- Inability to understand prescribed treatment

ASSOCIATED DISORDERS

This nursing diagnosis can occur in association with any medical diagnosis, procedure, or treatment. Keep in mind that mentally ill and developmentally disabled patients have a legal right to informed consent.

EXPECTED OUTCOMES

Initial outcome
- Patient requests information about treatment or procedure.

Interim outcome
- Patient can state the procedure, the person who will perform it, the potential for serious adverse effects, and the consequences of not having the procedure.

Discharge outcome
- Patient undergoes the treatment or procedure or expresses awareness of his right to refuse treatment without having other care or support withdrawn.

INTERVENTIONS AND RATIONALES

Initial interventions
- Ask the patient or the patient's guardian to describe his understanding of the procedure to be performed *to determine if the patient has been provided with adequate information.*
- Answer the patient's questions within the scope of your knowledge, using terms he understands. If you're unable to answer questions, refer the patient to the doctor *to uphold the patient's right to informed consent. The responsibility for obtaining informed consent rests with the person who will be carry-*

ing out the treatment or procedure, usually the attending doctor.
- If you're not comfortable providing requested information, document the patient's knowledge deficit in the medical record. Make sure the patient gets necessary information from his doctor. *If you're aware that the patient hasn't been sufficiently informed to give consent and assist with the procedure, you may be held liable.*

Interim interventions
- Make sure the patient or his legal guardian can name the procedure, the person who will perform it, the potential for serious adverse effects, and the consequences of not undergoing the procedure *to ascertain whether he has sufficient understanding to give consent.*
- Tell the patient that he has the right to refuse treatment, especially if he does not fully understand the procedure, *to protect his rights.*

Discharge intervention
- If the procedure is ongoing, continue to educate the patient about his care and his legal rights *to ensure continuity of care and ongoing respect for the patient's autonomy.*

EVALUATION STATEMENTS

Patient:
- can describe the treatment or procedure.
- knows the name of the person who will perform the procedure.
- can describe the potential harm or adverse effects that can result from the procedure or treatment.

- expresses satisfaction with his decision to proceed with the treatment or procedure.

DOCUMENTATION

- Patient's level of understanding of treatment or procedure
- Actions taken to ensure informed consent
- Patient's response to teaching provided by the nurse or doctor
- Signed consent form
- Evaluation statements.

Management of therapeutic regimen, ineffective

related to mistrust of health care personnel

DEFINITION

Failure to integrate the program for treating illness and its sequelae into daily routine

ASSESSMENT

Cultural status
- *Demographics:* age, sex, level of education, occupation, nationality, race, ethnic group
- *History:* beliefs, values, and attitudes about health and illness; health customs, practices, and rituals; attitudes and beliefs about health professionals; attitudes toward other cultures
- *Diagnostic tests:* Cultural Assessment Guide, Health Belief Model

Self-care status
- *History:* mental and physical ability to manage therapeutic regimen; strengths and weaknesses that affect ability to manage self-care; presence of neurologic, sensory, or psychological impairment; use of adaptive equipment, devices, or supplies; availability of family and social support
- *Observation:* functional ability (muscle tone, size, and strength; range of motion; coordination), daily activities (dressing, grooming, bathing, toileting, and hygiene)
- *Signs and symptoms:* decreased ability to carry out voluntary activities
- *Diagnostic tests:* Functional Ability Scale, Self-Care Assessment Tool

Psychological status
- *History:* motivation to perform care-related activities, reactions to illness and disability, impact of illness on function, treatment for psychiatric illness and patient's response
- *Attitude toward therapeutic regimen:* perception of effectiveness in managing therapeutic regimen, commitment to management of therapeutic regimen, life events interfering with management of therapeutic regimen

Physical status
- *History:* medical disorders; use of prescribed and over-the-counter drugs, including dosage and schedule; activity and exercise regimen; diet; personal habits; diagnostic test results

Family status
- *History:* family goals and values (especially as they relate to health and patient's illness), socioeconomic status,

coping patterns, family health history, usual patterns of managing illnesses

Defining characteristics

- Blunted affect
- Difficulty integrating prescribed treatment into lifestyle
- Exacerbation of illness
- Failure to take action to reduce risk factors for illness and sequelae
- Failure to take steps to incorporate treatment regimen into daily routine
- Inability or unwillingness to look directly at health care personnel when speaking
- Inappropriate choices regarding meeting the goals of treatment or prevention program
- Increased motor activity, such as agitation, pacing, inability to sleep
- Noncompliance with therapeutic regimen
- Refusal to participate in personal health care planning
- Unreasonable mistrust of health care personnel

ASSOCIATED DISORDERS

Any physical or psychiatric illness may be managed ineffectively by the patient. Common examples include acquired immunodeficiency syndrome, asthma, arthritis, bipolar disorders, cancer, chronic fatigue syndrome, chronic renal failure, diabetes mellitus, hearing loss, heart disease, hypertension, schizophrenia, and spinal cord injury.

EXPECTED OUTCOMES

Initial outcomes
- Patient expresses personal beliefs about illness and its management.
- Patient exhibits trust in one or more members of the health care team.

Interim outcomes
- Patient discusses strategies for managing his therapeutic regimen.
- Patient and family members describe a plan to integrate components of the therapeutic regimen, such as medications, activity, and diet, into pattern of daily living.

Discharge outcomes
- Patient selects daily activities to meet the goals of treatment or prevention program.
- Patient expresses intent to reduce risk factors for progression of illness.
- Patient and family members use available support services.

INTERVENTIONS AND RATIONALES

Initial interventions
- Review the patient's history and discuss his personal beliefs about illness *to establish the common understanding necessary for developing a plan to improve management of the therapeutic regimen.*
- Express your trust in the patient's ability to manage the therapeutic regimen, and praise his efforts. Maintain a consistently friendly attitude, making sure verbal and nonverbal messages are consistent. *Consistency helps the patient develop trust and establishes a pos-*

itive tone for the therapeutic relationship.

■ Demonstrate to the patient that you are trustworthy: Be sure to do as you say or explain why you cannot. Encourage other staff members to be consistent in words and deeds *to foster trust.*

■ Establish a predictable treatment schedule for the patient *to enhance his sense of control over his situation and thereby reduce feelings of mistrust.*

■ Try to control any of your own feelings of anxiety when you're with the patient. *Exhibiting anxiety may contribute to the patient's sense of anxiety and mistrust.*

■ Explore the patient's feelings about his and other people's behavior. Help him analyze why deviations from expected behavior occur. When he seeks to express his feelings, especially those relating to the illness, treatment regimen, and health care personnel, encourage him to use "I" statements, such as, "I am disappointed." *A patient capable of expressing his feelings is less likely to make generalizations, such as, "People are evil and can't be trusted," when others fail to live up to expectations. Although he may be disappointed, he is more likely to be able to cope.*

■ Help the patient relate specific feelings, such as anxiety, fear, helplessness, disappointment, or hurt, to specific events. Encourage him to avoid generalizing his feelings to unrelated events or people *to deter indiscriminate, pathologic feelings of mistrust.*

■ Offer assistance frequently and reinforce the efforts of other caregivers. Help the patient develop appropriate ways to ask for help. Work with him to develop a script for rehearsing how to

ask for help. Teach the patient that it's normal to ask for help when in need. *The patient may need assistance in describing his needs.*

■ Acknowledge the patient's right to manage the therapeutic regimen without interference from health care personnel. *If the patient perceives efforts to encourage compliance as an attempt to control his behavior, it may exacerbate mistrust.*

■ Let the patient know that when he's ready to explore strategies for integrating the therapeutic regimen into his daily life, you'll be available to assist him. *Expressing your availability and willingness to assist the patient promotes trust. Putting the patient in control of the process reinforces the notion that it's his choice to meet health-related goals.*

■ Avoid responding to the patient's questions with pat answers or speaking to him in platitudes, *which reinforces feelings of depersonalization. The patient needs to feel that you're truly interested in understanding his experiences and problems. If he feels you're not relating to him as an individual, he may become more mistrustful.*

■ Acknowledge and reinforce appropriate feelings of mistrust. Stress the importance of balancing trust with a healthy skepticism. *For the patient to make appropriate judgments, he must recognize that not everyone is worthy of his trust. Blind trust results in passivity, dependence, and excessive risk-taking.*

■ Consider enlisting the help of support personnel who share common experiences with the patient, for example, people with the same cultural background or the same illness. *The patient may be more willing to trust someone with characteristics or beliefs similar to his own.*

Interim interventions

- Provide the patient with literature about managing the therapeutic regimen. Make sure printed matter is consistent with his language and reading skills. Remind him that you're available to help with planning. *If the patient still doesn't trust you enough to discuss the therapeutic regimen, he may use the printed materials to help improve his health practices. Reminding the patient of your availability prevents him from interpreting use of printed material as evidence of your lack of interest in his progress.*
- When the patient expresses greater interest in care-related activities, assess his current knowledge and beliefs about managing his illness and provide new information as needed. *A review of basics will establish the common understanding needed to develop a plan for better health care.*
- Be aware of the patient's response to teaching. Watch for cues that the patient wants to continue. Let him decide when to terminate the session. *Acknowledging the patient's choice in initiating and ending teaching sessions fosters trust and a sense of control.*
- Explain the pathophysiology of illness and its relationship to the therapeutic regimen. *If the patient understands the underlying reasons for his treatment, he may be more willing to make adjustments to his lifestyle.*
- Work with the patient to clarify his values regarding his lifestyle and health care choices *to gain insight on*

conflicting values that may interfere with self-care.

- Help the patient and family members identify factors that interfere with self-care activities, such as social pressures, lack of family support, conflicting values and beliefs, and previous behavior patterns. Work with them to modify interfering factors *to enhance the level of care.*
- Assist the patient and family members in selecting appropriate options for managing the therapeutic regimen *to help them integrate potentially complicated and disruptive therapeutic interventions into their lifestyle.*
- Provide instructions on how to integrate health-promoting activities into the patient's lifestyle, for example, how to integrate the medication regimen into his daily routine *to encourage new behavior, now or in the future.*

Discharge interventions

- Refer the patient and family members to appropriate support services or self-help organizations *to empower them in taking control of their lives. Greater degrees of social support promote better health.*
- Help the patient and family plan for the future course of the illness. For example, they made need to make structural changes in the home to accommodate a wheelchair or hospital bed. *Planning ahead will enhance their ability to cope with change.*
- Provide the patient and family members with phone numbers and addresses of appropriate health resources so they can obtain additional assistance when needed. *Knowledge of community resources increases the likelihood that*

the family will plan ahead rather than wait for a crisis to develop.

EVALUATION STATEMENTS

Patient:
- expresses personal beliefs about illness and the therapeutic regimen.
- demonstrates trust in himself and members of the health care team.
- demonstrates appropriate levels of mistrust.
- participates in planning the integration of therapeutic regimens into his pattern of daily living.
- states intent to reduce risk factors for illness.

Patient and family members:
- successfully incorporate components of the therapeutic regimen into daily activities.
- contact appropriate support services.

DOCUMENTATION

- Patient's knowledge and beliefs about illness and therapeutic regimen
- Patient behaviors indicating mistrust of others
- Patient behaviors indicating greater willingness to trust health care personnel
- Patient's stated plans to improve the effectiveness of managing therapeutic regimens
- Nursing interventions to promote the patient's trust in himself and others
- Nursing interventions to improve patient and family management of therapeutic regimens
- Test results that indicate effectiveness of therapeutic regimens, such as urine drug levels, blood sugar levels, blood pressure
- Patient's response to nursing interventions
- Evaluation statements.

Noncompliance

related to cultural differences

DEFINITION

Failure, for cultural reasons, to follow through with treatment regimen established by health care professionals

ASSESSMENT

Cultural status
- *Demographics:* age, sex, level of education, occupation, marital status, cultural group
- *History:* beliefs, values, and attitudes about health and illness; health customs, practices, and rituals; use of folk remedies; attitudes toward time, personal space, work, and money; attitude toward members of other cultural groups; family and child-rearing beliefs and values; rules governing relationships with family members and with people outside family
- *Communication:* primary spoken language; use of art, music, or literature in healing rituals
- *Diet:* prohibited food, preferences, special preparation requirements, importance of food and nutrients to healing

Family status
- *Family roles:* formal and informal roles, role performance, degree of family agreement on roles, interrelationship of family roles
- *Family communication:* style and quality of communication, methods of conflict resolution
- *Socioeconomic factors:* economic status of family, sense of adequacy and self-worth, attitudes toward work
- *Coping patterns:* major life events and their meaning to each family member
- *Diagnostic test:* Family Genogram

Self-care status
- *Observation:* functional ability (muscle tone, size, and strength; range of motion; coordination), daily activities (dressing, grooming, bathing, toileting, and hygiene)
- *Diagnostic test:* Functional Ability Scale

Social status
- *History:* conversational and interpersonal skills; social network, ability to function in social settings

DEFINING CHARACTERISTICS

- Health care beliefs and personal habits that do not conform to norms of Western civilization
- Self-care habits, social patterns, or spiritual beliefs that impede adherence to health care regimen

ASSOCIATED DISORDERS

All medical diagnoses in which follow-up treatment and care is needed for health maintenance and restoration; for example, diabetes mellitus, chronic obstructive pulmonary disease, alcoholism, bipolar disorders (mania and depression), end-stage disease (renal, cardiac, or pulmonary)

EXPECTED OUTCOMES

Initial outcomes
- Patient describes usual health practices and methods of coping with disease or illness.
- Patient describes the recommended health care regimen.

Interim outcomes
- Patient integrates his traditional health practices with recommended health care regimen.
- Patient follows through with the recommended health care regimen and incorporates it into his daily activities.

Discharge outcome
- Patient values the health care regimen as evidenced by his verbal reports and behavior.

INTERVENTIONS AND RATIONALES

Initial interventions
- Assess the patient's primary spoken language and provide an interpreter if needed *to facilitate communication, reduce feelings of anxiety, and to ensure effective teaching.*
- Encourage the patient to talk about family, culture, beliefs, and rituals *to convey acceptance and to foster a caring therapeutic relationship.*
- Assess cultural influences on the patient's health care practices. *If the patient is having problems complying with*

the medical and nursing regimen, it may be because it conflicts with folk and popular health care practices.

- Ask the patient to describe his health care practices and those of his family and community, keeping in mind that he has the right to choose the health care options he believes are most appropriate, *to avoid stereotyping and to establish a basis for planning patient teaching.*
- Examine your own cultural biases *to determine how they may influence your view of the patient and his health status. Cultural norms largely determine our definition of health. For example, North American culture values thinness and considers heavier people unhealthy or unattractive. Another society may consider obesity a sign of good health and high economic and social status.*
- Within your teaching plan, recommend ways the patient's cultural practices can be adapted or incorporated into the health care regimen *to overcome cultural barriers by adapting practices that are not harmful into the treatment regimen.*

Interim interventions
- Encourage the patient and family members to bring in familiar objects from home, such as pictures, special blankets, or significant cultural items, *to reduce anxiety caused by unfamiliarity with health care setting.*
- Communicate to the patient that you do not wish to prevent him from participating in ritual healing or folk practices, but instead will try to find ways to modify or incorporate practices into the health care regimen *to demonstrate respect for the patient's culture and foster compliance.*

- When talking to the patient use simple terms and be careful to avoid abbreviations and jargon. Use drawings or demonstrations of equipment *to communicate specific information.*
- Monitor the patient's and family members' understanding of the health care regimen and provide follow-up teaching as needed *to reinforce learning.*
- Observe the patient's response to teaching for signs of lack of understanding or discomfort with the recommendations *to determine the need for revisions to the teaching plan.*
- If possible, observe the patient's incorporation of aspects of the recommended health care regimen into daily and weekly activities *to judge the effect of your teaching. Observation of changes in daily activities is more reliable than statements provided by the patient.*

Discharge interventions
- Find out what importance the patient and his family place on the health care regimen. *If patients and families come to value the treatment recommendations from the professional health care system, sustained compliance is more likely.*
- Monitor the patient's ongoing compliance with the health care regimen and make revisions to the plan of care as necessary. *Additional revision may be needed as you become more aware of the patient's lifestyle.*

EVALUATION STATEMENTS

Patient:
- describes the treatment recommended by health care professionals

- describes usual health practices and methods of coping with disease or illness.
- integrates traditional health practices with recommended health care regimen.
- incorporates recommended health care regimen into his daily activities.
- behaves and speaks in manner that suggests increased acceptance of the health care regimen.

DOCUMENTATION

- Evidence of failure to comply with health care regimen
- Patient's and family members' views about health and illness
- Patient's and family members' description of health care practices
- Patient's and family members' statements indicating their expectations of health care professionals
- Nursing interventions, include suggestions for incorporating nonharmful cultural practices into the treatment plan
- Patient's statements and behaviors indicating increased adherence to the medical and nursing regimen
- Evaluation statements.

Noncompliance

related to denial of chronic mental illness

DEFINITION

Unwillingness to practice health-related behaviors

ASSESSMENT

Family status
- *Marital status*
- *Family roles:* extent to which family members agree on roles, interrelationships of different roles
- *Family communication:* style and quality of communication, methods of conflict resolution
- *Developmental stage of family:* shifts in role responsibility over time, changes in problem-solving methods over time
- *Physical and emotional needs:* ability of family members to meet each other's essential physical, social, and emotional needs; disparities between patient's needs and family's willingness or ability to meet them
- *Family goals and values:* family members' goals and values; extent to which family permits individual members to pursue their own goals and values
- *Socioeconomic factors:* employment status, attitudes toward employment, religious identification, influence of religious beliefs on values and daily practices
- *Coping patterns:* usual coping patterns, family members' perception of effectiveness of coping patterns
- *Family health history:* presence of physiologic or psychiatric disorders, evidence of abuse
- *Diagnostic tests:* Family Environment Scale, Family Adjustment Device

Psychological status
- *Current illness:* changes in appetite, energy level, motivation, personal hygiene, self-image, self-esteem, sleep

pattern, sexual drive, or function; alcohol or drug abuse; recent life changes
- *Psychiatric history:* presence of psychiatric disorder, age at onset, type and severity of symptoms, impact on functioning, type of treatment, patient's response to treatment
- *Developmental history:* personality traits, relationships with peers and authority figures, religious or social group involvement, life events in childhood, scholastic performance, extracurricular activities, delinquency or criminal activity, military history, level of education, occupation, recreational activities, spirituality, reaction to mental illness or disability
- *Laboratory findings:* thyroid function tests, blood and urine drug toxicology screening
- *Diagnostic tests:* Brief Psychiatric Rating Scale, Hamilton Rating Scale for Depression

Self-care status
- *Personal habits:* compliance with medication and laboratory test regimen, participation in self-help groups, use of community resources
- *Physical examination:* presence of neurologic, sensory, or psychological impairment; ability to carry out voluntary activities
- *Diagnostic tests:* Functional Ability Scale, Self-Care Assessment Tool

Social status
- *Personal habits:* conversational and interpersonal skills, size of social network, quality of relationships, degree of trust in others, level of self-esteem, ability to function in social and occupational roles
- *Medications:* neuroleptics

- *Signs and symptoms:* withdrawal, lack of eye contact, intrusiveness, inappropriate responses, aggressiveness
- *Diagnostic test:* Social Adjustment Scale

DEFINING CHARACTERISTICS

- Denial of chronic mental illness
- Dysfunctional family
- Failure to adhere to treatment regimen (medication, laboratory work, dietary considerations, community resources, or self-help groups)
- Impaired cognitive functioning related to psychotic or depressive disorders, or drug or alcohol abuse
- Lack of a social network
- Lack of interpersonal skills as evidenced by withdrawal or aggressiveness
- Long-standing developmental deficits in functioning
- Low self-esteem
- Refusal of family members to accept patient's mental illness

ASSOCIATED DISORDERS

Anxiety disorders, delusional disorder, dementia due to human immunodeficiency virus or other cause, eating disorders, mood disorders, personality disorders, schizophrenia, substance-related disorders

EXPECTED OUTCOMES

Initial outcomes
- Patient identifies factors that influence noncompliance.
- Patient expresses feelings related to his psychiatric diagnosis.

Interim outcomes

- Patient and family members recognize that grieving normally accompanies a diagnosis of chronic mental illness, and allow themselves to grieve.
- Patient and family members describe the cause, signs and symptoms, usual course, and treatment of disorder.

Discharge outcome

- Patient and family demonstrate knowledge of and willingness to comply with treatment, including medication, laboratory follow-up tests, dietary considerations, follow-up appointments, and involvement with community support groups.

INTERVENTIONS AND RATIONALES

Initial interventions

- Listen to the patient's reasons for noncompliance. *Active listening communicates interest, promotes development of a therapeutic relationship, and helps the patient clarify concerns.*
- Encourage the expression of feelings about the psychiatric diagnosis. During discussions with the patient, reflect upon and restate his feelings *to validate his pain and communicate your acceptance.*

Interim interventions

- Explain to the patient and family members that grieving normally accompanies any loss. In this case, they must grieve for the loss of their previous self-concept (as individuals and as a family) and perceptions of the patient's premorbid functioning. *Placing the patient's and family's dis-*

tress within an understandable framework diminishes anxiety and helps them to express and overcome their grief.

- Provide opportunities (active listening and referral to support groups) for the patient and family to grieve. *The patient needs an environment that gives him permission to grieve.*
- Encourage compliance with the therapeutic regimen. *Medications and supportive measures can effectively treat mental disorders.*
- Teach the patient and family members about the cause, signs and symptoms, usual course, and treatment of the patient's disorder. *Patient education promotes better use of health care resources.*

Discharge interventions

- Educate the patient and family members about the plan of care following discharge. Try to address all their concerns *to help prevent future hospitalizations.*
- Assist the patient in making contacts with follow-up resources (such as assisted living programs, support groups, and community mental health centers) before discharge *to encourage use of community resources.*

EVALUATION STATEMENTS

Patient:
- discusses possible reasons for noncompliance.
- expresses feelings regarding psychiatric diagnosis.
- is able to explain the grieving process and relate it to his refusal to perform self-care activities necessitated by chronic mental illness.

- takes medications and attends therapeutic activities while in the hospital.
  Patient and family:
- discuss the cause, signs and symptoms, usual course, and treatment of patient's disorder.
- voice a willingness to comply with discharge plan and make contact with community resources, such as a local chapter of the National Alliance for the Mentally Ill.

DOCUMENTATION

- Patient's statements regarding health care activities
- Patient's expression of feelings regarding psychiatric diagnosis
- Observations of patient's mental status and self-care behavior
- Nursing interventions to promote compliance with treatment plan
- Patient's response to nursing interventions
- Evaluation statements.

Nutrition alteration: Less than body requirements

related to psychological factors

DEFINITION

Change in normal eating pattern that alters weight

ASSESSMENT

Cultural status
- *Demographics:* age, sex, level of education, occupation, nationality, race, ethnic group
- *History:* beliefs, values, and attitudes about health and illness; health customs, practices, and rituals

Nutritional status
- *Personal habits:* usual exercise pattern; eating habits; typical daily food intake; use of drugs, alcohol, or laxatives; changes in internal and external cues that trigger desire to eat, rate of food consumption, stated food preference
- *Medications:* iron and other minerals; multivitamins, vitamin B_{12}, or other nutritional supplements; diuretics
- *Physical examination:* height, weight, basal energy expenditure, anthropometric measurements, abdominal examination
- *Signs and symptoms:* cachexia, weight loss, nausea and vomiting, fainting, constipation, diarrhea, pallor, irritability, cravings, binging and purging, hoarding food
- *Laboratory tests:* hemoglobin and hematocrit; serum iron, serum albumin, total protein, serum transferrin, cholesterol, and triglyceride levels; total lymphocyte count; nitrogen balance; creatinine-height index
- *Diagnostic tests:* upper GI series, barium enema, barium swallow, intradermal skin tests

DEFINING CHARACTERISTICS

- Abdominal pain with or without pathology
- Aversion to eating
- Body weight 20% or more under ideal weight
- Diarrhea
- Lack of interest in food

- Less than recommended daily intake of essential nutrients
- Pale conjunctiva and mucous membranes
- Perceived inability to ingest food
- Poor muscle tone
- Reported inadequate food intake

ASSOCIATED DISORDERS

Anorexia nervosa, bipolar disorder (manic or depressive phase), bulimia nervosa, malabsorption syndrome, mood disorder, nutritional deficiencies

EXPECTED OUTCOMES

Initial outcome
- Patient consumes adequate calories daily (specify) to prevent further tissue breakdown.

Interim outcomes
- Patient gains adequate weight weekly (specify).
- Patient eats independently without being prodded.
- Patient identifies emotional and psychological factors that interfere with eating.

Discharge outcomes
- Patient develops a plan to monitor and maintain target weight.
- Patient states plan to use mental health resources to help cope with psychological conflict.

INTERVENTIONS AND RATIONALES

Initial intervention
- Observe and record the patient's intake (both liquid and solid) *to assess*

nutrient intake and determine what supplements, if any, the patient needs.

Interim interventions
- Determine the patient's food preferences and attempt to obtain preferred foods. Offer foods that appeal to olfactory, visual, and tactile senses *to enhance the patient's appetite.*
- Offer high-protein, high-calorie supplements, such as milk shakes, custard, or ice cream. *Such foods prevent body protein breakdown and provide caloric energy.*
- Serve foods that require little cutting or chewing *to help prevent malingering at meals.*
- Provide a pleasant environment at mealtime *to enhance the patient's appetite.*
- Keep snacks at the bedside *to give the patient some control over eating.*
- If necessary, begin with nutritious liquids and gradually introduce solids. *A severely malnourished patient may not be able to chew solid foods immediately.*
- Avoid asking whether the patient is hungry or wants to eat. Be positive in offering food. *A positive, undemanding attitude will help to avoid confrontation with the patient.*
- Provide opportunities for the patient to discuss reasons for not eating *to help assess the causes of the eating disorder.*
- Whenever possible, sit with the patient for a predetermined length of time during meals. *This inhibits the patient from dawdling during meals or from hiding or hoarding food.*
- Monitor and record elimination patterns. *The patient may be taking laxa-*

tives or diuretics to keep weight low in spite of eating.
- Weigh the patient at the same time every day. Reinforce weight gain with privileges or rewards. *This yields accurate data and gives the patient some control over food eaten and privileges or rewards gained.*

Discharge interventions
- Set the target weight and have the patient record daily weight *to involve in treatment.*
- Refer the patient and family members to an appropriate mental health professional. *An eating disorders commonly indicates unresolved psychological conflict. Treating the underlying issues may help prevent recurrence.*

EVALUATION STATEMENTS

Patient:
- consumes specified number of calories daily.
- gains specified amount of weight weekly.
- eats independently without constant encouragement.
- describes emotional and psychological factors that interfere with eating.
- states plan to monitor weight and maintain specific target weight after discharge.
- contacts support groups and mental health resources as needed.

DOCUMENTATION

- Patient's expressed attitudes toward food and eating
- Patient's expressed feelings about weight and body image

- Patient's daily intake (liquid and solid) and output (urine, stool, vomitus)
- Daily weights and progression of weight gain
- Nursing interventions to feed patient adequately
- Patient's response to nursing interventions
- Evaluation statements.

Nutrition alteration: More than body requirements

related to excessive intake

DEFINITION

Change in normal eating pattern that causes increase in weight

ASSESSMENT

Nutritional status
- *Personal habits:* usual exercise pattern; eating habits; typical daily food intake; use of drugs, alcohol, or laxatives; changes in internal and external cues that trigger desire to eat, rate of food consumption, stated food preference
- *Medications:* iron and other minerals, multivitamins, vitamin B_{12}, or other nutritional supplements
- *Physical examination:* height, weight, basal energy expenditure, anthropometric measurements, abdominal examination
- *Signs and symptoms:* weight gain, nausea and vomiting, fainting, constipation, diarrhea, pallor, irritability, cravings, binging and purging, hoarding food

- *Laboratory tests:* hemoglobin and hematocrit; serum iron, serum albumin, total protein, cholesterol, triglyceride, and serum transferrin levels; total lymphocyte count; nitrogen balance; creatinine-height index
- *Diagnostic tests:* upper GI series, barium enema, barium swallow, intradermal skin tests

DEFINING CHARACTERISTICS

- Body weight 10% or more over ideal weight
- Clinical obesity
- Dysfunctional eating patterns, such as concentrating food intake at end of day, eating in response to internal cue other than hunger (anxiety, for example), eating in response to such social cues as time of day and social situation, pairing food with other activities
- Observed use of food as a reward or comfort measure
- Reported or observed obesity in one or both parents
- Triceps skin fold greater than 15 mm in men and 25 mm in women

ASSOCIATED DISORDERS

Anxiety disorder, depressive disorder, diabetes mellitus, obesity, pickwickian syndrome

EXPECTED OUTCOMES

Initial outcomes
- Patient voices feelings about current weight.
- Patient identifies internal and external cues that increase food consumption.

Interim outcomes
- Patient states need to lose weight.
- Patient sets a realistic weekly weight-loss goal.
- Patient plans menus appropriate to prescribed diet.
- Patient adheres to prescribed diet.
- Patient loses a realistic and appropriate amount of weight weekly.
- Patient sets target weight before discharge.

Discharge outcomes
- Patient describes plan to monitor weight and maintain target weight.
- Patient participates in selected exercise programs weekly.

INTERVENTIONS AND RATIONALES

Initial interventions
- Help the patient identify eating habits and circumstances in which he turns to food. Encourage him to express feelings associated with eating and his current weight. *Permanent weight loss starts with examination of factors contributing to weight gain.*
- Discuss the patient's normal food preferences *to evaluate eating habits and include preferred foods in the diet.*
- Teach the patient about low-calorie, nutritious foods *to encourage him to eat foods that provide energy without causing weight gain.*

Interim interventions
- Help the patient set realistic goals for losing weight *to reduce frustration and help ensure a sense of accomplishment.*

- Have a dietician discuss meal planning with the patient *to help plan nutritious, satisfying meals.*
- Give the patient emotional support and positive feedback for adhering to the prescribed dietary regimen *to promote compliance.*
- Encourage nondietary rewards for desired behavior, such as the purchase of a new accessory or book, *to promote continuation of dietary plan and help the patient avoid using food as a reward.*
- Weigh the patient weekly or as prescribed *to monitor the effectiveness of the diet plan.*
- Set target weight with the patient and have him record his weight *to involve him in care and provide an opportunity for positive reinforcement.*

Discharge interventions
- Explore participation in Overeaters Anonymous or another support group or use an individual diet therapy plan *to ensure continued treatment and support after discharge.*
- If such a resource is available, refer the patient to a mental health professional for behavior modification *to help him change poor eating habits, thereby helping to ensure permanent weight loss.*
- Help the patient select an exercise program (walking, jogging, aerobics, swimming) that's appropriate to his age and physical condition. *Besides aiding weight loss, activities offer an alternative to eating to alleviate stress.*

EVALUATION STATEMENTS

Patient:
- expresses feelings about present weight.
- identifies cues that increase food consumption.
- expresses desire to lose weight.
- establishes weekly weight loss goal, in cooperation with health care team.
- adheres to prescribed diet.
- loses specified amount of weight weekly.
- summarizes plan to monitor weight and maintain specified target weight.
- participates in selected weekly exercise activities for a specified amount of time.
    Patient and family:
- plan menus within parameters of prescribed diet.
    Patient and health care professional:
- set target weight before discharge.

DOCUMENTATION

- Diagnostic test results and laboratory findings
- Patient's expressions of feelings about weight, eating, food, dieting
- Goals set by patient
- Record of weight
- Foods consumed by patient
- Strategies used to facilitate weight reduction
- Factors that impede weight reduction
- Evaluation statements.

Pain

related to psychological factors

DEFINITION

Sensation of discomfort derived from multiple sensory nerve interactions gen-

erated by physical, chemical, biological, or psychological stimuli

ASSESSMENT

Cultural status
- *Demographics:* age, sex, developmental stage, nationality, race, ethnic group
- *History:* beliefs, attitudes, and values about health and illness; methods of dealing with stress

Psychological status
- *History:* presence of psychiatric illness, body image, previous experience with pain, type of treatment and impact on function, anxiety level, type and severity of symptoms

Health status
- *History:* current illness; exposure to physical, biological, or chemical agents that may be the cause of pain; pain tolerance

DEFINING CHARACTERISTICS

- Absence or insufficient levels of physical, biological, or chemical agents to cause pain intensity experienced by patient
- Communication of painful sensation (verbal or behavioral)
- Distracting behavior, such as moaning, crying, pacing or restlessness, or seeking out people or activities
- Facial mask of pain, including lackluster eyes, fixed or scattered movement, grimacing, altered muscle tone (may range from listless to rigid)
- Guarded or protective behavior, such as favoring a body part

- Narrowed focus as evidenced by altered time perception, social withdrawal, impaired thought processes
- Description of pain that's difficult to associate with a physiologic condition

ASSOCIATED CONDITIONS

Psychiatric conditions, such as somatoform pain disorder, hypochondriasis, somatization disorder, or factitious disorder; psychological factors, such as stress, depression, and ineffective coping may intensify pain caused by physical, biological, or chemical agents.

EXPECTED OUTCOMES

Initial outcomes
- Patient identifies specific characteristics of pain.
- Patient reports satisfactory relief from pain within a reasonable time.
- Patient helps develop a plan for pain control.

Interim outcomes
- Patient acknowledges that physical pain may be associated with emotional stress.
- Patient requires less analgesics (specify).
- Patient uses alternative pain control techniques.

Discharge outcomes
- Patient reports satisfaction with pain management regimen.
- Patient contacts appropriate support groups or mental health care agencies.

INTERVENTIONS AND RATIONALES

Initial interventions

- Ask the patient to describe his pain and assess him for physical symptoms that indicate pain. *Continuous assessment allows for care plan modification as needed.*
- Administer prescribed pain medication *to provide pain relief.*
- Check the effectiveness of the medication after 30 minutes *to monitor pain relief and build a level of trust needed for a therapeutic relationship.*
- Acknowledge the patient's distress *so that he won't feel his pain is being minimized.*
- Ask the patient to help establish goals for pain relief (including reduction in his reliance on analgesics) and develop a plan for pain control *to give the patient a sense of control.*
- Spend at least 15 minutes each shift allowing the patient to express his feelings *to improve his sense of control, decrease his isolation, and foster trust.* When talking to the patient, emphasize his overall well-being *to help minimize focusing on a specific symptom.*
- Consult with a liaison nurse, if necessary, to explore your feelings about the patient's responses and to obtain a more objective view of the situation. *Having a colleague to consult with may help reduce your frustration when the expected outcomes seem impossible to attain.*

Interim interventions

- Encourage open communication *to help the patient identify emotional or environmental stressors.*

- Explain the possible relationship between stressors identified by the patient and the exacerbation of pain *to encourage him to explore emotional or environmental factors that may be linked to pain.*
- Plan distractions, such as reading, watching television, and family visits, *to help keep the patient from focusing on pain.*
- Teach the patient alternative pain control techniques, such as self-hypnosis, biofeedback, and relaxation *to reduce reliance on analgesics.*
- Have the patient keep a symptom diary *to explore further the connection between stress and the onset of illness.*
- Provide positive feedback as the patient makes progress toward established goals *to motivate him and encourage compliance.*

Discharge intervention

- Consult with a psychiatric liaison nurse when developing the discharge plan and refer the patient to appropriate support groups and mental health care agencies. *The patient may need additional help in dealing with anxiety or other psychological factors associated with pain.*

EVALUATION STATEMENTS

Patient:
- describes characteristics of pain, including location, duration, and frequency.
- reports achieving pain relief with analgesia or other measures.
- participates in developing his health care plan.
- acknowledges that pain may be related to emotional factors.

- lists stressors that may exacerbate pain.
- reduces use of pain medication.
- states satisfaction with pain management regimen.
- demonstrates motivation by seeking resources to understand his pain.
- cooperates with treatment plan.

DOCUMENTATION

- Patient's expressions of physical pain
- Patient's expressions of emotional pain
- Observations of patient's physical condition
- Nursing interventions for controlling pain
- Patient's response to interventions
- Evaluation statements.

Pain, chronic

related to physical disability

DEFINITION

Physical and emotional discomfort which lasts more than 1 year

ASSESSMENT

Cultural status
- *Demographics:* age, sex, level of education, marital status, occupation, nationality, race, ethnic group
- *History:* beliefs, values, and attitudes about health and illness; health customs, practices, and rituals

Neurologic status
- *History:* medical disorders; stress-related illness; food, drug, or environmental allergies; pain management methods
- *Medications:* pain medications, anxiolytic agents, antidepressants, alcohol, illicit drugs
- *Mental status:* appearance and attitude, level of consciousness, motor activity, thought and speech patterns, mood and affect, perceptions, orientation, memory, attention span, judgment and insight
- *Signs and symptoms:* lethargy, headache, vertigo, pain
- *Diagnostic test:* Folstein Mini-Mental Health Status Examination

Psychological status
- *Reactions to illness and disability:* age at onset; impact of condition on functioning; treatment and response; change in energy level, motivation, personal hygiene, self-image, self-esteem, or sexual drive; evidence of alcohol or substance abuse or withdrawal
- *Life events:* recent divorce, job loss, or loss of loved one; change of environment
- *Developmental history:* academic and occupational history, marital history, hobbies and recreation
- *Diagnostic tests:* Brief Psychiatric Rating Scale, Hamilton Rating Scale for Depression

Sleep status
- *History:* usual hours of sleep, energy level after sleep, sleep pattern disturbance or change, rest and relaxation pattern

- *Medications:* sleeping aids, caffeine, alcohol, amphetamines

Nutritional status
- *History:* eating disorder, nutrient deficiency, obesity
- *Personal habits:* exercise pattern, typical daily food intake
- *Signs and symptoms:* weight loss or gain, pallor

Social status
- *History:* interpersonal skills, quality of relationships, degree of trust in others, ability to function in social and occupational roles
- *Signs and symptoms:* withdrawal, inappropriate responses

Family status
- *History:* family composition, developmental stage, family roles, changes in roles or responsibilities over time, alliances and interactions among members, effects of alliances on family stability, support systems
- *Communication:* style and quality of communication, methods of resolving conflict and their effectiveness, usual coping patterns and their effectiveness
- *Needs fulfillment:* family's ability to meet patient's physical and emotional needs, disparities between patient's needs and family members' willingness and ability to meet them
- *Health history:* previous medical conditions, history of psychiatric disorders, including bipolar disorder, depressive disorder, or suicide in any family member

Spiritual status
- *History:* religious or church affiliation, influence of beliefs on values and practices, perceptions about life and suffering, support network, spiritual response to medical condition and change in body image

DEFINING CHARACTERISTICS

- Anxious or depressed mood
- Attention-seeking behavior related to pain
- Demands for immediate relief
- Dependence
- Disparity between reported discomfort level and expected level based on physical findings
- Expressions of despair or helplessness
- Insomnia
- Narrowed perception and awareness of surroundings
- Pain behavior such as crying, moaning, or pained facial expression
- Physical dysfunction
- Self-focusing
- Verbal and nonverbal indications of pain

ASSOCIATED DISORDERS

Chronic or terminal illness, injury, malingering, somatic disorder

EXPECTED OUTCOMES

Initial outcomes
- Patient expresses feelings of pain.
- Patient identifies sources of pain.
- Patient states needs openly and directly.
- Patient identifies relationship between pain and stress or conflict.

Interim outcomes
- Patient develops pain management program that includes activity and rest, exercise, and medication regimen that is not contingent on pain.
- Patient adjusts behavior and participates in activities to enhance social life.

Discharge outcomes
- Patient identifies factors that affect occurrence or severity of pain.
- Patient uses diversions and recreational activities to reduce pain.
- Patient uses noninvasive pain relief measures, such as relaxation or imagery.
- Patient describes how stress may exacerbate pain.
- Patient seeks ongoing treatment and counseling from support groups and community resources.

INTERVENTIONS AND RATIONALES

Initial interventions
- Establish a specific time to talk with the patient about pain and its psychological and emotional effects *to establish a trusting, supportive relationship and to foster open communication.*
- Assess the patient's daily activities and physical symptoms of pain, monitor and record effectiveness and adverse effects of medication, and correlate the patient's pain behavior with activities and time of day *to establish a baseline assessment for plan of care.*
- Note inconsistencies between pain behavior and verbal expressions of pain *to gauge the patient's perception of his pain.*
- Encourage the patient and family members to participate in planning a

reasonable, effective pain management strategy *to help the family understand pain-related behavior and to foster long-term, effective coping in the home setting.*

Interim interventions
- Develop a behavior-oriented plan of care that includes an activity schedule *to foster reduction of learned pain-related behavior through behavioral-cognitive therapy.*
– Instruct the patient to use relaxation techniques, music, or therapy to relieve pain *to provide an adjunct to medications and to foster self-help and independence.*
– Provide rewards for limiting pain-related talk and pain-related behavior *to help the patient focus less on pain.*
– Encourage the patient to develop a schedule of self-care activities *to increase his sense of control and reduce his dependence on others.*
- Work closely with staff and with the patient's family *to achieve the goals of the pain management program and to foster cooperation, which may help the patient function at optimal level.*

Discharge interventions
- Encourage the patient to accept limitations caused by pain and to use diversions, recreational activities, and noninvasive pain relief measures *to enhance his quality of life.*
- Provide a written and verbal summary of the pain management plan *to provide reinforcement and increase adherence to the plan.*
- Provide a list of community resources for ongoing treatment and counseling *to reduce the patient's sense of isola-*

tion and to foster continued care after discharge.

EVALUATION STATEMENTS

Patient:
- identifies factors or events that trigger pain.
- manages pain with appropriate techniques, such as recreation, diversions, music, or imagery.
- accepts inevitability of some pain.
- receives information about community resources for ongoing treatment and counseling.

DOCUMENTATION

- Diagnostic test results
- Patient's description of physical pain, and feelings about pain
- Effect of pain on patient's behavior and affect
- Relationship between activities and time of day and reports of pain
- Comfort measures initiated by nurse, patient, or family
- Nursing interventions to control chronic pain
- Response to nursing interventions
- Response to medications
- Discharge plan
- Evaluation statements.

Parenting alteration, high risk for

related to mental illness

DEFINITION

Potential deficit in parenting skills resulting from mental illness

ASSESSMENT

Cultural status
- *Demographics:* age, sex, level of education, occupation, nationality, race, ethnic group
- *History:* beliefs, values, and attitudes about health and illness; health customs, practices, and rituals; religious identification; influence of religious beliefs on values and daily practices

Family status
- *History:* patient's marital status; family roles; previous nurturing experience with children, pets, siblings
- *Family communication:* style and quality of communication, methods of conflict resolution
- *Physical and emotional needs:* family's ability to meet the patient's physical and emotional needs
- *Family goals, values, and aspirations:* extent to which family members understand and articulate family goals and values, extent to which family permits pursuit of individual goals and values
- *Socioeconomic factors:* economic status of family, sense of adequacy and self-worth of family members, em-

ployment status, attitudes toward work

- *Evidence of abuse:* history of violence; physical, emotional, or sexual abuse
- *Family health history:* psychiatric, stress-related, or medical illness; suicide; substance abuse; mental retardation in any family member
- *Diagnostic tests:* Family Genogram, Holmes and Rahe Social Readjustment Rating Scale, Family Environment Scale, Parenting Stress Index

Social status
- *History:* conversational skills, interpersonal skills, size of social network, quality of relationships, degree of trust in others, level of self-esteem, ability to function in social and occupational roles, use of alcohol or drugs
- *Diagnostic test:* Social Adjustment Scale

Neurologic status
- *Mental status:* appearance and attitude, level of consciousness, motor activity, thought and speech, mood and affect, perceptions, orientation, memory, general information, calculations, capacity to read and write, visual-spatial ability, attention span, abstraction, judgment and insight
- *Physical examination:* motor and sensory function, reflexes, presence of tardive dyskinesia or other adverse effects of medication
- *Prior medical conditions:* head injury, fetal or infant distress, seizure disorder
- *Laboratory tests:* complete blood count; electrolyte, blood urea nitrogen, creatinine, and glucose levels; tuberculosis, human immunodeficiency virus, and syphilis screening; alcohol and illicit drug screening panel; medication plasma levels
- *Diagnostic tests:* electroencephalography (EEG), Abnormal Involuntary Movement Scale, cranial nerve assessment, electrocardiography, magnetic resonance imaging (MRI), Cognitive Capacity Screening Examination

Psychological status
- *Current illness:* evidence of cognitive disorder (hallucinations, delusions, bizarre behaviors); evidence of mood disorder (depression, mania, labile mood swings, diminished or grandiose self-esteem); motivation and attention to parenting; feelings regarding each child; past hospitalizations or institutionalizations; response to supportive people and agencies
- *Childhood development:* developmental milestones, intelligence quotient, personality traits, behavior, school performance, relationships with peers, experience of being nurtured
- *Adolescent development:* involvement in religious organizations or social clubs; recreational interests; relationship with parents, authority figures, or therapists; sexual activities; academic and social comfort and performance; level of independence; ability to connect emotionally with other people; treatment of animals
- *Adult development:* level of independence; social activities; sexual behaviors; housing situation; relationship with fellow parent; capacity to empathize, love, and accept responsibility; socioeconomic status and support; degree of isolation or involvement with support systems; self-es-

teem; reality orientation; ability to accurately assess condition and seek assistance when needed; understanding of mental illness, medications, and therapy
- *Medication history:* use of neuroleptics, antimanic agents, anticonvulsants, anxiolytics, sedative-hypnotics, anticholinergics, or antidepressants; response to medications; compliance with medication regimen; past and current use of alcohol, cigarettes, illicit drugs
- *Diagnostic tests:* Wechsler Adult Intelligence Survey, Minnesota Multiphasic Personality Inventory

RISK FACTORS

- Abnormal EEG or MRI results
- Acting out (violence, isolation, or projection) used as a means to cope with frustrations or disordered thoughts
- Change in sleep and activity patterns
- Evidence of sexual, physical, or emotional abuse in family (one or both parents may have been abused as a child)
- Family history of psychiatric illness
- Impaired thinking, orientation, or mood
- Lack of knowledge regarding child development, including developmental milestones, appropriate behaviors, and physical, emotional, social, and spiritual needs of children
- Limited insight
- Low self-esteem
- Noncompliance with therapy or appointments with social service agencies
- Poor communication skills
- Poor motivation

- Positive alcohol or drug screening tests
- Presence of disabilities in children (children with disabilities are more likely to be abused)
- Psychotropic medication serum levels outside of therapeutic range
- Suicidal or homicidal thoughts
- Thought disturbances, such as command hallucinations or delusions involving the children

ASSOCIATED DISORDERS

Brief psychotic disorder, dementia and other cognitive disorders, intermittent explosive disorder, mood disorders, obsessive-compulsive disorder, personality disorders, posttraumatic stress disorder, schizophrenia, substance-related disorders

EXPECTED OUTCOMES

Initial outcomes
- Staff member assesses patient's health and psychiatric status, therapy needs, and compliance with medication regimen.
- Patient identifies individuals with whom he can safely confide.
- Patient expresses feelings regarding his parenting skills.
- Patient identifies areas where his parenting skills need improvement.
- Patient admits that he needs help and support to improve parenting skills.
- Patient expresses understanding that all family members need therapy and support.

Interim outcomes

- Patient identifies factors that may contribute to his difficulty complying with the medication regimen.
- Patient discusses the possibility of increasing his network of contacts.
- Patient describes his feelings regarding each of his children.
- Patient explores his own learning deficiencies and emotional needs.
- Patient agrees that including all family members in therapy is an important goal.
- Patient describes frustrations associated with parenting.

Discharge outcomes

- Patient states commitment to comply with therapy, including medication regimen, medical care, and psychiatric treatments.
- Patient states plans to expand his network of personal contacts, for example, social service agencies, day care services, church or synagogue groups, or the National Alliance for the Mentally Ill.
- Patient focuses on needs of each child.
- Patient gathers information relevant to child care needs.
- Patient arranges for family members to attend family therapy sessions.
- Patient agrees to attend group therapy for support in parenting.

INTERVENTIONS AND RATIONALES

Initial interventions

- Provide a safe environment, whether treating the patient on an inpatient or outpatient basis, *to lessen the patient's anxiety.*

- Point out to the patient that people with chronic mental illness have a tendency to become isolated *to educate him about risks inherent in his condition.*
- Let the patient know that you accept him as a person and a parent *to promote trust in the therapeutic relationship.*
- Praise the patient when he honestly identifies learning needs *to communicate that asking for help is a positive step.*
- Explain family therapy sessions. Tell the patient that all members of the family are required to participate. *Knowing what to expect may help the patient succeed in treatment.*
- Determine the parent's ability to participate in group therapy. Assess his orientation, commitment to attend the full schedule, ability to be physically close to others, willingness to discuss feelings and behaviors, capacity to trust, empathy, and desire to share feedback *to determine if group therapy is an appropriate treatment option.*

Interim interventions

- Help the patient evaluate the consequences of his behaviors *to help him feel responsible and to encourage responsible behavior.*
- Encourage the patient to express fears about increasing social contacts. *Fear may come from embarrassment or, in a patient with a cognitive disorder, delusions. Understanding his fear may help the patient reach out to others when ready.*
- Determine the patient's ability to meet the physical and emotional needs of his children. Tell him that morally and legally he is required to

care for them. *Being honest reinforces the patient's need to assume responsibility. If the patient cannot provide child care, appropriate steps need to be taken.*

- Tell the patient that the therapist will have an ongoing relationship with social services personnel *to promote the best interests of the child* and that any suspected child abuse or neglect will be reported. *Awareness of these facts may help the patient cope better in times of crisis.*

- Teach the patient about child care needs and parenting skills *to promote an intellectual and emotional understanding of parental responsibility.*

- Conduct family therapy sessions. Make sure all members of the family are present. *Family therapy provides an opportunity to assess family dynamics, reinforce areas of strength, initiate discussion of conflicts, and role-play communication skills.*

- If assessment indicates that group therapy is an appropriate treatment option for the patient, make sure the group is suited to the patient's developmental stage and emotional needs. Also tell him what is expected of him in therapy and ask him to sign a contract to participate. *Informing the patient of expectations in therapy and asking him to sign a contract reinforces his feelings of control and helps to emphasize the value of therapy.*

Discharge outcomes

- Tell the patient the times of treatment appointments and reinforce this information with a written schedule. *Providing verbal and visual reinforcement helps to ensure that the patient will keep appointments.*

- Inform the patient that you or a caseworker will call and visit to evaluate his status and remind him of appointments. *Follow-up visits promote timely evaluation and convey your concern.*

- Help the patient make contact with appropriate individuals or agencies and evaluate the quality of ensuing relationships regularly through follow-up interviews. *For chronically mentally ill patients, most personal contacts are made by either social service personnel or family members. Increasing the patient's support network helps to decrease isolation, improve self-esteem, and promote increased support for fulfilling parental responsibilities. It also increases the child's exposure to adults who can monitor his status and provide healthy role models.*

- Reinforce appropriate child-rearing behaviors. *If lessons are repeated, the patient is more likely to retain them and put them to practice.*

- Provide printed or taped materials about such subjects as communication, discipline, appropriate expressions of anger, nutrition, immunizations, and pediatric medical care. *Visual and auditory reinforcement promotes retention of information.*

- Help the patient make contact with people or agencies that can assist with parenting tasks, including the school principal, the teachers, a primary care doctor, a family nurse practitioner, a child and family psychotherapist, an advanced practice psychiatric nurse, a social worker, or a hospital case manager *to strengthen the patient's support system.*

- Assess family members' behavior during family therapy sessions. Provide support as they express their feelings *to foster improvement in family coping.*

■ Help family members identify trigger behaviors that lead to acting out or family conflict *to help them deal honestly with each other and better understand family dynamics.*

■ Institute child care contingency plans to be used if the patient relapses. *Acknowledging that the patient may have episodes of relapses demystifies mental illness and gives the child permission to contact others for help.*

■ Encourage the patient to become involved in group therapy. Help him understand behavioral expectations within the group. Advise him to be open in discussing his experiences with group members and to identify parenting concerns. *Active participation in therapy will provide the patient with healing emotional experiences in a group setting, decrease isolation, increase trust and socialization, and provide an opportunity to learn additional parenting skills. Group therapy may also provide a safe environment to bring up difficult subjects, such as birth control and genetic counseling.*

EVALUATION STATEMENTS

Patient:
■ discusses medication regimen, including expected results, potential adverse reactions, and need for periodic laboratory tests of plasma levels.
■ allows social services personnel to visit his home.
■ increases contacts with others and reports he is adjusting to increased contact with support people.

■ describes developmental and physical needs of his children and identifies appropriate means to fulfill his children's needs.
■ attends group therapy sessions and expresses feelings about the sessions.
■ acknowledges improvement in his condition and identifies areas in which he still needs help.

Family members:
■ attend family therapy sessions.
■ report increased understanding of family dynamics and the patient's psychological condition.
■ identify caretakers and therapists to contact in case the patient relapses.

DOCUMENTATION

■ Diagnostic test results
■ Patient teaching regarding medications
■ Evidence of site visits or telephone calls by therapist or caseworker
■ Progress notes reflecting patient's telephone or personal contact with support personnel
■ Social service reports, school records, immunization records, and medical records of children
■ Family's contingency plans in case the patient has a relapse or recurrence of symptoms
■ Group therapy records including attendance and progress notes
■ Patient's charted medication compliance
■ Individual, family, and group therapy participation
■ Evaluation statements.

Personal identity disturbance

related to a history of sexual abuse

DEFINITION

Uncertainty about personal identity brought about by childhood sexual abuse

ASSESSMENT

Cultural status
- *Demographics:* age, sex, marital status, nationality, education, occupation
- *History:* beliefs, values, and attitudes about health and illness; health customs, practices, and rituals
- *Diagnostic test:* Cultural Assessment Guide

Family status
- *Family roles:* formal and informal roles and role performance
- *Family rules:* rules that foster stability, maladaptive rules, methods of modifying family rules
- *Family communication:* quality of communication, methods of conflict resolution
- *Family subsystems:* family alliances, affect of alliances of family stability
- *Family needs:* ability of family to meet the patient's physical and emotional needs
- *Socioeconomic factors:* economic status of family; sense of belonging to racial, cultural or ethnic group; influence of religious beliefs on daily life
- *Evidence of abuse:* evidence of physical, sexual, or emotional abuse within family (victims and victimizers)

- *Family health history:* psychiatric disorders, substance abuse, incarceration of family members
- *Diagnostic tests:* Family Genogram, Index of Family Relations

Psychological status
- *History:* mood; eating habits; sleeping habits; decision-making ability; self-esteem; social interaction; grooming; body weight; feelings about identity, career choice, friendships, religion, sexual behavior
- *Childhood development:* personality traits, adaptive and maladaptive behaviors, memories, academic performance, relationships with peers, religious and social group involvement, life events in childhood, evidence of antisocial behavior, recreational activities
- *Adolescent development:* reaction to puberty and sexuality, relationships with authority figures, scholastic performance, occupational choices, peer relationships, extracurricular activities, delinquency, situational crises
- *Adult development:* academic, military, and occupational history; dating and marital history; hobbies and recreational activities; spirituality
- *Signs and symptoms:* anxiety; depression; regressive behavior, such as loss of interest in friends, school, or activities; phobias; repetitive nightmares; feelings of shame or humiliation; poor grooming; excessive or inadequate body weight
- *Diagnostic tests:* Brief Psychiatric Rating Scale, Hamilton Rating Scale for Depression, Self-Rating Anxiety Scale

DEFINING CHARACTERISTICS

- Altered family roles, such as daughter acting as family caretaker
- Change in eating habits
- Conflicts regarding career choice, friendship patterns, religious identification, patterns of sexual behavior and moral issues
- Cultural values that support abusive behavior, such as belief that children are property of parents or wife is property of husband
- Denial of sexual abuse
- Disturbed body image
- Disturbed mood or affect
- Dysfunctional personal relationships
- History of drug or alcohol abuse
- Irritability and lack of impulse control
- Lack of trust, low self-esteem, or excessive dependence on others
- Marital conflict, single parent home, or overcrowded household during childhood; passive, sick, absent, or incapacitated mother; father with psychiatric problem or substance abuse
- Poor decision making, judgment, and insight; poor orientation to reality
- Poor family communication and functioning
- Poor grooming
- Recurring nightmares or sleep disturbance
- Social isolation
- Traumatic interpersonal experiences

ASSOCIATED DISORDERS

Alcohol- or drug-related disorder, borderline personality disorder, eating disorder, mood disorder, posttraumatic stress disorder, schizophrenia, schizophreniform disorder, sexual arousal disorder, sexual desire disorder, stress-related illnesses such as headache, ulcer, or other GI disturbance

EXPECTED OUTCOMES

Initial outcomes
- Patient acknowledges disturbance in personal identity.
- Patient demonstrates increased comfort with feelings of rage and sadness.
- Patient discusses problems and feelings with nurse and other health care professionals.

Interim outcomes
- Patient explores feelings associated with sexual abuse.
- Patient discusses past experiences of abuse that have influenced self-concept and behavior.
- Patient helps make decisions about treatment.
- Patient expresses positive feelings about self.

Discharge outcomes
- Patient expresses increased understanding of effects of sexual abuse on identity.
- Patient demonstrates increased ability to establish short- and long-term goals.

INTERVENTIONS AND RATIONALES

Initial interventions
- Establish a trusting relationship by conveying acceptance and respect *to provide a safe environment for the patient to express distressing feelings.*

- Help the patient identify a psychological impairment that may be affecting her ability to function *to foster recognition of problems, causes, and contributing factors.*
- Encourage the patient to identify and discuss such feelings such as anger and hostility *to facilitate the grieving process and to help her cope with unresolved issues.*
- Tell the patient that expressing negative feelings toward an abuser is essential in the healing process *to alleviate any feelings of guilt.*
- Praise the patient for her efforts to identify problems, verbalize feelings, and develop new coping methods *to increase her sense of control and reduce her feelings of powerlessness.*

Interim interventions
- Encourage the patient to express feelings through writing, crying, art therapy, music therapy, pet therapy, or other ways that are comfortable to her *to help her identify and express feelings and to facilitate the grieving process. Abused patients are not always able to communicate emotions verbally and may benefit from alternative forms of expression.*
- Help the patient understand the relationship between past experiences of abuse and present emotions *to provide increased perception and insight into present difficulties. For example, a female patient sexually abused by a male might have difficulty with sexual arousal that causes her to feel sexually inadequate.*
- Help the patient explore how her experiences of abuse influence her behavior and self-concept *to determine*

sources of anxiety and to assess impact of traumatic experiences.
- Demonstrate appropriate behaviors through role playing and role reversal. For example, a woman abused during childhood might need to role-play situations involving authority figures that generate anxiety. *Role playing may help to decrease anxiety and to encourage effective problem solving.*
- Encourage the patient to make decisions, and provide positive feedback when she takes responsibility for solving problems *to foster effective decision making and to increase her self-esteem.*

Discharge interventions
- Help the patient identify support systems *to reduce her feelings of isolation.*
- Encourage the patient to identify positive and negative aspects of options for her future *to reinforce feelings of control and to increase effective decision making.*
- Provide positive feedback for continued verbalization of feelings and for continued decision making *to reinforce successful new behaviors and to increase self-confidence and self-esteem.*
- Refer the patient to an appropriate support agency *to ensure continued healing.*

EVALUATION STATEMENTS
Patient:
- acknowledges disturbance in personal identity.
- participates in care decisions.
- communicates feelings about experience of sexual abuse.
- expresses positive feelings about self.

- develops better understanding of effects of sexual abuse.
- demonstrates increased ability to make decisions about short- and long-term goals.
- identifies available sources of support.
- recognizes that choices are available and describes options for future.
- expresses need for continued care and agrees to receive further treatment.

DOCUMENTATION

- Results of diagnostic tests
- Patient's statements indicating personal identity disturbance
- Nursing interventions to help patient identify emotional distress and feelings associated with sexual abuse
- Nursing interventions to enhance patient's self-esteem and self-confidence
- Patient's responses to nursing interventions
- Referrals to specialized professionals, agencies, and support groups
- Evaluation statements.

Personal identity disturbance

related to the presence of alternate personalities

DEFINITION

Difficulty integrating personality components early in life to cope with an overwhelmingly hostile and punitive environment

ASSESSMENT

Cultural status

- *Demographics:* age, sex, level of education, occupation, nationality, race, ethnic group
- *History:* beliefs, values, and attitudes about current illness; routine health practices; lifestyle
- *Diagnostic test:* Cultural Assessment Guide

Family status

- *Family roles:* formal and informal roles and role performance, degree of family agreement on roles, interrelationships of roles
- *Family rules:* rules that foster stability, maladaptive rules, family's methods of modifying rules
- *Family communication:* style and quality of communication, methods of conflict resolution
- *Developmental stage:* lengths of relationships in family, how family adapts to change, shifts in role responsibility
- *Family subsystems:* conflict between family members, supportive relationships, effect of family alliances on family stability
- *Socioeconomic factors:* economic status of family, sense of adequacy and self-worth, employment status, attitudes toward work
- *Coping patterns:* major life events and their meaning to each family member, usual coping patterns, family members' perceptions of effectiveness of coping patterns
- *Evidence of abuse:* physical and behavioral indicators
- *Family health history:* medical and psychiatric disorders

Neurologic status

■ *Mental status examination:* appearance, attitude, level of consciousness, motor activity, thought and speech, mood and affect, perceptions, judgment, insight, orientation, memory, abstraction, calculations, concentration
■ *Signs and symptoms:* severe headaches or migraines, excessive use of analgesics

Psychological status

■ *History:* changes in appetite, self-image, self-esteem, sleep pattern, or sexual drive; substance abuse; recent life changes
■ *Psychiatric history:* presence of illness, age at onset, type and severity of symptoms, impact on patient's function, type of treatment, response to treatment

DEFINING CHARACTERISTICS

■ Amnesic periods, during which patient experiences loss of time and identity
■ Avoidance of or seeking out physical contact
■ Extreme mood swings
■ Flashbacks
■ Frequent changes of therapists
■ History of aggressive acting out
■ History of psychiatric hospitalizations with little alleviation of symptoms
■ Low self-esteem
■ Nightmares
■ Presence of alternate personalities of which the patient may or may not be aware
■ Psychiatric complications, such as sexual dysfunctions, sleep disorders, substance abuse, suicidal ideation or behavior, eating disorders
■ Regular wakening at certain times of the night
■ Reports hearing voices from inside his head
■ Self-mutilation or other self-destructive behavior

ASSOCIATED DISORDERS

Borderline personality disorder, dissociative identity disorder, substance-related disorders

EXPECTED OUTCOMES

Initial outcome

■ Patient does not harm himself.

Interim outcomes

■ Patient establishes trusting relationship with caregiver.
■ Patient focuses on the goals of treatment and does not preoccupy himself with minor mishaps and misunderstandings.
■ Staff members provide consistent care even if alternate personalities assert themselves.

Discharge outcome

■ Patient participates in outpatient counseling and support groups.

INTERVENTIONS AND RATIONALES

Initial intervention

■ Assess the patient's potential for suicide or self-inflicted injury at the beginning of each shift and as needed; institute necessary safety measures. *Pa-*

tient safety is the most important nursing consideration.

Interim interventions

- Assign consistent staff to care for the patient *to foster trust.*
- Develop a contract with the patient that specifies reasons for admission, expectations regarding cooperation with unit regulations, specific nursing interventions, and criteria for discharge. *This provides the patient with a sense of control and focus and decreases the potential for staff conflict and division.*
- If the patient becomes preoccupied with minor unit mishaps and misunderstandings, refocus his attention on the goals of the admission. Avoid reacting defensively or allowing staff divisions. *Because past traumatic relationships have distorted the patient's perspective, he is likely to overreact to events. By not being drawn into a reenactment of past relationships, staff members can provide a corrective emotional experience.*
- Accept the presence of alternate personalities, but do not change your behavior when confronted with alternative personalities *to maintain a consistent and therapeutic environment.*
- Explain unit expectations to the patient and ask him to comply with reasonable limits. If alternate personalities emerge, explain expectations and limits to the new personalities. *Limits reinforce the notion that the patient can remain in control of his impulses.*

Discharge intervention

- Encourage the patient to participate in outpatient counseling and support groups, recognizing that behavior

change will be a long-term process. *This discourages unrealistic expectations and validates the need for a long-term commitment to therapy.*

EVALUATION STATEMENTS

Patient:
- doesn't harm himself.
- communicates openly with caregiver.
- achieves goals established in admission contract.
- maintains appropriate behavior at all times, including during the appearance of alternate personalities.
- expresses commitment to outpatient psychotherapy.

DOCUMENTATION

- Diagnostic test results
- Patient's statements related to his level of safety
- Patient's description of his identity
- Patient's reports of flashbacks, fears, amnesic periods
- Observations of changes in the patient's mood, voice, or behavior
- Headaches and eating or sleep disturbances reported by the patient
- Nursing interventions performed to strengthen the patient's identity
- Patient's response to nursing interventions
- Evaluation statements.

Posttrauma response

related to assault

DEFINITION

Sustained painful response to an unexpected life event

ASSESSMENT

Cultural status
- *Demographics:* age, sex, level of education, occupation, nationality

Psychological status
- *History:* circumstances of the assault, available support systems, patient's perceptions of the event, coping patterns, effect of trauma on social interactions, grief reaction
- *Signs and symptoms:* changes in appetite, self-image, sleep pattern, sexual drive or competence; problems with concentration, memory, orientation, mood, behavior

DEFINING CHARACTERISTICS

- Psychic numbing, including confusion, constricted affect, difficulty with interpersonal relationships, impaired reality interpretation, phobia, poor impulse control
- Reexperience of trauma, including exaggerated startle response, excessive or minimal verbalization of traumatic event, flashbacks, excessive alertness, intrusive thoughts, nightmares, verbal reports of guilt and self-recrimination

ASSOCIATED CONDITIONS

This nursing diagnosis can occur in any patient hospitalized with injuries from physical assault. Examples include battered spouses, physically abused children and elderly persons, victims of gunshot wounds or stabbings, prisoners of war, and hostages.

EXPECTED OUTCOMES

Initial outcomes
- Patient achieves maximum possible recovery from physical injuries.
- Patient expresses feelings related to the assault.
- Patient reports feeling safe.

Interim outcomes
- Patient uses effective coping mechanisms to reduce fear.
- Patient contacts sources of support and seeks professional help when necessary.

Discharge outcome
- Patient reestablishes and maintains adaptive interpersonal relationships.

INTERVENTIONS AND RATIONALES

Initial interventions
- Follow the prescribed medical regimen to manage physical injuries. *Recovery from injury will help reduce the patient's anxiety.*
- Visit the patient frequently *to promote trust and reduce fear of being left alone.*
- Listen to the patient's fears and concerns *to demonstrate empathy and encourage open expression of feelings.*

- Communicate to the patient that you accept his feelings and behavior *to reassure him that his feelings and behaviors are appropriate and valid.*
- Reassure the patient of his safety and take appropriate measures to ensure it. For example, keep the patient's location in the hospital confidential, notify the police, and report cases of child or elder abuse to social services *to reduce fear of repeated assaults.*
- Avoid activities and environmental stimuli that can intensify symptoms, such as loud noises, bright lights, abruptly entering the room, or painful procedures or treatments. *Trauma may be intensified by misinterpreting procedures or environmental factors as repeated assaults.*
- Monitor the patient's mental status. When necessary, reorient the patient to his surroundings and interpret reality *to alleviate psychic numbing.*

Interim interventions
- Teach the patient one or more fear-reducing behaviors, for example, seeking support from others when frightened. *This helps the patient develop a sense of control over his emotions.*
- Encourage family members and friends to express their feelings *to help reduce their anxiety.*
- Teach family members the phases of crisis and describe the patient's probable reactions to them *to promote understanding and lessen anxiety.*

Discharge intervention
- Provide referrals to community resources, such as clergy, mental health professionals, social services, and support groups for victims of assault. *Contact with individuals that under-*

stand the patient's experience will help reduce feelings of isolation and encourage constructive coping patterns.

EVALUATION STATEMENTS

Patient:
- recovers from injuries to the greatest extent possible.
- resumes normal daily activities to the greatest extent possible.
- expresses feelings of anger, blame, fear, and guilt.
- spends less time recriminating.
- reports feeling safe inside the hospital.
- demonstrates one or more fear-reducing behaviors.
- uses available support groups.
- resumes usual social activities.

DOCUMENTATION

- Patient's stated perception of event
- Observations of patient's behavior
- Observations of patient's interaction with others
- Nursing interventions to prevent or reduce fear of repeated assaults
- Patient's response to interventions
- Referrals to sources of support
- Evaluation statements.

Posttrauma response
related to history of childhood incest

DEFINITION

A sustained painful response to childhood incest

ASSESSMENT

Cultural status
- *Demographics:* age, sex, level of education, occupation, sexual orientation, marital status, nationality, race, ethnic group, religion
- *History:* beliefs, values, and attitudes about health and illness; health customs, practices, and rituals
- *Diagnostic test:* Cultural Assessment Guide

Family status
- *History:* family roles, family rules, communication patterns, coping patterns, ability of family to meet physical and emotional needs of its members, socioeconomic status, support systems, health history (medical and psychiatric), history of abuse (sexual, emotional, or physical), alcohol and drug use
- *Interfamily relationships:* family alliances, intense parent-child relationships, parent-children role reversal, prepubertal sexual play and exploration, ability of family members to maintain appropriate boundaries, tolerance for individuality among family members
- *Signs and symptoms:* overcrowded living conditions, dysfunctional family structure, social isolation, lack of contacts outside the family, family history of mental illness, poor communication within the family, presence of disturbed violent adult with partner unable to protect children, inappropriate sexual behavior within family, (exhibitionism, peeping, explicit sexual discussions, touching, caressing), fused boundaries, loss of individuality

- *Diagnostic tests:* Family Genogram, Index of Family Relations

Social status
- *History:* conversational skills, interpersonal skills, size of social network, quality of relationships, degree of trust in others, level of self-esteem, ability to function in social and occupational roles, use of alcohol or drugs
- *Diagnostic test:* Social Adjustment Scale

Psychological status
- *Childhood development:* personality traits, maladaptive behaviors, early memories, continuous memories, academic performance, relationships with siblings and peers, religious and social group involvement, life events, evidence of antisocial behavior, separation anxiety, recreational activities
- *Adolescent development:* history of poor impulse control, alcohol or drug use, reaction to puberty and sexuality, quality of authority relationships, scholastic performance, choices of occupation, relationships with peers, extracurricular activities, delinquency, situational crises
- *Adult development:* dating and marital history, promiscuity or celibacy, abusive partners, homosexual or lesbian relationships, reactions to illness and disability, impulse control, cognitive deficiency, homicidal or suicidal ideation or attempt, drug and alcohol use, issues related to suspicion, paranoia, or trust
- *Signs and symptoms:* emotional pain, self-blame, shame, sadness, vulnerability, helplessness, hyperalertness or hypervigilance, anxiety, panic, in-

tense distress at reminders of the trauma (for example, anniversaries)
- *Diagnostic tests:* Brief Psychiatric Rating Scale, Hamilton Rating Scale for Depression, Self-Rating Anxiety Scale, Minnesota Multiphasic Personality Inventory

DEFINING CHARACTERISTICS

- Dissociation or amnesia
- Feelings of detachment or alienation
- Impaired memory or inattentiveness
- Irritability
- Lack of interest in activities
- Psychic numbing as evidenced by confusion, constricted affect, difficulty with interpersonal relationships, impaired interpretation of reality, phobia, poor impulse control
- Reexperience of trauma, including exaggerated startle response, flashbacks, intrusive thoughts, repetitive dreams or nightmares, excessive or minimal discussion of traumatic events, verbalized guilt and self-recrimination
- Rigid adherence to role or stereotypical behavior
- Self-destructive behavior, such as substance abuse or attempted suicide
- Vagueness in recollecting childhood incest

ASSOCIATED DISORDERS

Adjustment disorder, borderline personality disorder, depressive disorder, dissociative disorders (dissociative amnesia, dissociative fugue, dissociative identity disorder, depersonalization disorder), eating disorders, factitious disorder, malingering, mood or anxiety disorders, panic disorder, pain disorders, schizophrenia, sexual arousal disorders, substance-related disorders, suicidal ideation or attempt

EXPECTED OUTCOMES

Initial outcomes
- Patient establishes a therapeutic alliance with nurse.
- Patient acknowledges that incest occurred during childhood.
- Patient begins to express feelings, such as fear, anger, and guilt.

Interim outcomes
- Patient reports experiencing less anxiety, fear, or guilt when remembering episodes of incest that occurred during childhood.
- Patient states increased acceptance of losses caused by an abusive sexual relationship.
- Patient comes to terms with her past in the way she feels is best.
- Patient begins to take steps to pursue personal goals.

Discharge outcomes
- Patient identifies and contacts appropriate sources of support.
- Patient participates in planning follow-up care.

INTERVENTIONS AND RATIONALES

Initial interventions
- Establish a therapeutic relationship with the patient. Remain nonjudgmental and convey your acceptance of the patient. *Communicating acceptance is important to avoid reinforcing the incest survivor's tendency to blame herself for her past.*

- Be careful to maintain appropriate boundaries in your relationship with the patient. Keep in mind that she may have trouble relating to authority figures, feel threatened easily, or test your ability to maintain boundaries. *Patients with posttrauma response have problems related to trust, acceptance, authority, and limits for appropriate behavior.*
- Encourage the patient to talk about incest and her perception of it. *Discussion helps the patient develop an understanding of her experience with incest.*
- Listen while the patient talks about her feelings. Help her clarify feelings and encourage expressions of anger, rage, or guilt. *Listening conveys empathy and acceptance and communicates to the patient that her feelings are valid and appropriate.*
- Monitor the patient's mental status. Reorient the patient to her surroundings and interpret reality as often as necessary. *This alleviates psychic numbing, a characteristic symptom of assault.*

Interim interventions

- Assess for indications of substance abuse, eating disorders, somatic complaints, mood disturbances, sexual dysfunction, anxiety, or other signs that the patient is having difficulty coping. *The patient may develop dysfunctional behavior patterns in an attempt to suppress or release emotions related to incest.*
- Teach the patient positive coping strategies, such as techniques for stress management and relaxation and assertiveness skills, *to enhance self-confidence and the ability to cope with stress.*
- Help the patient as she explores more deeply her experience with in-

cest. Help her understand that circumstances that led to incest were not her fault and, therefore, she could not protect herself *to relieve her sense of guilt and to promote healing.*
- Discuss ways to recognize and manage emotional reactions to anniversary dates marking traumatic episodes of incest. Explain that the reoccurrence of disturbing thoughts and feelings at these times is normal *to help the patient recognize recurrence of traumatic feelings and cope with them constructively.*
- Encourage the patient to make realistic plans for the future. Suggest that she write down a list of options for the near future. *The patient may feel undeserving of a happy future or incapable of making choices about her life. Making plans for the future is an important step in resolution of the grieving process.*

Discharge interventions

- Provide information about community resources and support groups. *Recovering from trauma can be a prolonged process and follow-up therapy can help the patient work through the grieving process. Support groups provide a safe setting for the patient to explore issues related to incest. By offering support and help to other group members, the patient may increase her sense of self-worth.*
- Help the patient schedule follow-up therapeutic treatment. *The patient will require additional therapy to help her fully confront the effects of the trauma and integrate the experience into her life.*

EVALUATION STATEMENTS

Patient:
- participates a therapeutic relationships with the nurse.
- acknowledges her history of incest and expresses her feelings about it.
- exhibits fewer symptoms of trauma.
- works to achieve resolution of past trauma in the manner that she feels is best.
- identifies and uses sources of support.
- reports developing a more positive self-image.
- participates in planning ongoing care.

DOCUMENTATION

- Diagnostic test results
- Patient's description of history of incest
- Dysfunctional coping patterns developed in response to history of abuse (as described by patient)
- Nursing interventions performed to help the patient identify and express feelings associated with childhood incest
- Nursing interventions performed to improve coping skills and help the patient manage stress
- Patient's response to nursing interventions
- Referrals to psychiatrist, psychologist, community services, support groups
- Evaluation statements.

Posttrauma response

related to parent's alcoholism

DEFINITION

Impaired behavior and emotions following prolonged exposure to parent's alcoholism

ASSESSMENT

Family status
- *Family functions:* parent's ability to meet family's emotional and physical needs; family members' perceived roles; communication styles; methods of conflict resolution; behaviors associated with alcoholism; behaviors during periods of abstinence; physical, emotional, or sexual abuse; family's values and goals
- *Social factors:* socioeconomic level; social interaction; family's involvement with relatives, friends, and community
- *Diagnostic tests:* Family Genogram, Parental Stress Inventory

Social status
- *History:* conversational skills, interpersonal skills, size of social network, quality of relationships, degree of trust in others, level of self-esteem, ability to function in social and occupational roles, use of alcohol or drugs
- *Diagnostic test:* Social Adjustment Scale

Spiritual status
- *History:* religious affiliation, current religious practices and beliefs, support

network, effects of religious belief on management of stress and maintenance of self-esteem

Neurologic status

- *History:* head injury, especially secondary to violence or accidents
- *Physical examination:* mental status examination, motor and sensory functions, reflexes
- *Laboratory tests:* complete blood count; electrolyte, creatinine, and glucose levels; human immunodeficiency virus and syphilis tests
- *Diagnostic tests:* electroencephalography, magnetic resonance imaging, glucose tolerance test, endocrine function studies, urinalysis

Psychological status

- *Current illness:* presenting complaints; signs and symptoms; recent psychiatric treatment or hospitalization; effect of illness on sleep pattern, appetite, sexual function
- *Personal factors:* alcohol or drug use or abuse; self-esteem; perception of level of independence and competence; issues surrounding control, trust, and boundaries; interpersonal relationships; defense mechanisms; ability to express feelings
- *Childhood development:* age when parents abused alcohol; severity and duration of alcohol abuse; personality traits; adaptive behaviors; maladaptive behaviors; coping skills; academic performance; interactions with peers, siblings, and parents; recreational activities; religious education
- *Adolescent development:* adult role models; peer interactions; dating history; experimentation with alcohol or drugs; academic performance; rela-

tionship with parents, siblings, extended family, and authority figures; recreational and social interests; perceived family role
- *Adult development:* dating and marriage history, characteristics of interpersonal relationships, coping strategies, alcohol and drug use or abuse, military history, employment history, leisure activities, depression or anxiety, nurturing abilities
- *Medication history:* anxiolytics, antidepressants, antipsychotics, sedative-hypnotics, analgesics, hormone replacements, or antimanic agents; medications for physiologic disorder
- *Diagnostic tests:* Minnesota Multiphasic Personality Inventory, Wechsler Adult Intelligence Survey, Family Environment Scale, Myers-Briggs Type Indicator, Fundamental Interpersonal Relations Orientation-Behavior, State-Trait Anxiety Inventory, Michigan Alcoholism Screening Test

DEFINING CHARACTERISTICS

- Absence of parents due to hospitalization or incarceration
- Covert drinking by parents
- Denial of adult child of alcoholic (ACOA) trauma
- Difficulty in interpersonal communication
- Difficulty resolving conflicts
- Exaggerated startle response
- Family enmeshment or estrangement
- History of physical, sexual, or emotional abuse
- Hypervigilance
- Inability to express feelings
- Inconsistent behavior and responses by parents

- Intensification of symptoms when exposed to situation that resembles the original trauma
- Lack of healthy role models
- Lack of support from healthy adults during childhood and adolescence
- Maladaptive behaviors such as arguing or being manipulative
- Multigenerational family history of alcoholism
- Psychic numbing or isolation
- Reliving of trauma through intrusive thoughts
- Survivor guilt or depression

ASSOCIATED MEDICAL DIAGNOSES

Adjustment disorder, anxiety disorders, dissociative disorders, eating disorders, mood disorders, personality disorders, substance-related disorders

EXPECTED OUTCOMES

Initial outcomes
- Patient expresses feelings of depression, anxiety, anhedonia, or other symptoms.
- Patient discusses difficulties in establishing interpersonal relationships.
- Patient identifies specific effects of ACOA trauma.
- Patient states reasons for seeking treatment.
- Patient expresses need for emotional support.

Interim outcomes
- Patient discusses his history and acknowledges that he is an ACOA.
- Patient explores behaviors and emotions associated with being an ACOA, including shame, guilt, or denial.

- Patient expresses his feelings regarding family enmeshment or estrangement; negative parental role modeling; and physical, sexual, or emotional abuse.
- Patient appraises his current situation.
- Patient learns of available treatment options.
- Patient obtains information about group therapy.

Discharge outcomes
- Patient agrees to continue to learn about the psychological effects of being raised as a child of alcoholic parents.
- Patient expresses increased awareness of the effect of being an ACOA on personal relationships.
- Patient states plan to continue treatment and participate in group therapy.
- Patient expresses desire to improve his life situation.
- Patient reports benefits of participating in ACOA Anonymous.

INTERVENTIONS AND RATIONALES

Initial interventions
- Assess patient's physical, psychological, social, intellectual, and spiritual status *to facilitate diagnosis and treatment.*
- Provide emotional support and a safe environment while discussing the patient's condition *to overcome fears about remembering trauma.*
- Encourage the patient to identify factors that led him to seek therapy *to help him view stressors and conflicts as motivating forces.*

- Inform the patient about treatment options, including group therapy, *to empower him in determining his course of therapy.*
- Reassure the patient that feelings of loneliness, shame, and guilt are normal responses to the trauma of growing up with an alcoholic parent *to reduce his feelings of shame.*

Interim interventions
- Describe the dynamics of ACOA trauma. *Helping the patient understand he suffers from a specific disorder may reduce feelings of uncertainty and guilt.*
- Discuss specific symptoms of ACOA trauma that are manifest in the patient's emotions and behavior. *Treatment should acknowledge the patient's unique feelings and emotions.*
- Help the patient establish the connection between ACOA trauma and his current life situation *to help the patient assume responsibility for personal growth.*
- Assess the patient's readiness to improve personal relationships. *Pushing the patient too quickly may cause panic and retreat.*
- Provide information about ACOA Anonymous, a 12-step program for children of alcoholics *to encourage participation in the program, thereby reducing isolation. The patient may also have fears about attending a 12-step program that must first be addressed.*
- Consult with group therapists about the patient's participation in group therapy. Educate the patient about what to expect regarding the format and expectations of therapy *to further educate him about treatment options. Unlike ACOA Anonymous, group thera-py will be led by a professional therapist and will provide specific therapeutic agendas. The therapist may help the patient work in-depth on psychological conflicts regarding such issues as control, dependence, anger, and establishing boundaries. The therapist may also employ behavioral and cognitive techniques to help the patient.*

Discharge interventions
- Inform the patient that working through ACOA issues is an ongoing process *to encourage him to allow adequate time for therapy and care.*
- Encourage the patient to commit to therapy until he feels an improvement in self-esteem and a decrease in symptoms *to give the patient permission to work on himself and to help him perceive his well-being as the treatment outcome.*
- Affirm the connections made by the patient between past ACOA trauma and his current situation *to promote therapeutic healing, decrease feelings of isolation, and increase his empathy for other children of alcoholic parents.*
- Reassure the patient of the value of ACOA Anonymous. Explain that participating is a lengthy but finite process *to promote participation.*
- Work with the patient on meeting interpersonal and other life goals gradually *to allow time to internalize information, help him stay motivated, and accomplish change.*
- Encourage the patient to use a combination of treatments, for example, ACOA Anonymous and group therapy. *The most effective treatment may be a combination of professional care and peer-group support.*

EVALUATION STATEMENTS

Patient:
- expresses understanding of ACOA trauma and its characteristic traits.
- describes how ACOA traits are manifested in his own personality and behavior.
- acknowledges relationship between his current situation and history of ACOA trauma.
- defines negative feelings and behaviors as motivators for change.
- identifies goals of treatment.
- states intention to attend ACOA Anonymous.
- participates in group therapy for a specified number of sessions.
- discusses behaviors and cognitive techniques taught in group therapy.

DOCUMENTATION

- Diagnostic test results
- Assessment data
- Nursing interventions
- Patient's response to nursing interventions
- List of goals defined by patient and supported by his therapist
- Patient's statements about current feelings and behaviors and future goals
- Group therapy attendance records and progress notes
- Patient's evaluation of techniques to decrease symptoms, such as thought blocking, relaxation exercises, guided imagery, daily exercise program, reframing negative perceptions, and diminishing all-or-none thinking
- Evaluation statements.

Powerlessness

related to health care environment

DEFINITION

Perceived lack of control and perception that one's actions won't significantly affect an outcome

ASSESSMENT

Cultural status
- *Demographics:* age, sex, level of education, occupation
- *History:* beliefs, values, and attitudes about health and illness; health practices; previous hospitalization

Family status
- *History:* marital status, family alliances and impact on family stability, interactions and conflicts, major life events, impact of life events on each family member
- *Communication:* style and quality of communication, conflict resolution methods and effectiveness, usual coping patterns and effectiveness

Health status
- *History:* neurologic, sensory, or psychological impairment; current medical condition; knowledge and understanding of physical condition; physical, mental, and emotional readiness to learn; use of adaptive devices; medication regimen; possible adverse effects
- *Hospital environment:* equipment and supplies, health care staff, privacy,

space, lighting, noise level, location of personal belongings

Social status
- *Social interactions:* conversation and interpersonal skills, degree of trust in others, self-esteem, ability to function in social role
- *Signs and symptoms:* withdrawal, lack of eye contact, intrusiveness, inappropriate responses, aggressiveness

Spiritual status:
- *History:* religious affiliation, influence of religious beliefs on values and daily practices, perceptions about life and suffering, responses to chronic or terminal illness, change in body image
- *Signs and symptoms:* crying, despair, withdrawal

DEFINING CHARACTERISTICS

- Anger, apathy, fear, guilt, irritability, resentment, sadness, or crying
- Dependence or passivity
- Discomfort
- Dissatisfaction and frustration over inability to perform tasks or activities
- Dissatisfaction with health care environment
- Doubt about role performance
- Perceived lack of control or influence over self-care or current situation

ASSOCIATED DISORDERS

Conditions that restrict or confine patient, such as blindness, confinement to intensive care or cardiac care unit, isolation, multiple intravenous lines, multisystem trauma, paralysis, or traction; dependence on ventilator; language barrier

EXPECTED OUTCOMES

Initial outcomes
- Patient identifies feelings of powerlessness associated with environment.
- Patient describes modifications or adjustments to environment that increase feeling of control.
- Patient identifies factors that are beyond his control.

Interim outcomes
- Patient participates in self-care activities.
- Patient reports increased feeling of control.

Discharge outcome
- Patient discusses future plans, such as discharge.

INTERVENTIONS AND RATIONALES

Initial interventions
- Assess and monitor the patient for a change in status *to provide a basis for a change in the care plan.*
- Help the patient identify factors that contribute to his feeling of powerlessness *to increase his sense of control over expectations.*
- Determine the patient's strengths and limitations *to foster realistic care planning.*
- Acknowledge the importance of the patient's space by verbally delineating it and, if he is immobilized, by asking for instructions regarding placement of personal belongings *to enhance his potential for regaining a sense of power.*
- Place the call light, television controls, bedside table, telephone, urinal, and other items within easy reach *to*

reduce his frustration over an inability to reach nearby items and to increase his feeling of control over self-care.
- Explain all treatments and procedures and encourage the patient to participate in planning his care. Provide choices regarding when and how activities, such as bathing, eating, and getting out of bed, will occur *to increase his feeling of empowerment and to reduce his passivity and dependence on caregiver.*
- Allow the patient to take control over decisions, such as position, injection site, and visiting, *to reduce maladaptive coping behaviors.*

Interim interventions
- Provide consistent staffing as much as possible *to foster a trusting relationship, which increases predictability and comfort level, and to encourage adaptation to the situation.*
- Increase effective communication with the patient by providing time for questions and answers *to increase his sense of control.*
- Encourage the patient to initiate and perform self-care measures as much as possible *to foster his independence and sense of control.*
- Encourage the patient to express feelings about regaining control *to promote healthy adjustment and hope for future.*

Discharge intervention
- Provide referrals to appropriate community resources and encourage patient to make plans for obtaining needed assistance following discharge *to ensure continuity of care.*

EVALUATION STATEMENTS

Patient:
- expresses feelings about lack of control over the health care environment.
- reports increased feelings of control after adaptive changes in surroundings.
- participates in self-care to the greatest extent possible.
- makes plans to ensure continuity of care.

DOCUMENTATION

- Patient's expressions of anger, frustration, and lack of control
- Patient's interest in surroundings and participation in self-care
- Patient's understanding of medical diagnosis
- Nursing interventions to reduce the patient's perceptions of powerlessness
- Response to interventions
- Evaluation statements.

Powerlessness

related to homelessness

DEFINITION

Loss of control over the ability to meet present and future needs for housing, food, and physical care

ASSESSMENT

Cultural status
- *Demographics:* age, sex, level of education, nationality, race, ethnic group, past occupation, marital status and

history, circumstances leading to homelessness; available resources, including family, extended family, friends, community and social support; personal strengths
- *History:* beliefs, values, and attitudes about health and illness

Neurologic status
- *Mental status:* appearance and attitude, level of consciousness, judgment, mood and affect, perceptions, memory, coping abilities, evidence of psychotic thinking, delusions, drug or alcohol intoxication
- *Physical examination:* motor function, cerebellar function, sensory system, reflexes
- *Medical conditions:* head injury, dementia, epilepsy, human immunodeficiency virus (HIV), acquired immunodeficiency syndrome, other sexually transmitted diseases
- *Medications:* anticonvulsant, neuroleptic, and other psychoactive drugs; analgesics; alcohol and illicit drugs
- *Laboratory tests:* drug toxicology screening, enzyme-linked immunoabsorbent assay for HIV infection, venereal disease research laboratory test
- *Diagnostic test:* Folstein Mini-Mental Health Status Examination

Nutritional status
- *Physical examination:* height and weight, skin color and turgor, nutritional deficiencies, cachexia
- *Signs and symptoms:* nausea, vomiting, fainting, constipation, diarrhea, pallor, irritability
- *Laboratory tests:* hemoglobin, hematocrit, cholesterol, triglyceride, serum iron, serum albumin, and electrolyte levels

Psychological status
- *History:* past violence, legal problems; episodes of mental illness, hospitalizations, drug or alcohol dependency; affective state; orientation and level of cognition; quality of thought and memory; brief family history; medication history
- *Diagnostic tests:* Brief Psychiatric Rating Scale, Hamilton Rating Scale for Depression or Zung Self-Rating Depression Scale

Self-care status
- *History:* ability to carry out voluntary activities, resources (family, friends, church, homeless companions), living conditions (shelter, safety, adequate clothing), vulnerability to abuse, use of medical resources

DEFINING CHARACTERISTICS

- Apathy, depression, decreased self-esteem
- Expressions of helplessness, anger, despair, victimization
- Homelessness due to loss of benefits, loss of or estrangement from family and friends, recent migration, release from prison, or relocation
- Inability to focus attention or plan for the future
- Low educational level
- Mental illness, alcohol and drug abuse

ASSOCIATED DISORDERS

Amnestic and other cognitive disorders, bipolar disorder, delirium, dementia, personality disorders, schizophrenia, substance- or alcohol-related disorders. The nursing diagnosis also may be associated with untreated physical conditions, such as diabetes and skin disorders, aggravated by the patient's limited access to care.

EXPECTED OUTCOMES

Initial outcomes
- Patient develops enough trust in staff members to cooperate in his evaluation and accept emergency shelter, food, and health care.
- Patient expresses feelings of powerlessness and associated feelings, such as loss, anger, depression, and guilt.

Interim outcomes
- Patient accepts treatment for medical and psychiatric conditions.
- Patient's nutritional status improves.
- Patient sets and attains a small goal each day.
- Patient responds positively to emotional support offered by nurses and social services staff members.

Discharge outcomes
- Patient willingly contacts health care agencies, mental health services, social service agencies, and community resources.
- Patient expresses a greater sense of control over some facet of life.

INTERVENTIONS AND RATIONALES

Initial interventions
- Demonstrate patience and respect as you explain the reasons for interview questions, examinations, and tests *to reduce the patient's distrust.*
- Meet the patient's basic needs for food, comfort, and safety *to ensure his well-being and promote trust.*

Interim interventions
- Explain all treatments (using special care if the patient shows paranoia) *to help him reduce feelings of being overwhelmed and to regain control over his diet and medications.*
- Help the patient contact family or community resources, such as emergency shelters, soup kitchens, and welfare agencies that provide food, medical, and income assistance. *According to Maslow's hierarchy of needs, such needs as shelter, food, and safety must be addressed before the patient can regain a sense of control.*
- Encourage the patient to join group activities in the hospital *to help him develop self-esteem, coping strategies, and connections with others.*
- Teach the patient problem-solving skills and how to improve dress and hygiene. Prepare the patient for contact with social service agency personnel through role playing and written instruction *to enhance his self-esteem and encourage his active participation (essential in combating powerlessness).*
- Encourage the patient to set manageable goals and then to take small steps to regain control of his life *to keep him from becoming paralyzed by overwhelming problems.*

Discharge interventions
- Help the patient identify alternative sources of support, such as church and community groups, extended family, Alcoholics Anonymous,

abused women's shelter, state employment counseling services, and veteran's assistance services. *The homeless patient may be cut off from family and friends and unfamiliar with community resources.*
- Encourage the patient to participate in all aspects of care, including meeting physical and hygiene needs and contacting appropriate social service agencies *to empower the patient and enhance self-esteem.*

EVALUATION STATEMENTS

Patient:
- cooperates in his evaluation and treatment.
- expresses feelings related to homelessness and powerlessness.
- demonstrates a decrease in his distrust of others.
- expresses positive feelings about contacting sources of support.
- establishes manageable goals.
- becomes an active participant in care.

DOCUMENTATION

- Results of diagnostic tests
- Patient's expression of feelings related to his homeless status
- Information about patient's family or contacts within the community
- Observations of the patient's response to treatment
- Patient's perceptions of treatment plan and discharge plan
- Evidence of an increased sense of empowerment
- Evaluation statements.

Powerlessness

related to physical, sexual, or emotional abuse by partner

DEFINITION

Perceived lack of control over life events and belief that one's actions will not affect outcomes

ASSESSMENT

Cultural status
- *Demographics:* age, sex, level of education, occupation, religion, nationality, race, ethnic group
- *Diagnostic test:* Cultural Assessment Guide

Family status
- *History:* marital status; developmental stage; family roles; family rules; communication patterns; coping patterns; family alliances; family's willingness and ability to meet patient's physical and emotional needs; socioeconomic status; support systems; history of sexual, emotional, or physical abuse; family health history
- *Diagnostic tests:* Family Genogram, Index of Family Relations

Psychologic status
- *History:* beliefs, values, and attitudes about health and illness; alcohol or drug use
- *Current crisis:* description of sexual, emotional, or physical abuse; feelings of powerlessness; effect on personality; effect on daily functioning; feelings of dependence on others

- *Childhood development:* personality traits, coping methods, adaptive and maladaptive behaviors, earliest memories, continuous memories, academic performance, relationships with peers, religious or social group involvement, life events in childhood, evidence of passive behavior, recreational activities
- *Adolescent development:* reactions to puberty and sexuality, relationships with authority figures, scholastic performance, occupational choices, peer relationships, extracurricular activities, delinquency, situational crises
- *Adult development:* military history, higher education, occupation and job changes, dating and marital history, hobbies and recreational activities, spirituality, reactions to illness and disability
- *Signs and symptoms:* feelings of loss of control possibly accompanied by apathy, anxiety, uneasiness, resignation, or anger; aggressive behavior; acting-out behavior; withdrawal and depression; reported dissatisfaction or frustration over inability to control situation or to perform previous tasks or activities; passivity; refusal to participate in self-care or decision making; difficulty seeking information regarding care; expressions of doubt regarding role performance; reluctance to express true feelings due to fear of alienation from caregivers; irritability, resentment, anger, or feelings of guilt related to dependence on others; statements such as, "It won't do any good" or, "It won't make any difference"
- *Diagnostic tests:* Brief Psychiatric Rating Scale, Automatic Thoughts Questionnaire, Fear Questionnaire, Problem Solving Inventory, Self-Rating Anxiety Scale

DEFINING CHARACTERISTICS

- Denial of seriousness of abuse
- Fear of continued abuse
- Fear of disapproval from others
- Feelings of shame or humiliation about abuse
- History of childhood abuse
- Ineffective coping mechanisms
- Lack of positive feedback or consistent negative feedback
- Lack of resources for support
- Low self-esteem
- Perceived helplessness
- Social isolation
- Unmet dependency needs

ASSOCIATED DISORDERS

Anxiety disorder; cognitive disorder; dementia; dependent personality disorder; head trauma; mood disorder; physical injuries related to abuse, such as fractures, bruises, hematomas; post-traumatic stress disorder

EXPECTED OUTCOMES

Initial outcomes
- Patient identifies feelings of powerlessness.
- Patient identifies risks to personal safety.

Interim outcomes
- Patient makes choices related to care and becomes involved in care.
- Patient identifies life situations over which she has no control.
- Patient identifies life situations over which she does have control.

Discharge outcome
- Patient develops plan and methods to take control of life and decrease feelings of powerlessness.

INTERVENTIONS AND RATIONALES

Initial interventions
- Determine whether the patient is safe from personal harm. *Ensuring the patient's safety is your first nursing responsibility. For example, consider referring the patient to a women's shelter if warranted. If the patient is hospitalized, consult with social services.*
- Discuss the patient's relationship with her abusive partner. Help her to identify feelings of powerlessness as well as circumstances that lead to such situations *to help her recognize situations that threaten her sense of control and to provide a basis for developing problem-solving techniques.*
- Help the patient recognize her use of manipulative behavior to manage feelings of powerlessness, distrust of others, fear of disapproval, and feelings of shame. Encourage her to discuss her needs openly and to develop mutually agreeable ways *to help her overcome manipulative behavior. For example, an abused woman may enlist support from friends or family, resulting in increased attention and caring, but she continues to stay in the abusive relationship despite recommendations to leave it.*

Interim interventions
- Contact social services and make sure they speak with the patient *to ensure that she will receive legal and financial support as needed after discharge.*

- Allow the patient to take as much responsibility for self-care as possible by setting her own care goals and establishing an activity schedule. Support her efforts to develop a realistic plan, take action, and reach goals. Provide choices and allow her to make decisions without caregiver influence. For example, provide information about women's support groups, but allow the patient to decide whether she wants to become involved *to increase her feelings of control over herself, decrease feelings of powerlessness, and decrease use of manipulation to get attention and care.*
- Help the patient identify factors that are not within her control, such as other people's feelings and behavior, *to enable the patient to cope with unresolved issues and accept what cannot be changed.*
- Help the patient recognize situations where she exhibited determination and control over her life *to reinforce past successes and to develop a basis for establishing future goals.*
- Help the patient identify situations that can be controlled and assess benefits and consequences of available alternatives *to reduce her feelings of powerlessness and increase her ability to solve problems.*

Discharge interventions
- Help the patient set realistic goals and suggest periodic review of goal achievement *to reduce the likelihood of failure and feelings of powerlessness.*
- Help the patient identify activities in which she can achieve success, and provide positive feedback for participating in these activities. Encourage her to think productively and positive-

ly and to take responsibility for her thoughts, feelings, and actions *to enhance the patient's self-esteem and empower her.*

- Refer the patient to a women's shelter *to ensure her continued safety after discharge.*
- Refer the patient to a women's support group and psychotherapist *to ensure ongoing treatment for mental health needs.*

EVALUATION STATEMENTS

Patient:
- identifies feelings of powerlessness.
- identifies risks to personal safety posed by living with an abusive partner.
- verbalizes feelings associated with lack of control.
- demonstrates improved problem-solving skills.
- demonstrates ability to make effective choices in an effort to regain control over life situation.

DOCUMENTATION

- Results of diagnostic tests
- Physical or psychological evidence of abuse
- Patient acknowledgment of abuse
- Nursing interventions
- Patient responses to nursing interventions
- Referrals to specialized professionals, agencies, and support groups
- Evaluation statements.

Rape-trauma syndrome: Compound reaction

DEFINITION

Trauma syndrome that develops after rape or attempted rape in which the patient undergoes an acute phase of disorganization and a long-term reorganization. In a compound reaction, the patient experiences drastic changes in behavior, psychological equilibrium, and ability to function as a consequence of rape.

ASSESSMENT

Physical status
- *Demographics:* age, sex
- *History of traumatic event:* circumstances surrounding trauma
- *Signs and symptoms:* injuries sustained, including genitourinary, integumentary, musculoskeletal, and neurologic injuries

Psychological status
- *History:* problem-solving and coping techniques used in the past, self-concept, spirituality, emotional reactions to rape
- *Support systems:* family, friends, spouse or companion, clergy
- *Signs and symptoms:* changes in mood, behavior, appetite, energy level, sleep pattern; expressions of guilt

DEFINING CHARACTERISTICS

Acute phase
- Aggressive behavior
- Alcohol or drug dependence

- Anger or desire for revenge
- Embarrassment or humiliation
- Fear of physical violence or death
- Homicidal ideation
- Hysterical outbursts
- Multiple physical signs and symptoms, such as GI irritability, genitourinary discomfort, muscular tension, sleep-pattern disturbance
- Reactivated symptoms of preexisting conditions, such as physical or psychiatric illness
- Self-blame
- Suicidal ideation

Long-term phase
- Changes in lifestyle, including change of residence
- Repetitive nightmares
- Seeking of support from family and social network

ASSOCIATED CONDITIONS

Incest, rape, sexual assault, spouse abuse

EXPECTED OUTCOMES

Initial outcome
- Patient achieves optimal recovery from physical injuries.

Interim outcomes
- Patient expresses feelings about the rape.
- Patient reports feeling safe.
- Patient begins process of recovering from trauma.

Discharge outcomes
- Patient contacts appropriate sources of support.

- Patient states desire to reestablish and maintain interpersonal relationships.

INTERVENTIONS AND RATIONALES

Initial interventions
- Follow the medical regimen to manage physical injuries. *This is the first step in meeting the patient's hierarchy of needs. The degree of care required depends on the extent of physical injury and intensity of the patient's psychological response.*
- Follow hospital protocol regarding legal responsibilities. Be aware that you may be called as a witness in any legal proceedings. Document and report the rape *to protect the patient's legal rights.*
- When interviewing the patient, ask open-ended questions and listen intently *to encourage the patient to talk about the trauma and to express her feelings, both verbally and through behavior.*
- Show the patient that you accept her feelings, but set limits on aggressive behavior. *Demonstrating acceptance reassures the patient that her response is valid. Setting limits on behavior provides the patient with necessary structure.*

Interim interventions
- Intervene to reassure the patient of her safety; for example, approach her carefully with open hands, stay with her, and have female staff conduct the interview and physical examination. *Safety measures help reduce the patient's anxiety and fear of another assault.*

- Direct the patient to perform purposeful activities, such as taking medications and following instructions of health care personnel. *Completing tasks helps to reduce the patient's anxiety and restore her sense of control.*
- Describe the many possible responses to trauma. *The patient with a compound reaction may feel that the extreme emotional turmoil she experiences after rape is abnormal. Helping her understand that her reactions are no different than others who have undergone similar experiences may reassure her and reduce feelings of isolation.*
- Encourage family members to express their reactions to the trauma. Explain the compound reaction to rape and the patient's response *to help them cope with the trauma and prepare to support the patient.*

Discharge interventions
- Provide the patient with referrals to appropriate support people, such as clergy, mental health professionals, or a rape counselor. Encourage participation in support or therapy groups provided by a rape counseling center. *The patient may need long-term care to cope with the psychological consequences of rape.*
- Provide ongoing emotional support as the patient struggles to regain psychological equilibrium. Encourage her efforts to renew involvement in usual activities. *To achieve long-term personality reorganization, the patient will require time, consistent support, and ongoing counseling.*

EVALUATION STATEMENTS

Patient:
- recovers from physical injuries.
- resumes normal or near-normal activities.
- expresses feelings associated with the rape.
- reports feeling safe.
- participates in long-term counseling or joins a support group.
- reports improved ability to cope with psychological consequences of the rape.
- reestablishes social ties and interactions.

DOCUMENTATION

- Patient's expressions of feelings related to trauma
- Observations of patient's behavior and interactions with others
- Nursing interventions
- Patient's response to interventions
- Referrals for further counseling
- Evaluation statements.

Rape-trauma syndrome: Silent reaction

DEFINITION

Trauma syndrome that develops after rape, attempted rape, or sexual assault, in which the patient undergoes an acute phase of disorganization and a long-term process of reorganization. In a silent reaction, the patient doesn't tell anyone about the rape or deal with her feelings about it.

ASSESSMENT

Physical status
- *Demographics:* age, sex, occupation
- *History of the traumatic event:* circumstances surrounding the trauma
- *Signs and symptoms:* injuries sustained, including genitourinary, integumentary, musculoskeletal, neurologic injuries

Psychological status
- *History:* problem-solving techniques used by the patient, self-concept, spirituality, emotional response to trauma
- *Support systems:* family, friends, companion, clergy
- *Signs and symptoms:* changes in mood, behavior, appetite, energy level, sleep pattern; expressions of guilt

DEFINING CHARACTERISTICS

- Abrupt change in relationships with men
- Increase in frequency of nightmares
- Increased anxiety during interview evidenced by blocking of associations, stuttering, physical distress
- No admission that rape, attempted rape, or sexual assault occurred
- Pronounced changes in sexual behavior
- Signs and symptoms of posttraumatic response, such as numbness, impaired concentration, disbelief, panic, extreme detachment, severe anxiety, anger, depersonalization
- Sudden onset of phobic reactions

ASSOCIATED CONDITIONS

Incest, rape, sexual assault, spouse abuse

EXPECTED OUTCOMES

Initial outcome
- Patient discloses that rape, attempted rape, or sexual assault occurred.

Interim outcomes
- Patient achieves optimal recovery from physical injuries.
- Patient expresses willingness to address emotional problems associated with traumatic experience.

Discharge outcome
- Patient contacts support groups or seeks professional counseling.

INTERVENTIONS AND RATIONALES

Initial interventions
- Establish an atmosphere of trust *to help the patient overcome her unwillingness to talk about the rape or sexual assault.*
- Confront the patient directly but gently with the question of whether she is a victim of rape or sexual assault. *A patient with a silent reaction needs patience and encouragement to overcome anxiety about disclosing rape or sexual assault.*
- Explain the nature of rape and sexual assault. For example, the patient may believe that sexual assault did not occur if no intercourse occurred or if the attacker was a boyfriend, spouse, or family member. Explain that sexual assault can take different forms and

that all forms are traumatic. *This will clear up misconceptions the patient may have concerning rape and sexual assault and help her more clearly define the traumatic event.*

Interim interventions
- If the patient remains unwilling to talk about the attack, tell her that you'll continue to be available to help. Encourage her to contact you any time she needs to talk. *This demonstrates compassion, provides the patient with a resource for future help, and maintains open communication.*
- If the patient starts to discuss the attack, respond in a caring and nonjudgmental manner *to cultivate trust and cooperation.*
- Follow the medical regimen to manage physical injuries (if rape or sexual assault was recent) and follow hospital protocol for documenting and reporting the assault to authorities *to ensure the patient's physical well-being and protect her legal rights.*
- Ask open-ended questions and listen intently *to encourage the patient to talk about the trauma.*
- If the patient is withdrawn, be understanding and supportive when gathering information and allow her to proceed at her own pace *to build a trusting relationship and encourage complete disclosure.*
- Emphasize that the patient was in no way responsible for the attack. *The patient with a silent reaction may feel intense guilt and shame over the assault.*
- Describe the variety of common emotional responses to trauma, including suicidal ideation, disorientation, confusion, extreme detachment, nightmares, flashbacks, guilt, and de-

pression. *The patient may believe that her emotional turmoil is abnormal. Learning that others have experienced similar reactions may make her feel less isolated, encourage her to talk about symptoms, and motivate her to seek follow-up care.*

Discharge intervention
- Provide appropriate referrals to support people, such as mental health professionals, a rape counselor, or clergy. A rape crisis center can provide information about local support or therapy groups. If assault was an isolated incident, short-term counseling may be sufficient. However, if the patient has endured repeated sexual assaults (common in incest), long-term psychotherapy may be required. *Appropriate referrals help ensure that the patient receives necessary care.*

EVALUATION STATEMENTS

Patient:
- discloses that rape, attempted rape, or sexual assault occurred.
- recovers from physical injuries to the extent possible.
- resumes normal or near-normal activities.
- contacts rape counselor and agrees to participate in therapy group.
- acknowledges that the assault was not her fault.
- acknowledges her need to deal with psychological consequences of the assault.

DOCUMENTATION

- Evidence that rape or sexual assault occurred, including observations of

the patient's behavior and physical evidence
- Efforts to help the patient discuss the assault and her response
- Nursing interventions
- Patient's response to interventions
- Referrals for further care
- Evaluation statements.

Role performance alteration

related to changed health status

DEFINITION

Disruption in the ability to perform usual social, vocational, or family roles because of illness

ASSESSMENT

Cultural status
- *Demographics:* age, sex, marital status, level of education, occupation, nationality
- *History:* beliefs, values and attitudes about health and illness; health customs, practices, and rituals

Family status
- *Family roles:* formal roles and role performance, informal roles and role performance, degree of family agreement on roles, interrelationships of various roles
- *Family rules:* rules that foster stability, maladaptive rules, methods of modifying family rules
- *Family communication:* style and quality of communication, methods of conflict resolution

- *Developmental stage:* changes in relationships between family members, problems adapting to change, shifts in role responsibility over time, changes in problem-solving over time
- *Family subsystems:* effect of family alliances on individual members and family as a unit
- *Physical and emotional needs:* ability of family to meet patient's physical and emotional needs, disparities between patient's needs and family's willingness or ability to meet them
- *Family goals and values:* extent to which family permits pursuit of individual goals and values
- *Socioeconomic factors:* economic status of family; sense of adequacy and self-worth; employment status; attitudes toward work; sense of belonging and identity to racial, cultural, or ethnic group; religious identification, influence of religious beliefs on values and practices
- *Coping patterns:* major life events, meaning of life events to each family member, usual coping patterns, family's perception of effectiveness of coping patterns
- *Family health history:* bipolar disorder, depressive disorder, suicide, schizophrenia, mental retardation, substance abuse, stress-related illness, medical illness, evidence of abuse

Psychological status
- *Drug history:* illicit drugs or alcohol, over-the-counter drugs, prescription medications
- *Current illness:* patient's perception of condition, signs and symptoms, impact on functioning, coping methods

DEFINING CHARACTERISTICS

- Change in perception of role (by self and others)
- Change in physical capacity to resume role
- Change in usual responsibilities
- Conflict among vocational, family, and social roles
- Denial of role or responsibility
- Lack of knowledge about roles and responsibilities

ASSOCIATED DISORDERS

This diagnosis may be associated with any illness that results in long-term disability or incapacitation. Examples include chronic obstructive pulmonary disease, coronary artery disease, dementias, personality disorders, quadriplegia, recurrent mood disorders, rheumatoid arthritis, schizophrenia, and substance-related disorders.

EXPECTED OUTCOMES

Initial outcomes
- Patient expresses feelings about diminished capacity to perform usual roles.
- Patient recognizes limitations imposed by illness and expresses feelings about these limitations.

Interim outcomes
- Patient makes decisions regarding course of treatment and management of illness.
- Patient identifies his strengths and opportunities to continue to make meaningful contributions.

Discharge outcome
- Patient continues to function in usual roles to the greatest extent possible.

INTERVENTIONS AND RATIONALES

Initial interventions
- If possible, assign the same nurse to the patient each shift *to establish rapport and foster development of a therapeutic relationship.*
- Spend an ample amount of time with the patient each shift *to foster a sense of safety and decrease loneliness.*
- Provide opportunities for the patient to express thoughts and feelings *to help him identify how altered role performance has affected his life.*
- Convey your belief in the patient's ability to develop necessary coping skills. *By projecting a positive attitude, you can help the patient gain confidence.*
- Be aware of the patient's emotional vulnerability and allow open expression of all emotions. *An accepting attitude will help the patient deal with the effects of chronic illness and loss of functioning.*

Interim interventions
- Provide opportunities for the patient to make decisions, and encourage him to maintain personal responsibilities to the extent possible. *Showing respect for the patient's decision-making ability enhances his feelings of independence.*
- Encourage the patient to participate in self-care activities, keeping in mind physical and emotional limitations, *to promote optimal functioning.*
- Assess the patient's knowledge of illness, and educate him about his condi-

tion, treatment, and prognosis. *Education will enable the patient to cope with the effects of illness more effectively.*

- Encourage the patient to be aware of personal strengths and to use them *to help maintain optimal functioning and foster a healthier self-perception.*
- Encourage the patient to continue to fulfill life roles within the constraints posed by his illness *to help him maintain a sense of purpose and preserve connections with other people.*
- Encourage the patient to participate in his care as an active member of the health care team *to foster the establishment of mutually accepted goals between the patient and caregivers. The patient who participates in care is more likely to take an active role in other aspects of his life.*

Discharge interventions

- Assist family members in identifying their feelings about the patient's decreased role functioning. Encourage participation in a support group. *Relatives of the patient may need social support, information, and an outlet for ventilating feelings.*
- Offer the patient and family a realistic assessment of the patient's illness. *Education helps promote patient safety and security and enables family members to plan for future health care requirements.* Communicate optimism for the future without conveying false hope.
- Educate the patient and family about managing illness, controlling environmental factors that affect the patient's health, and redefining roles *to promote optimal functioning. If family members understand the patient's*

condition, they may be better able to help him adjust to role changes.

EVALUATION STATEMENTS

Patient:

- shares feelings about illness and altered role performance in a constructive manner.
- demonstrates increased functioning by making decisions related to health care.
- participates in the planning and implementation of aspects of personal care.
- demonstrates ability to perceive options and uses options to adapt to role changes and illness.
- expresses feeling of having made a productive contribution to self-care, to others, or to the environment.

  Patient and family:
- express understanding of role changes that are occurring because of chronic illness.

DOCUMENTATION

- Observations of the patient's physical, emotional, and mental status
- Patient's expression of thoughts and feelings regarding illness and diminished role capacity
- Nursing interventions performed to help patient change in role functioning
- Patient's response to nursing interventions
- All health teaching, counseling, and precautions taken to maintain or enhance the patient's level of functioning
- Referrals to sources of support for patient and family
- Evaluation statements.

Role performance alteration

related to guilt brought on by transmission of HIV infection

DEFINITION

Inability to perform usual social, vocational, or family roles because of guilt over the transmission of human immunodeficiency virus (HIV) infection

ASSESSMENT

Cultural status
- *Demographics:* age, sex, level of education, occupation, nationality
- *History:* beliefs, values and attitudes about health and illness; sense of identity with racial, cultural, or ethnic group
- *Diagnostic test:* Cultural Assessment Guide

Family status
- *Marital status:* current status, length of marriage or relationship, degree of mutual faithfulness
- *Family roles:* role performance, shifts in role responsibility over time
- *Family communication:* style and quality of communication, methods of conflict resolution
- *Family needs:* ability of family to meet patient's emotional needs, disparities between patient's needs and family's willingness or ability to meet them, extent to which family permits pursuit of individual goals
- *Diagnostic tests:* Family Adjustment Device, Family Genogram

Psychological status
- *Current illness:* signs of problems with self-image, self-esteem, or self-worth
- *Developmental history:* birth order, number of siblings, personality traits, relationships with peers, religious or social group involvement, sexuality, dating and marital history
- *Diagnostic tests:* Brief Psychiatric Rating Scale, Hamilton Rating Scale for Depression

Sexuality status
- *History:* attitudes toward sex, sexual orientation, previous sexual response patterns, exposure to sexually transmitted diseases
- *Diagnostic tests:* enzyme-linked immunoabsorbent assay, venereal disease research laboratory, cultures from infection site (urethra, cervix, rectum, or pharynx)

Social status
- *History:* social skills, quality of relationships, level of self-esteem
- *Signs and symptoms:* withdrawal, self-blame
- *Diagnostic test:* Social Adjustment Scale

Spiritual status
- *History:* religious affiliation; current views about faith and religious practices; support network including family, clergy, and friends
- *Signs and symptoms:* crying, expressions of guilt and despair
- *Diagnostic tests:* Spiritual and Religious Concerns Questionnaire, Spiritual Well-Being Scale

DEFINING CHARACTERISTICS

- Altered role, as perceived by patient and others
- Change in usual religious or spiritual beliefs or behaviors
- Change in relationships with family members or partner
- Self-blame for transmission of HIV infection

ASSOCIATED DISORDERS

Acquired immunodeficiency syndrome, HIV infection, HIV encephalopathy, Kaposi's sarcoma, *Pneumocystis carinii* pneumonia

EXPECTED OUTCOMES

Initial outcomes
- Patient discusses feelings about changes in role performance.
- Patient discusses guilt over HIV transmission.
- Patient identifies source of guilt.

Interim outcomes
- Patient recognizes extent to which guilt interferes with his ability to function.
- Patient seeks counseling and spiritual support to deal with guilt.
- Patient begins to improve his coping skills by realizing the irrational basis of his feelings of guilt.
- Patient's family members and spouse or companion express understanding that acquired immunodeficiency syndrome (AIDS) is a disease, not a punishment.

Discharge outcome
- Patient exhibits less guilt.

INTERVENTIONS AND RATIONALES

Initial interventions
- Help the patient discuss feelings about difficulty performing usual roles *to help him see how altered role performance has affected his life.*
- Help the patient recognize the source of the guilt. *This is the first step in addressing and alleviating guilt.*

Interim interventions
- Assist the patient in identifying attitudes underlying his guilt (such as shame regarding I.V. drug use or homosexuality or regret about unsafe sexual practices). Encourage him to distinguish attitudes based on personal beliefs and values from attitudes based on arbitrary social norms *to help him understand the cause of his feelings.*
- Help the patient cope with the feelings of being ostracized. *The stigma associated with HIV infection is a reality that the patient must learn to deal with.*
- Tell the patient that despite other people's misconceptions and prejudices, the virus is an illness and not a punishment *to help him regain a healthful view of reality, which in turn, will strengthen his self-image.*
- If the patient has transmitted the disease to her child, be aware that guilt may be especially strong. She may also encounter increased social disapproval and feel abandoned by friends and family. Help her realize that by fulfilling her role as a mother she can make her child's remaining time more valuable. Refer her for professional counseling and provide support. *Ongoing*

intervention and unconditional support are crucial.

▪ Encourage the patient to list his good attributes. *This will help him realize his life is more significant than the disease and its transmission.*

▪ Refer the patient to a support group for HIV-positive people. *Discussing concerns with others often decreases feelings of isolation and foster new coping skills.*

▪ Discuss AIDS with the patient's family members, spouse, or companion *to help them realize that it is a disease, not a punishment. The family members' acceptance of the patient will help to strengthen his self-esteem.*

Discharge intervention

▪ Encourage the patient to continue to fulfill usual roles as much as possible *to help him maintain a sense of purpose, to get maximum enjoyment out of his remaining time, and preserve relationships with others.*

EVALUATION STATEMENTS

Patient:
▪ reports feelings of guilt associated with HIV transmission.
▪ requests help in developing more effective ways of dealing with guilt.
▪ seeks out appropriate support groups for assistance.
▪ reports less guilt associated with illness.
▪ receives more support from family, spouse, or companion.

DOCUMENTATION

▪ Diagnostic test results

▪ Patient's expressions of feelings of guilt
▪ Family members', spouse's, or companion's statements about AIDS
▪ Nursing interventions to facilitate changes in patient's self-perception and family members' attitudes toward illness
▪ Patient's response to nursing interventions
▪ Evaluation statements.

Self-care deficit: Bathing and hygiene

related to perceptual or cognitive impairment

DEFINITION

Inability to carry out bathing and hygiene

ASSESSMENT

Cultural status
▪ *Demographics:* age, sex, level of education, occupation, nationality, ethnic group
▪ *History:* beliefs, values, and attitudes about health and illness; health customs, practices, and rituals

Self-care status
▪ *History:* neurologic, sensory, or psychologic impairment; ability to carry out voluntary activities; use of adaptive equipment, devices, or supplies
▪ *Diagnostic test:* Self-Care Assessment Tool

Neurologic status

- *History:* environmental exposure to lead or other toxins, pain management, safety practices
- *Medications:* anticonvulsants, neuroleptics, anxiolytic agents, antidepressants, antimanic agents, barbiturates, pain medications, antiparkinsonian agents, alcohol, illicit drugs
- *Mental status:* appearance and attitude, level of consciousness, motor activity, thought and speech, mood and affect, perceptions, orientation, memory, general information, calculations, capacity to read and write, visual-spatial ability, attention, abstraction, judgment and insight
- *Motor system:* muscle tone, strength, and symmetry; gait; cerebellar function; cranial nerve function
- *Sensory system:* cortical function (position sense, stereognosis, two-point discrimination, and extinction), dermatome, peripheral sensory system (pain, position, and vibration), paresthesia
- *Reflexes:* deep tendon (biceps, triceps, brachioradialis, quadriceps, Achilles), superficial (abdominal, cremasteric, plantar), pathological (palmar grasp, Babinski's, Moro's, tonic neck); pupillary response
- *Laboratory findings:* drug toxicology, thyroid function, serotonin and electrolyte levels
- *Signs and symptoms:* lethargy, restlessness, stupor, headache, vertigo, seizures, syncope, aura, tremors, paresthesia, paresis, incoordination, numbness and tingling, tics, falls, myoclonus, fasciculation, chorea, pain
- *Diagnostic tests:* computed tomography, lumbar puncture, magnetic resonance imaging, positron emission to-

mography, cerebral arteriography, Doppler ultrasound, digital subtraction angiography, electroencephalography, evoked potential studies, Glasgow Coma Scale, Folstein Mini-Mental Health Status Examination, Abnormal Involuntary Movement Scale

Musculoskeletal status

- *History:* exercise and activity patterns, use of mobility aids
- *Medications:* aspirin, anti-inflammatory agents, muscle relaxants
- *Physical examination:* range of motion of all joints; joint and muscle symmetry; evidence of swelling, masses, or deformity; pain or tenderness on movement; coordination and gait; muscle size, strength, and tone; functional mobility
- *Diagnostic tests:* Functional Mobility Scale, Muscle Strength Scale

DEFINING CHARACTERISTICS

- Clinical evidence of perceptual or cognitive impairment
- Impaired short- or long-term memory
- Inability to carry out personal hygiene
- Inability to obtain or get to water source
- Inability to regulate water temperature or flow

ASSOCIATED DISORDERS

Acquired immunodeficiency syndrome, alcoholism, Alzheimer's disease, autism, bipolar disease (manic or depressive phase), brain tumor, cerebrovascular accident, dementia, head injury,

Huntington's disease, Laënnec's cirrhosis, mental retardation, movement disorders, multiple sclerosis, organic brain syndrome, Parkinson's disease, psychotic disorders, schizophrenia, substance- and alcohol-related disorders, tardive dyskinesia, temporal lobe epilepsy, transient ischemic attacks

EXPECTED OUTCOMES

Initial outcome
- Barriers to patient's bathing and hygiene needs are identified.

Interim outcomes
- Complications are avoided or minimized.
- Patient or caregiver carries out self-care program daily.
- Patient communicates feelings related to self-care deficit.

Discharge outcomes
- Patient or family member carries out written bathing and hygiene regimen.
- Patient or family member identifies resources to help cope with problems after discharge.

INTERVENTIONS AND RATIONALES

Initial interventions
- Observe, document, and report the patient's perceptual or cognitive abilities daily *to detect deficits that may interfere with his ability to perform bathing and hygiene.*
- Assess the patient's bathing and hygiene skills *to determine appropriate interventions.*

Interim interventions
- Perform the prescribed treatment for the underlying condition. Monitor progress and report favorable and adverse responses. *Therapy must be consistently applied to aid the patient's independence.*
- Allow the patient to express frustration, anger, or feelings of inadequacy *to help him cope with the emotional consequences of functional deficits.*
- Provide privacy *to enhance the patient's compliance; he may not be comfortable being observed.*
- Remind the patient of what he must accomplish and monitor his progress. Offer praise. *Reinforcement and rewards may encourage the patient to perform self-care.*
- Allow ample time for the patient to perform bathing and hygiene. *Rushing creates unnecessary stress and promotes failure.*
- Teach the patient bathing and hygiene measures, using simple instructions given one at a time *to aid comprehension.*
- Assist with daily bathing and hygiene only when the patient has difficulty *to encourage independence and self-reliance.*
- Give written instructions on bathing and hygiene techniques to the patient's family members, caretaker, or companion, and supervise their return demonstration. *A return demonstration identifies problem areas and increases the caretaker's self-confidence.*
- When the patient is bathing, reassure him with such statements as, "You're in the tub" and "The water is only 3" deep" *to guard against panic reaction caused by fear of being drowned.*

Discharge intervention

- Refer the patient to a psychiatric liaison nurse, support group, or home health care agency, as needed, to provide ongoing reinforcement for activities planned to meet the patient's needs.

EVALUATION STATEMENTS

Patient:
- reports that self-care needs are met with help of staff.
- does not experience infection, skin integrity alteration, or other complications of altered self-care.
- expresses feelings about self-care deficit.
- seeks assistance from family member, companion, or staff within 24 hours, if unable to meet own needs.
    Patient, family member, or companion:
- becomes more active in carrying out self-care program; need for staff assistance decreases.
- identifies and contacts available support resources as needed.

DOCUMENTATION

- Diagnostic test results and laboratory findings
- Patient's, family member's, or companion's expression of feelings and concern about self-care deficits
- Observations of patient's impaired ability to perform bathing and hygiene
- Patient's response to treatment for underlying condition
- Nursing interventions to provide supportive care
- Patient's response to nursing interventions

- Instructions to patient, family member, or companion, their understanding of the instructions, and demonstrated skill in carrying out self-care functions
- Evaluation statements.

Self-esteem, chronically low

related to mood disturbance

DEFINITION

Long-standing, negative evaluation or feelings about oneself or one's capabilities

ASSESSMENT

Cultural status

- *Demographics:* age, sex, level of education, occupation, nationality, race, ethnic group
- *History:* beliefs, values, and attitudes related to current illness; health practices

Neurologic status

- *History:* medical problems, medications, mental status, appearance, mood, affect
- *Laboratory tests:* drug toxicology screening, thyroid function test, serotonin and electrolyte levels, liver function test
- *Diagnostic tests:* Mini–Mental Status Examination, electroencephalography

Psychological status
- *History:* drug use, mental illness, significant life events or losses, abuse (physical, sexual, or emotional)
- *Signs and symptoms:* depression, changes in appetite, energy, motivation, or mood
- *Diagnostic tests:* Hamilton Rating Scale for Depression, Beck Depression Inventory, Minnesota Multiphasic Personality Inventory, Wechsler Adult Intelligence Survey

Self-care status
- *History:* ability to perform activities of daily living (ADLs), work or school attendance

Social status
- *History:* social and occupational interaction, communication skills, marital status, ability to have intimate relationships
- *Signs and symptoms:* social isolation, withdrawal, lack of eye contact

DEFINING CHARACTERISTICS

- Chronic medical problems
- Chronic mental health problems, such as depression or suicidal ideation
- Difficulty making decisions
- Expressions of shame or guilt
- Extreme conformity or dependence on the opinions of others
- Frequent expression of negative thoughts about self
- Hesitation to try anything new
- Inability to provide self-care
- Need for excessive reassurance
- Nonassertive or passive tendencies
- Perceived failures in work or personal life
- Perceived loss of control over important aspects of life

ASSOCIATED DISORDERS

Acquired immunodeficiency syndrome, anxiety disorders, bipolar disorders, depressive disorders, diabetes mellitus, disabilities or deformities, personality disorders, psychoactive substance disorders

EXPECTED OUTCOMES

Initial outcomes
- Patient remains safe while in the hospital.
- Patient performs ADLs with assistance.

Interim outcomes
- Patient acknowledges personal strengths.
- Patient verbalizes feelings related to self-esteem.
- Patient identifies unrealistic personal expectations.
- Patient exhibits fewer symptoms of depression or anxiety.

Discharge outcomes
- Patient participates in decision-making regarding discharge and outpatient care.
- Patient agrees to attend appropriate outpatient treatment, for example Alcoholics Anonymous or therapy.

INTERVENTIONS AND RATIONALES

Initial interventions
- Provide for uninterrupted noncare-related time, engaging the patient in

conversation *to encourage self-explora-tion.*

■ Listen to the patient and respond with nonjudgmental acceptance, genuine interest, and sincerity *to improve his self-awareness and reduce any perceived threat.*

■ Assess suicide risk, as indicated. *Extremely low levels of self-esteem may lead to suicide.*

■ Remove any dangerous items from the patient *to prevent him from injuring himself.*

■ Communicate and demonstrate concern for the patient's physical appearance and health. *This shows the patient that he is worthwhile and deserving of attention and care.*

■ Help the patient perform ADLs, as needed. *Patients with low self-esteem may neglect the fundamentals of self-care.*

Interim interventions

■ Help the patient identify personal strengths *to help improve his self-esteem and foster a realistic self-perception.*

■ Encourage him to express negative feelings such as anger. *Expressing unpleasant emotions makes them seem less threatening.*

■ Encourage him to identify unrealistic expectations *to prevent feelings of inadequacy and a further lowering of self-esteem.*

■ Promote his participation in individual or group counseling. *Discussing thoughts, feelings, and behaviors helps the patient assume more responsibility for himself.*

Discharge interventions

■ Help the patient develop decision-making skills *to enhance his sense of self-confidence.*

■ Provide information about outpatient therapies appropriate for his needs *to ensure continuity of treatment.*

■ Involve the patient in decisions about the treatment plan *to improve his self-confidence and sense of control.*

EVALUATION STATEMENTS

Patient:
■ exhibits increased self-confidence.
■ participates in discharge planning.
■ performs ADLs.
■ describes available outpatient meetings and resources.
■ no longer exhibits signs of major depression or anxiety.

DOCUMENTATION

■ Diagnostic test results
■ Behaviors and verbal reports indicating low self-esteem
■ Medication history
■ Evidence of participation in ADLs
■ Signs and symptoms of depressive or anxiety disorders
■ Suicide assessment, nursing interventions, and patient's response
■ Patient's response to interventions
■ Behaviors and verbal reports indicating improved self-esteem
■ Evaluation statements.

Self-esteem, situational low

related to life events

DEFINITION

Negative self-evaluation or feelings that develop in response to loss or change in an individual who previously had a positive self-evaluation

ASSESSMENT

Cultural status
- *Demographics:* age, sex, developmental stage

Family status
- *History:* physical and mental health of family members, methods of conflict resolution, family roles, ability of family to meet essential needs, socioeconomic status, evidence of abuse

Neurologic status
- *History:* medical problems, medications, orientation, appearance, mood, affect, judgment
- *Laboratory tests:* drug toxicology screening, thyroid and liver function tests, serotonin and electrolyte levels
- *Diagnostic tests:* Mini–Mental Status Examination, electroencephalography

Psychological status
- *History:* presence of psychiatric illness, coping skills, ability to carry out voluntary activities, sense of adequacy and self-worth, recent losses or stressors

- *Signs and symptoms:* depression, anxiety, negative statements about self, inability to make decisions, psychological impairment, drug and alcohol abuse

Social status
- *History:* marital status, social network, ability to perform social and occupational roles, work or school attendance

Self-care status
- *History:* ability to perform activities of daily living (ADLs), grooming, dietary habits, exercise patterns

DEFINING CHARACTERISTICS

- Evidence of abuse
- Inability to make decisions
- Lack of family support
- Loss of self-care abilities
- Mental illness
- Multiple life stressors or losses
- Poor coping skills

ASSOCIATED DISORDERS

Depressive disorders, generalized anxiety disorder, major depressive disorders, posttraumatic stress disorder

EXPECTED OUTCOMES

Initial outcomes
- Patient identifies factors that harm self-esteem.
- Patient refrains from making negative statements about himself.
- Patient performs ADLs.
- Patient participates in unit activities.

Interim outcomes

- Patient identifies personal strengths.
- Patient describes past methods of coping.
- Patient explores realistic goals and self perceptions.
- Patient identifies new coping strategies and methods of gaining self-confidence.

Discharge outcome

- Patient and family acknowledge the need for ongoing therapy.

INTERVENTIONS AND RATIONALES

Initial interventions

- Establish a trusting relationship with the patient *to build rapport. Establishing a positive relationship is the first step in helping the patient overcome low self-esteem.*
- Provide a safe and supportive environment *to reduce the patient's anxiety.*
- Encourage the patient as he performs ADLs *to foster a positive self-image and sense of control.*
- When the patient discusses life events, help him view perceived mistakes in a realistic context. Correct him when he expresses distorted perceptions and unrealistic expectations *to reduce his anxiety and negative thinking.*
- Teach him to recognize negative thoughts and statements about himself. *Negative thought patterns and statements harm the patient's self-image.* Encourage him to consciously substitute self-affirming thoughts.
- Encourage his participation in unit activities *to decrease isolation.*

Interim interventions

- Encourage the patient to identify personal strengths, assets and accomplishments *to help instill self-confidence and begin the process of self-acceptance.*
- Advise him to list coping skills that enabled him to get through other difficult times. Identify how these coping skills might apply to his current situation *to encourage him to use his own resources.*
- Encourage the patient to make a scrapbook of pictures showing meaningful events, successes, hobbies, family, friends, or pets. Include in this scrapbook a list of strengths and accomplishments as well as inspirational articles and quotations *to provide him with a long-term project that will foster feelings of self-worth.*
- Encourage him to make decisions about treatment *to help build his confidence.*
- Provide positive reinforcement when he expresses realistic, positive thoughts and comments about himself. *Reinforcement helps promote desirable behavior.*

Discharge interventions

- Involve family members in teaching sessions and patient care *to help the patient feel secure about leaving the hospital.*
- Praise the patient as he attempts to function more independently and gain greater control over life decisions *to provide support.*
- Provide appropriate references and referrals *to reinforce progress initiated in the hospital.*

EVALUATION STATEMENTS

Patient:
- demonstrates the ability to recognize negative thinking patterns.
- reframes feelings about losses and perceived mistakes in a more realistic perspective.
- describes a realistic mental image of himself.
- sets goals and participates in decision making.

DOCUMENTATION

- Behaviors demonstrating low self-esteem, such as indecision, lack of eye contact, and lack of self-care
- Behaviors indicating improved self-esteem, such as smiling, proper self-care, relaxed demeanor, social interaction, and decision making
- Family participation in patient care
- Indications of cognitive distortions
- Nursing interventions to strengthen the patient's self-esteem
- Patient's response to nursing interventions
- Realistic goals developed by patient
- Referrals provided
- Evaluation statements.

Self-mutilation, high risk for

related to psychological disturbance

DEFINITION

State in which an individual is at risk for performing a deliberate act of self-harm intended to produce immediate tissue damage

ASSESSMENT

Cultural status
- *Demographics:* age, sex, level of education, occupation, nationality, ethnic group
- *History:* beliefs, values and attitudes about health and illness; health customs, practices, and rituals

Neurologic status
- *Mental status:* appearance and attitude, level of consciousness, motor activity, thought and speech, mood and affect, perceptions, orientation, memory, general information, calculations, capacity to read and write, visual-spatial ability, attention span, abstraction, judgment and insight

Psychological status
- *History:* reaction to losses, personality traits, maladaptive behaviors, earliest memories, current stressors, coping skills
- *Evidence of self-mutilation:* incisions, scars, lesions
- *Diagnostic tests:* Hamilton Rating Scale for Depression, Beck Depression Inventory, Minnesota Multiphasic Personality Inventory

Social status
- *History:* degree of trust in others, level of self-esteem, ability to function in social situations
- *Signs and symptoms:* withdrawal, lack of eye contact, inappropriate responses

RISK FACTORS

- Aggressive feelings or behavior
- Borderline personality disorder

- Depressive disorder
- Dysfunctional family dynamics
- History of physical, sexual, or emotional abuse
- History of using self-injury as coping mechanism
- Inability to cope with increased stress
- Lability of affect
- Poor self-esteem, sense of identity, coping patterns, self-image
- Poor social network, isolation, inability to function in social roles
- Psychotic disorder
- Unstable interpersonal relationships

ASSOCIATED DISORDERS

Autistic disorder, borderline personality disorder, developmental disability, dissociative disorders, factitious disorder with predominantly physical signs and symptoms, malingering, personality disorder, posttraumatic stress disorder, sexual masochism

EXPECTED OUTCOMES

Initial outcomes
- Patient does not harm himself while hospitalized.
- Patient expresses self-destructive or suicidal thoughts.
- Patient expresses feelings of anger, pain, and frustration.

Interim outcomes
- Patient participates in therapeutic milieu.
- Patient discusses causes of his anger, pain, and frustration.
- Patient explores adaptive methods of coping with anger, frustration, and thoughts of self-inflicted harm.

- Patient participates in social interaction while hospitalized.

Discharge outcomes
- Patient no longer expresses self-destructive or suicidal thoughts.
- Patient reports being able to cope better with disorganization, aggressive impulses, anxiety, or hallucinations.
- Patient reports improved self-esteem and sense of security.
- Patient experiences few or no dissociative states.
- Patient describes community resources that can provide assistance when he feels out of control.

INTERVENTIONS AND RATIONALES

Initial interventions
- Remove potentially hazardous items (such as razor blades, glass objects, belts) from the patient's environment *to promote safety.*
- Limit the number of staff members that interact with the patient *to ensure continuity of care and to improve the patient's sense of security.*
- Have staff members make frequent, short visits with the patient *to provide reassurance without stifling the patient's sense of independence.*
- Administer psychotropic medications, if prescribed, *to reduce tension, impulsive behavior, hallucinations, and panic.*
- Ask the patient directly, "Are you considering suicide?" If so, ask, "What do you plan to do?" *to identify need for additional precautions.*
- Make short-term verbal contracts with the patient in which he agrees not to harm himself. *This demon-*

strates positive regard for the patient and helps him understand that he is responsible for his personal safety and capable of guaranteeing it.
- Encourage the patient to talk about his feelings, especially anger, anxiety, pain, and frustration *to begin the process of revealing true feelings and possible causes.*

Interim interventions
- If the patient enters a dissociative state or hallucinates, move him to a quiet room with fewer stimuli. If restraints are necessary, remain with the patient and provide reassurance *to calm and orient him to reality.*
- If the patient harms himself, calmly care for the injury without conveying judgment, and encourage the patient to talk about the feelings that prompted the injury. Help him clearly define any disclosed feelings. *Talking at this time may help the patient identify feelings that precede self-destructive acts. It is also an opportunity to discuss alternative ways of dealing with negative thoughts and feelings.*
- If self-destructive behavior persists, consider developing a behavior-modification program that rewards self-control, for example, with personal attention or desired materials *to reinforce self-control.*
- Conduct frequent team meetings *to ensure patient safety and treatment that is consistent with the patient's current behavior.*
- Teach the patient cognitive techniques for managing fear, anxiety, and depression and adaptive coping methods for managing anger, frustration, and pain. *Cognitive techniques help the patient minimize destructive impulses.*

Adaptive coping methods (such as regular exercise, relaxation techniques, or talking about feelings with a friend) are basic skills that will help him cope with difficult feelings when they occur.

Discharge outcomes
- Include members of the patient's family when teaching coping techniques. *Family members can help the patient practice adaptive methods of coping with self-destructive feelings.*
- Provide the patient and family members with referrals to appropriate community resources *to reduce feelings of isolation and help them cope with stress and anxiety.*
- If the patient is participating in therapy, discuss the patient's risk of self-harm with community members *to enhance protection and promote psychological support.*

EVALUATION STATEMENTS

Patient:
- remains free from injury during hospitalization.
- fulfills terms of verbal contracts not to harm himself.
- describes circumstances and feelings that precede self-destructive behavior.
- describes techniques that improve his ability to cope with hallucinations and feelings of aggression, anger, anxiety, depression, disorganization, frustration, or emotional pain.
- exercises regularly.
- demonstrates relaxation techniques.
- describes community resources that can provide help in managing self-destructive impulses.

DOCUMENTATION

- Diagnostic test results
- Observations of the patient's behavior
- Evidence of suicidal ideation
- Expression of feelings of depression, hopelessness, helplessness, rejection, isolation
- Terms of verbal contracts
- Patient behaviors or statements that indicate a change in perspective
- Demonstrations of improved ability to cope with feelings associated with self-destructive behavior
- Nursing interventions, including teaching topics, and patient and family responses
- Evaluation statements.

Sensory or perceptual alteration

related to hallucinations

DEFINITION

Perceptions or sensations that occur in the absence of external stimuli

ASSESSMENT

Cultural status
- *Demographics:* age, sex, level of education, occupation, nationality, ethnic group, religion
- *History:* values and beliefs concerning health care

Neurologic status
- *History:* sleep pattern, nutritional status, insight regarding hallucinations

- *Mental status:* insight, judgment, abstract thinking, general information, mood, affect, recent and remote memories, orientation (person, place, time)
- *Laboratory tests:* urinalysis, blood chemistry, and drug toxicology screening
- *Diagnostic tests:* Folstein Mini Mental Health Status Examination, computed tomography, electroencephalography

Psychological status
- *Current illness:* reason for hospitalization, patient's perception of problem, level of anxiety, recent stressors, changes in somatic functioning, circumstances surrounding onset of hallucinations, duration and diurnal nature of experiences, delusional beliefs, ability to perform activities of daily living
- *Medical history:* medications (response, effectiveness, adverse reactions), episodes of substance abuse (type, effect on mental status)
- *Personal history:* coping mechanisms, willingness to cooperate with treatment, support systems, communication skills (verbal and nonverbal), social interaction

DEFINING CHARACTERISTICS

- Acting out hallucinatory experiences (command hallucinations)
- Disorientation, dissociation
- Images that occur in the absence of external stimuli (visual hallucinations)
- Perceived body sensations of unknown origin, including misconceptions about body parts (tactile hallucinations)

- Perceived odors of specific or unknown origin (olfactory hallucinations)
- Perceived tastes of unknown origin (gustatory hallucinations)
- Perceived voices or sounds that are not heard by others and are unrelated to objective reality (auditory hallucinations)
- Preoccupation, lack of awareness of surroundings
- Restlessness
- Talking to self, watchfulness, or the appearance of listening in the absence of external stimuli

ASSOCIATED DISORDERS

Auditory nerve damage, delirium, dementia, hallucinogen-induced disorders, mood disorders, personality disorders (borderline, schizoid, paranoid, schizophreniform), schizophrenia, substance-induced disorders (intoxication or withdrawal)

EXPECTED OUTCOMES

Initial outcomes
- Patient remains free from injury during hospital stay.
- Patient expresses feelings provoked by hallucinations.

Interim outcomes
- Patient maintains orientation to surroundings (people, place, time).
- Patient demonstrates awareness that hallucinations are caused by internal stimuli.
- Patient describes and practices methods of testing reality at onset of hallucinations.
- Patient reports less anxiety.

Discharge outcomes
- Patient demonstrates an understanding of the prescribed medication regimen, including dosage, schedule, and possible adverse reactions.
- Patient states his intention to use community resources for support.

INTERVENTIONS AND RATIONALES

Initial interventions
- Provide a safe and structured environment. Identify and reduce as many stressors as possible. Be honest and consistent in all interactions with the patient. *These measures help reduce the patient's anxiety.*
- Encourage the patient to express feelings related to experiencing hallucinations. *This promotes a better understanding of the hallucinatory experience and lets the patient vent emotions, which helps reduce his anxiety.*
- Encourage the patient to identify and initiate anxiety-reducing measures *to give him a sense of control.*

Interim interventions
- In organic hallucinations, orientation and factual information help the patient cope. Explain that the hallucinations result from organic causes that can be effectively treated. *This helps maintain the patient's orientation and reduces his stress and anxiety.*
- In nonorganic hallucinations, do not attempt to reason with the patient or challenge hallucinations as they occur. Instead, ensure the patient's safety and provide comfort and support. *Attempts to reason with the patient only increase his anxiety, thereby exacerbating the hallucinations.*

- Use directive statements when speaking to the patient, for example, "Look at me and pay attention; try not to listen to the voice right now," *to help the patient to focus on you rather than internal stimuli.*
- Schedule regular periods of physical activity that require concentration and exertion *to distract the patient from internal stimuli.*
- Help the patient identify situations that evoke hallucinatory experiences *to increase self-awareness and enable him to take steps to avoid hallucinations.*
- Teach the patient ways to intervene during hallucinations. For example, encourage him to speak out using statements such as, "Go away; you're not real." *Responding directly to the hallucinatory experience fosters a sense of control, which reduces the frequency and duration of hallucinations.*
- Teach the patient to use consensual validation of perceptual experiences to test reality. *Having other people validate experiences improves the patient's orientation to reality.*
- As the patient's anxiety level decreases, encourage him to participate in group activities at the hospital and after discharge *to improve his level of functioning.*

Discharge interventions
- Provide the patient and family members with a clear, concise explanation of prescribed medications, including their intended effect, dosage, schedule, and possible adverse effects, *to reduce anxiety, ensure the patient's safety, and promote compliance.*
- Refer the patient and family members to appropriate psychiatric professionals for counseling and provide information about available support services in the community *to provide ongoing care and support for the patient and family.*

EVALUATION STATEMENTS

Patient:
- remains free from injury during hospitalization.
- demonstrates improved orientation to reality.
- describes hallucinatory experiences and expresses feelings associated with them.
- identifies situations that increase anxiety or evoke hallucinations.
- employs self-control strategies to reduce hallucinations.
- describes the proper administration of prescribed medications.
- reports a reduction in hallucination intensity and frequency within two weeks.
- demonstrates improved social skills.

DOCUMENTATION

- Diagnostic test results
- Patient's description of type, frequency, and intensity of hallucinations
- Environmental factors that precipitate or influence hallucinations
- Patient's level of anxiety
- Identified stressors
- Nursing interventions to help the patient cope with hallucinations
- Patient's response to nursing interventions
- Referrals to psychiatric counselors
- Evaluation statements.

Sensory or perceptual alteration

related to sensory deprivation

DEFINITION

Impaired response to surroundings caused by diminished stimuli

ASSESSMENT

Cultural status
- *Demographics:* age, sex, level of education, occupation, nationality, race, ethnic group
- *History:* beliefs, values, and attitudes about health and illness; health customs, practices, and rituals

Neurologic status
- *History:* medical disorders; food, drug, or environmental allergies; current environment; pain management
- *Mental status:* appearance and attitude, level of consciousness, motor activity, thought and speech patterns, mood and affect, perceptions, orientation, memory, general information processing, visual-spatial ability, attention span, judgment and insight
- *Motor system:* muscle tone, strength, and symmetry; gait; pupillary response; reflexes
- *Speech pattern:* characteristics of self-expression, adaptations to speech impediments
- *Signs and symptoms:* lethargy, restlessness
- *Laboratory tests:* electrolyte levels

- *Diagnostic tests:* electroencephalography, computed tomography, Folstein Mini-Mental Status Examination

Psychological status
- *Psychiatric history:* signs and symptoms, change in appetite or energy level, alcohol or drug abuse
- *Laboratory test:* blood glucose level

Sensory status
- *History:* visual acuity, auditory acuity, use of hearing aid or glasses
- *Environment:* equipment, lighting, noise level, privacy level, space allocation, location of patient's personal belongings

Family status
- *History:* family composition, family roles, alliances and interactions among members, support systems

DEFINING CHARACTERISTICS

- Apathy and altered posture
- Changed behavior pattern
- Decreased problem-solving abilities
- Disorientation to person, place, or time
- Fatigue
- Hallucinations
- Impaired ability to conceptualize and inappropriate responses
- Isolation
- Reported or measured change in sensory acuity

ASSOCIATED DISORDERS

Acquired immunodeficiency syndrome, bipolar disease (depressive phase), blindness, brain tumor, cerebrovascular accident, dementia, depressive disorder, encephalopathy, head injury, hemianopsia, hospitalization of elderly patient, isolation, movement disorder, multiple sclerosis, organic brain syndrome, Parkinson's disease, schizophrenia, substance- or alcohol-related disorder, temporal lobe epilepsy, transient ischemic attacks

EXPECTED OUTCOMES

Initial outcomes
- Patient's expresses fears, thoughts, and anxieties.
- Patient uses adaptive devices, such as glasses or hearing aid, as needed.

Interim outcomes
- Patient accurately identifies time, place, situation, himself, and others.
- Patient is able to distinguish reality from hallucinations.
- Patient receives adequate environmental stimulation.

Discharge outcome
- Family, friends, or caregivers continue the process of orienting the patient to reality.

INTERVENTIONS AND RATIONALES

Initial interventions
- Assess and monitor the patient's condition *to detect changes in his status.*
- Establish a therapeutic setting by approaching the patient calmly, confidently, and firmly *to help calm him.*
- Assist or encourage the patient to use adaptive devices, such as eyeglasses or a hearing aid, *to increase sensory stimuli.*

- Establish a positive therapeutic relationship with the patient *to increase his trust in caregivers.*
- Be an active listener and encourage the patient to verbalize his fears, thoughts, and anxieties *to reduce tension.*
- Arrange the patient's environment to offset his deficit by placing him in a room with a maximal view of his surroundings. Encourage his family to provide personal articles, such as books, cards, and photos. Keep his possessions in the same place *to promote a sense of identity.* Use safety precautions such as a night light when needed *to reduce sensory deprivation and to assure safety.*

Interim interventions
- Discuss the patient's response level with his family and the staff, and update the care plan as needed *to determine his sensory deprivation status and to provide a basis for evaluating response to stimuli.*
- Reorient the patient to reality using the following techniques:
– calling him by name and telling him your name
– orienting him frequently to time, place, and date
– orienting him to his environment, including sights and sounds
– providing visual contrast in his environment
– using large signs as visual cues
– posting the patient's own photograph on his door if he is ambulatory and disoriented *to increase his sensory stimuli.*
- Provide verbal stimuli by talking with the patient while providing care, by encouraging his family and friends

to discuss past and present events with him, and by interacting with him at predetermined times each day *to reduce isolation and to improve his reality orientation.*

- Turn on a television or radio for short periods of time based on the patient's interests *to provide additional stimuli and to orient him to reality.*
- Hold the patient's hand when talking, discuss interests with him and his family, and provide special items such as talking books *to increase his exposure to various forms of sensory stimuli.*

Discharge intervention

- Encourage the patient and his family members or friends to plan short trips outside the hospital and provide information about mobility, toileting, feeding, and other details *to facilitate continuing care after discharge.*

EVALUATION STATEMENTS

Patient:
- uses adaptive equipment to increase sensory stimuli.
- demonstrates ability to recall people, places, and past events.
- demonstrates ability to identify current events and correct time.
- uses safety precautions to remain free of injury.
- responds to environmental stimuli.
- expresses understanding of sensory stimulation exercises.
- identifies and uses techniques to prevent sensory deprivation.

DOCUMENTATION

- Diagnostic test results
- Laboratory findings

- Adaptive devices used
- Patient's and family members' questions and concerns
- Statements indicating fear, anxiety, or other emotions
- Observations of patient's orientation to person, place, and time and response to environmental stimuli
- Sleep patterns
- Nursing interventions
- Responses to nursing interventions
- Participation in activities of daily living
- Diversional activities
- Evaluation statements.

Sensory or perceptual alteration

related to sensory overload

DEFINITION

Impaired response to environment resulting from excessive or changed stimuli

ASSESSMENT

Cultural status

- *Demographics:* age, sex, level of education, occupation, nationality, race, ethnic group
- *History:* beliefs, values, and attitudes about health and illness; health customs, practices, and rituals

Neurologic status

- *History:* medical disorders; food, drug, or environmental allergies; current environment; pain management
- *Mental status:* appearance and attitude, level of consciousness, motor

activity, thought and speech patterns, mood and affect, perceptions, orientation, memory, general information processing, visual-spatial ability, attention span, and judgment and insight
- *Motor system:* muscle tone, strength, and symmetry; gait; pupillary response; reflexes
- *Speech pattern:* characteristics of self-expression, adaptations to speech impediments
- *Signs and symptoms:* lethargy, restlessness
- *Laboratory tests:* electrolyte levels
- *Diagnostic tests:* electroencephalography, computed tomography, Folstein Mini-Mental Health Status Examination

Psychological status
- *Psychiatric history:* signs and symptoms, changes in appetite or energy level, alcohol or drug abuse
- *Laboratory test:* blood glucose level

Sensory status
- *History:* visual acuity, auditory acuity, use of hearing aid or glasses
- *Environment:* equipment, lighting, noise level, privacy, space allocation, location of patient's personal belongings

Family status
- *History:* family composition, family roles, alliances and interactions among members, support systems

DEFINING CHARACTERISTICS
- Altered communication patterns
- Anxiety
- Bizarre thinking

- Change in behavior pattern or withdrawal
- Change in problem-solving abilities
- Clinical evidence of sensory overload
- Disorientation to person, place, or time
- Exaggerated emotional responses
- Hallucinations
- Impaired ability to conceptualize and inappropriate responses
- Irritability, restlessness, and sleep pattern disturbances
- Visual or auditory distortions

ASSOCIATED DISORDERS AND TREATMENTS

Acquired immunodeficiency syndrome, alcohol withdrawal, anxiety disorder, bipolar disease (manic phase), brain tumor, dementia, encephalopathy, head injury, hospitalization in intensive care unit due to major trauma or surgery, metabolic alkalosis, multiple sclerosis, Parkinson's disease, schizophrenia, substance- or alcohol-related disorder, temporal lobe epilepsy, transient ischemic attacks

EXPECTED OUTCOMES

Initial outcome
- Patient expresses decreased anxiety and irritability.

Interim outcomes
- Patient communicates in a lucid manner.
- Patient recognizes when sensory stimuli is excessive.
- Patient reestablishes usual sleep cycle.

- Patient states measures to reduce sensory overload.
- Patient demonstrates positive coping behavior during sensory overload.

Discharge outcome
- Family members, friends, or caregiver expresses understanding of measures to reduce sensory overload.

INTERVENTIONS AND RATIONALES

Initial interventions
- Assess and monitor the patient's condition *to detect changes in status.*
- Establish a therapeutic setting by approaching the patient calmly, confidently, and firmly *to help calm him.*
- Be an active listener and allow the patient to verbalize fears, emotions, ideas, and anxieties *to help establish a therapeutic relationship.*
- Provide the patient with a safe, quiet, low-stimulation environment *to decrease his experience of sensory disturbance.*

Interim interventions
- Accept the patient's perceptions of stimuli, including hallucinations or delusions. *Forcing the patient to admit that his perceptions are in error will not work.*
- Explain procedures, tests, special equipment, and unusual sounds *to increase the patient's knowledge base, which reduces sensory overload.*
- When sensory overload occurs, instruct the patient to use coping methods, such as turning off the television or leaving a stimulating environment, *to enhance his sense of control and limit sensory overload.*

- Encourage the patient to establish a regular sleep pattern and receive sufficient rest *to improve his tolerance to stimuli.*

Discharge interventions
- Encourage family or friends to visit frequently and to maintain consistent contact with the patient *to improve his orientation to reality.*
- Describe to family, friends, and caregivers interventions to reduce sensory overload. Provide referrals to appropriate social service agencies *to ensure continuity of care.*

EVALUATION STATEMENTS

Patient:
- experiences no injury.
- demonstrates ability to correctly identify people, places, and time and to recall past events.
- reports feeling less irritable and anxious.
- communicates clearly.
- recognizes when sensory stimuli are becoming excessive and requests time in quiet area.
- reestablishes usual sleep cycle.
- identifies and demonstrates measures to avoid sensory overload.

DOCUMENTATION

- Diagnostic test results
- Laboratory findings
- Safety precautions implemented
- Observations of orientation to reality, anxiety level, and sleep pattern
- Instructions regarding coping with sensory overload
- Responses to nursing interventions
- Evaluation statements.

Sexual dysfunction

related to altered body structure or function

DEFINITION

Reported sexual problems that the patient attributes to a medical condition

ASSESSMENT

Cultural status

- *Demographics:* age, sex, marital status, level of education, occupation, nationality, race, ethnic group, religion
- *History:* beliefs, values, and attitudes about health and illness; attitudes about sex; influence of religious beliefs on attitudes about sex

Family status

- *Family roles:* degree of family agreement on roles, interrelationships of family roles
- *Family subsystems:* family alliances, family conflicts, influence of family alliances on family stability
- *Coping patterns:* major life events, usual coping patterns
- *Evidence of abuse:* physical and behavioral indicators

Neurologic status

- *Personal habits:* pain management; use of medications such as neuroleptics or barbiturates; alcohol use
- *Mental status:* appearance and attitude, level of consciousness, motor activity, thought and speech, mood and affect, perceptions, orientation, memory, general information, calcula-

tions, capacity to read and write, visual-spatial ability, attention span, abstraction, judgment and insight
- *Physical examination:* motor system, sensory system
- *Signs and symptoms:* lethargy, stupor, vertigo, syncope, paresthesia, incoordination, fasciculation, chorea, pain
- *Diagnostic tests:* cerebral arteriography, electroencephalography

Musculoskeletal status

- *History:* degenerative joint disorders; neuromuscular or skeletal accident or trauma
- *Observation:* ability to carry out activities of daily living
- *Physical examination:* range of motion of all joints, evidence of swelling, deformity, coordination and gait, functional mobility
- *Signs and symptoms:* limited range of movement, muscle weakness, joint deformity, muscle atrophy

Psychological status

- *Life changes:* recent divorce, job loss, or loss of loved one
- *Effect of illness:* age at onset; type and severity of symptoms; impact upon functioning; type of treatment and response; changes in mood, behavior, or affect
- *Alcohol or drug abuse:* type of substance, evidence of abuse or withdrawal, impact upon functioning
- *Signs and symptoms:* changes in energy level, motivation, personal hygiene, self-image, self-esteem, sleep patterns, sexual drive, feelings of competence

Sexuality status
- *History:* changes in sexual behavior, sexual dysfunction, physiology, and body image
- *Medications:* oral contraceptives, antihypertensives, neuroleptics, sedatives, tranquilizers
- *Signs and symptoms:* vaginismus, impotence, decreased or increased libido, dyspareunia, premature ejaculation

Social status
- *History:* interpersonal skills, quality of relationships, degree of trust in others, level of self-esteem
- *Signs and symptoms:* withdrawal, inappropriate responses, aggressiveness, lack of eye contact

Spiritual status
- *Prior medical conditions:* illnesses that cause a change in body image
- *Signs and symptoms:* crying, withdrawal

DEFINING CHARACTERISTICS
- Actual or perceived limitation imposed by disease or therapy
- Alterations in relationship with spouse or partner
- Change of interest in self and others
- Inability to achieve desired satisfaction
- Insecurity about sexual desirability
- Preoccupation with sexual performance

ASSOCIATED DISORDERS AND TREATMENTS
Acquired immunodeficiency syndrome; brain tumor; chronic renal failure with hemodialysis; conditions requiring colostomy, coronary artery bypass, ileostomy, ostomy, pelvic surgery, radiation therapy, radical abdominal surgery, mastectomy, or ureteroileostomy; dementias; diabetes mellitus; drug therapy; endometriosis; genitourinary problems; multiple sclerosis, myocardial infarction; Parkinson's disease, pelvic inflammatory disease; rheumatoid arthritis; spinal cord injury; pregnancy; recent child birth; substance-related disorders; surgery; tardive dyskinesia; transient ischemic attack, trauma

EXPECTED OUTCOMES

Initial outcomes
- Patient acknowledges a problem in sexual function.
- Patient states reason for dysfunction.
- Patient identifies any stressors that may contribute to the dysfunction.

Interim outcomes
- Patient voices feelings about changes in sexual function.
- Patient discusses concerns related to sexuality openly.
- Patient and his partner explore alternative avenues of communication and sexual expression.
- Patient expresses understanding of limitations caused by illness or injury.

Discharge outcomes
- Patient reports decreased anxiety about sexual functioning.
- Patient acknowledges the need for psychotherapy if sexual dysfunction is compounded by psychological problems.

INTERVENTIONS AND RATIONALES

Initial interventions

- Encourage the patient to discuss his sexual problem and provide a non-threatening atmosphere *to help him overcome feelings of embarrassment.*
- Provide answers to specific questions about illness and sexuality *to help the patient focus on specific issues and clarify misconceptions.*
- Suggest that the patient discuss concerns with his spouse or partner *to foster sharing of concerns and strengthening of interpersonal relationships.*

Interim interventions

- As the patient becomes more comfortable discussing issues of sexuality, be especially careful to remain nonjudgmental *to foster communication and help eliminate shame.*
- Facilitate discussion between the patient and his partner *to foster communication.*
- Provide emotional support for the patient's spouse or partner through active listening *to communicate concern, interest, and acceptance.*
- Educate the patient and his spouse or partner about limitations imposed by his physical condition or treatment *to help him avoid complications or injury.* Answer any questions they may have and clarify any misconceptions *to avoid misunderstandings.*
- Educate the patient and his spouse or partner about alternative methods of sexual expression *to promote intimacy.*

Discharge intervention

- Suggest referral to a sex counselor, mental health professional, or another appropriate professional *to ensure continued therapy.*

EVALUATION STATEMENTS

Patient:
- acknowledges existence of problem in sexual function.
- expresses anxiety, anger, depression, or frustration over changes in sexual function.
- explains relationship between illness or treatment and sexual dysfunction.
- expresses willingness to obtain counseling.
- acknowledges the need for psychotherapy if the sexual dysfunction is compounded by other psychological issues.

DOCUMENTATION

- Patient's description of problem
- Comments made by patient indicating difficulty coping with change in structure or function
- Observations of patient's behavior
- Nursing interventions performed to assist the patient and spouse or partner
- Response to nursing interventions
- Evaluation statements.

Sexual dysfunction

related to decreased libido caused by depression

DEFINITION

Presence of physiologic or emotional factors that alter one's usual sexual performance

ASSESSMENT

Cultural status
- *Demographics:* age, sex, level of education, occupation, nationality, race, ethnic group
- *History:* beliefs, values, and attitudes about health and illness; customs, practices, and rituals.

Psychological status
- *History:* body image; self-esteem; expressions of guilt; change in energy, sleep pattern, or appetite; suicidal ideation; history of substance abuse
- *Medication history:* antidepressants, including tricyclic antidepressants or monoamine oxidase (MAO) inhibitors

Sexuality status
- *History:* sexual orientation; sexual desire, enjoyment, and performance; sexual responsiveness of partner

DEFINING CHARACTERISTICS

- Decreased or absent desire for sexual activity
- Decreased or absent sexual fantasies
- Symptoms of mood disorder, including depression, crying, fatigue, feelings of worthlessness, weight gain or loss, decreased pleasure in usual activities, insomnia, hypersomnia, psychomotor agitation or retardation

ASSOCIATED DISORDERS

Bipolar disorder (depressive phase), cyclothymic disorder, dysthymic disorder, hypoactive sexual desire disorder, major depressive disorder (single episode or recurrent), major depressive episode (melancholic type), sexual aversion disorder

EXPECTED OUTCOMES

Initial outcomes
- Patient acknowledges depressive episode and problem in sexual function.
- Patient voices feelings about decreases in sexual desire.

Interim outcomes
- Patient identifies ways to enhance pleasure and improve interpersonal communication with partner.
- Patient regains sexual desire with recovery from depression.

Discharge outcome
- Patient accepts referral for sex therapy if necessary.

INTERVENTIONS AND RATIONALES

Initial interventions
- Initiate a trusting therapeutic relationship with the patient. Make the purpose, nature, and parameters of this relationship clear *to help him feel secure and develop trust.*
- Educate the patient and his partner about the nature of depression, its treatment, and its effect on sexual desire. *Understanding the link between depression and sexual desire may diminish feelings of guilt and worthlessness and help raise self-esteem.*
- Allow the patient to express feelings openly in a nonthreatening, nonjudgmental atmosphere *to foster communication and help him cope with unresolved issues.* Offer feedback *to validate his feelings and promote self-esteem.*

Interim interventions

- Include the patient and his partner in planning care and interventions *to enhance feelings of control for both partners.*
- Reinforce compliance with the treatment plan for depression *even though tricyclic antidepressants and MAO inhibitors may diminish sexual desire.*
- Discuss with the patient and his partner alternative expressions of affection, such as hugging and nonsexual cuddling, *to enhance their relationship during treatment and help them preserve intimacy during temporary loss of libido.*

Discharge intervention

- Refer the patient for sex counseling or therapy if low sexual desire persists after resolution of depression. *Sexual desire should return to its usual level after successful treatment for depression. If it does not, professional therapy is required.*

EVALUATION STATEMENTS

Patient:
- describes depressive episode, treatment plan, and effects on sexual desire.
- expresses concerns to staff and partner.
- identifies at least three activities to enhance pleasure and communication with partner.
- reports the return of sexual fantasies and desire for sexual activity.
- communicates willingness to follow through with referral for sex therapy.

DOCUMENTATION

- Patient's statements indicating concern regarding loss of desire
- Observation of patient's behavior, including indications of depression or suicide
- Nursing interventions to assist the patient and his partner
- Patient's and partner's responses to nursing interventions
- Evaluation statements.

Sexual dysfunction

related to impotence

DEFINITION

Presence of physiologic or emotional factors that render a man unable to attain or maintain penile erection sufficient to complete intercourse

ASSESSMENT

Cultural status

- *Demographics:* age, level of education, occupation, nationality, race, ethnic group
- *History:* beliefs, values, and attitudes about health and illness; health customs, practices, and rituals

Family status

- *History:* relationship with parents, presence of family or social pressures
- *Coping patterns:* major life events and their meaning to each family member

- *Family communication:* style and quality of communication, methods of conflict resolution
- *Family roles:* formal and informal roles and performance, degree of family agreement on roles, interrelationships of family roles
- *Physical and emotional needs:* family's ability to meet the patient's physical and emotional needs

Physiological status

- *Signs and symptoms:* anatomic anomalies of penis, medical conditions, frequency of impotence, premature ejaculation, spontaneous morning erections

Sexuality status

- *History:* patient's perception of sexual performance, sexual drive, sexual orientation, relationships, and extramarital affairs; homosexual experiences; positive coital experiences; use of erotica for stimulation; professional counseling or sex therapy; medication history
- *Type of impotence:* organic (anatomic or central nervous system defect), functional (physiologic alterations in nervous and cardiovascular systems), psychogenic (emotions inhibit neural transmission from brain to sexual organs), primary (no previous satisfactory erection for coitus), secondary (at least one previously successful coitus)
- *Signs and symptoms:* desire for an erection, anger, guilt, shame, hostility, or disgust toward partner

DEFINING CHARACTERISTICS

- Anger, guilt, hostility, shame

- Expressions of concern about sexual performance
- Expressions of desire for an erection
- History of relationships with family members or previous sexual partners that adversely affect sexuality
- Inability to attain and maintain an erection throughout sexual intercourse
- Poor communication with partner
- Use of drugs that interfere with sexual performance

ASSOCIATED DISORDERS AND TREATMENTS

Alcohol- or substance-related disorders, cardiovascular disease (penile circulatory problem), diabetes mellitus, drug therapy with antihypertensives or beta blockers, endocrine dysfunction (low testosterone or high prolactin levels), male erectile disorder, male orgasmic disorder, premature ejaculation

EXPECTED OUTCOMES

Initial outcomes

- Patient acknowledges problem with sexual function.
- Patient discusses his sexual problems openly.
- Patient and partner discuss their feelings and perceptions about changes in sexual performance.

Interim outcomes

- Patient uses alternative methods of enhancing sexual pleasure for himself and his partner.
- Patient continues to communicate with partner about sexual issues and needs.

Discharge outcomes
- Patient agrees to sexual evaluation and therapy, if warranted.
- Patient develops and maintains a positive attitude about his sexuality and sexual performance.

INTERVENTIONS AND RATIONALES

Initial interventions
- Establish a therapeutic relationship with the patient *to provide a safe and comfortable atmosphere for discussing sexual concerns.*
- Encourage the patient to discuss feelings and perceptions about his sexual dysfunction *to help validate his perceptions and reduce emotional distress.*
- Encourage the patient's partner to discuss feelings and perceptions *to help clarify issues and improve communication.*

Interim interventions
- Teach the patient and his partner alternative ways of expressing sexual intimacy and affection. *Alternative expressions of intimacy can raise the patient's self-esteem during evaluation and treatment of impotence.*
- Encourage the patient and his partner to use sexual fantasies and erotica to enhance sexual stimulation and erection. *These stimuli can reduce inhibitions and intensify sexual response.*

Discharge intervention
- Encourage the patient to seek evaluation and therapy from a qualified professional. *Besides being necessary for proper diagnosis and treatment, professional therapy can help the patient increase his sexual pleasure during treatment.*

EVALUATION STATEMENTS

Patient:
- reports feeling comfortable discussing his sexual concerns.
- expresses feelings about diminished sexual performance.
- identifies and uses specific methods to enhance sexual pleasure with his partner.
- participates in sexual evaluation and therapy, if warranted.
- makes positive comments about himself.

Patient and partner:
- communicate with each other about their sexual relationship.

DOCUMENTATION
- Patient's perception of sexual problem
- Remarks made by patient indicating difficulty coping with impotence
- Observations of patient's behavior in response to his sexual dysfunction
- Nursing interventions
- Patient's and partner's response to interventions
- Evaluation statements.

Sexual pattern alteration
related to hypersexuality caused by mania

DEFINITION

Presence of physiologic or emotional factors that alter usual sexual behavior; episodes of sexual acting out associated with mania

ASSESSMENT

Cultural status
- *Demographics:* age, sex, marital status, level of education, occupation, nationality, race, ethnic group
- *History:* beliefs, values, and attitudes about health and illness; health customs, practices, and rituals

Psychological status
- *History:* appetite, energy level, level of motivation, personal hygiene, self-image, self-esteem
- *Substance abuse:* use of psychosis-inducing drugs (phencyclidine, amphetamines), use of disinhibiting drugs (alcohol, amphetamines, cocaine), effects on mood and behavior, evidence of withdrawal, impact on functioning,
- *Life changes:* recent divorce, illness, job loss, or loss of loved one
- *Psychiatric history:* age at onset of illness, type and severity of symptoms, impact on functioning, type of treatment, patient's response to treatment
- *Medications:* prescribed and over-the-counter medications (dosage, effectiveness, adverse reactions)
- *Signs and symptoms:* hypersexuality, intrusiveness, grandiosity, lack of impulse control, loose association, flights of fancy, extreme levels of energy, lack of sleep, poor nutrition, poor judgment, elevated mood, expansiveness, pressured and rapid speech, strained interpersonal relationships

Sexual status
- *History:* attitude toward sex, sexual orientation, sexual response patterns, partners, appropriateness of sexual behavior, sexual remarks or gestures

DEFINING CHARACTERISTICS
- Excessive motor activity
- Excessive or impulsive sexual activity
- Frustration and anger if sexuality is hindered
- Inability to adapt sexual behavior to social norms
- Inappropriate and provocative sexual comments
- Inappropriate and excessive physical closeness and touching with peers
- Periods of excessive elation or cycles of elation and depression
- Poor perception of reality caused by psychotic disorder
- Sexual encounters that are self-destructive

ASSOCIATED DISORDERS

Bipolar disorder (manic phase), substance-induced psychotic disorder

EXPECTED OUTCOMES

Initial outcome
- Patient reduces or eliminates harmful sexual behaviors.

Interim outcomes
- Patient refrains from making inappropriate remarks to staff.
- Patient discusses the difference between a social and a therapeutic relationship.
- Patient exhibits fewer symptoms of mania.
- Patient discusses impact of his behavior on others.

Discharge outcomes
- Patient meets sexual needs in a socially appropriate manner.

- Patient explores feelings underlying hypersexual behavior.

INTERVENTIONS AND RATIONALES

Initial interventions

- Set limits on the patient's sexual acting out, such as attempting to have sex with other patients or making suggestive remarks to patients or staff. Explain the expectations and consequences if limits are violated *to help him control his behavior.*
- Make sure that limitations regarding the patient's sexual acting out are understood and agreed upon by all staff. Tell staff to set limits when the patient begins to flirt or make sexual advances and not to wait until he is out of control. Help the staff understand that hypersexual behavior is part of the patient's illness. *The patient will not be able to control his behavior if consequences are not consistently administered.*
- Administer antimanic and neuroleptic medication as prescribed. *These medications provide rapid relief of symptoms of mania, including hypersexuality.*

Interim intervention

- If the patient makes sexual remarks to you, ignore them. *Lack of feedback may decrease these behaviors.*
- When the patient exhibits a decrease in symptoms of mania, explore the significance of sexual remarks by asking the following questions *to clarify the patient's misconceptions:*
  – What was the intent of your remark?
  – How do you view our relationship?

– What is the difference between a social relationship and a therapeutic relationship?
– Tell me about one sexual relationship you've had. How is our relationship different? How is it similar?
- Discuss with the patient the effect of his hypersexual behavior on others *to foster a sense of responsibility.*

Discharge interventions

- Encourage the patient to express sexual urges in socially acceptable ways (including masturbation in private) *to promote positive methods of relieving sexual tension.*
- Talk to the patient about his hypersexual behaviors and any associated feelings *to help him develop insights about his behavior.*
  – Provide an opportunity for the patient to express his feelings about his sexual behavior. Determine if he is troubled by impulsive sexual acts.
  – Ask the patient what types of feelings precede impulsive sexual behavior. Does stress, anxiety, or loneliness trigger sexual fantasy or activity?
  – Discuss the quality of the patient's interpersonal relationships. Does he feel isolated from others?
  – What benefits does the patient derive from impulsive sexual acts? Do they provide a relief from anxiety, or a feeling of power, or a feeling of connection with others?
- Provide referral for ongoing psychiatric treatment. *Indiscriminate and impulsive hypersexuality may indicate physical or psychiatric illness that requires further evaluation and treatment.*

EVALUATION STATEMENTS

Patient:
- does not make inappropriate sexual remarks or advances to other patients or staff.
- recognizes his hypersexual urges and his inability to cope with them.
- expresses understanding of the difference between a social and a therapeutic relationship.
- states his desire to express sexuality in a socially acceptable manner.
- reports finding opportunities for sexual release that are not harmful.
- explores feelings underlying sexual acting out.
- expresses willingness to participate in appropriate psychiatric care or sex therapy.

DOCUMENTATION

- Observations of patient's behavior, including inappropriate expressions of sexuality
- Comments made by patient with sexual content
- Nursing interventions to help patient set limits on hypersexuality
- Patient's response to interventions
- Evaluation statements.

Sexual pattern alteration

related to psychological distress

DEFINITION

Sexual behavior that leads to persistent or recurrent distress and sense of conflict

ASSESSMENT

Cultural status
- *Demographics:* age, sex, marital status, level of education, occupation, nationality, race, ethnic group, religion
- *History:* beliefs, values, and attitudes about health and illness; health customs, practices, and rituals; beliefs, attitudes, and values about sexual behavior; influence of religious beliefs on values and practices

Family status
- *History:* family composition, developmental stage of family, family alliances, affect of alliances on family stability, drug and alcohol use among family members
- *Family roles:* degree of family agreement about roles, interrelationships among roles
- *Family needs:* ability of family to meet patient's essential physical and emotional needs, willingness of family to allow members to pursue individual goals
- *Diagnostic tests:* Family Genogram, Index of Family Relations

Parental status
- *History:* parent's level of education, knowledge of normal growth and development in children, usual coping mechanisms, disciplinary measures, stability of parental relationship, attitudes toward sex, willingness to discuss sex with children, influence of religious beliefs on attitudes about sex

Sexuality status
- *History:* attitudes about sex, sexual orientation, sexual response patterns, exposure to sexually transmitted dis-

eases, content of sexual fantasies, contraceptive practices, triggers for sexual acting out

- *Behavior:* sexual obsessions, solicitation of prostitutes, exchange of sexual favors for money, chronic masturbation, repeated and obsessive phone sex, sadomasochism, heterosexual or homosexual affairs, obsessive use of pornography, repeated visits to massage parlors or adult bookstores, persistent violent sexual fantasies, cross-dressing, sexual addiction, anonymous sexual encounters in public places, exhibitionism, voyeurism, use of drugs during sexual activity, incest, pedophilia, fetishism, stalking, knowing and repeated participation in unsafe sex, self-erotic asphyxiation, rape, bestiality
- *Consequences of sexual behavior:* separation, divorce, incarceration, financial losses, sexually transmitted disease, damage to self-image and self-esteem, admission to psychiatric institution
- *Diagnostic tests:* Index of Sexual Satisfaction, Sexual Behavior Inventory

Psychological status

- *History:* values and beliefs about sex, self-concept, means and ability to meet emotional and sexual needs, history of rejection, abusive partners, compulsive behaviors, success in role performance, purpose or direction in life
- *Developmental history:* birth order, number of siblings, development milestones, reactions to illness, losses through separation or death
- *Childhood development:* gender identification, cross-dressing, feelings about anatomic characteristics, school

attendance, family relationships, peer relationships, role models of sexual behavior, knowledge about human sexuality, traumatic emotional or sexual experiences

- *Adolescent development:* reaction to puberty, sexual orientation, dating history, use of sexual activity to relieve anxiety, relationships with peers and authority figures, situational crises, traumatic emotional or sexual experiences
- *Signs and symptoms:* anxiety; unmet needs; feelings of tension, helplessness, hopelessness, inadequacy, or uncertainty; insomnia; focus on self; difficulties, limitations, or changes in sexual behaviors or activities; disorientation about sense of self; altered role performance associated with psychological distress

DEFINING CHARACTERISTICS

- Participation in sexual activity or fantasy that is perceived by the patient to be emotionally distressing
- Participation in sexual activity that can place the patient or others in serious emotional, legal, or medical jeopardy
- Reported difficulties, limitations, or changes in sexual behaviors

ASSOCIATED DISORDERS

Adult gender identity disorder, anxiety disorder, borderline personality disorder, exhibitionism, fetishism, mood disorder, pedophilia, sexual abuse of children, sexual arousal disorders, sexual dysfunction disorders, sexual masochism, sexual sadism, substance-related disorder, transvestic fetishism, voyeurism

EXPECTED OUTCOMES

Initial outcomes

- Patient identifies personal sexual concerns.
- Patient acknowledges distress over sexual behavior pattern.

Interim outcomes

- Patient communicates feelings about aspects of sexual behavior that are troubling to him.
- Patient expresses understanding of how personal background affects sexual behavior pattern.
- Patient works on ceasing dangerous sexual practices.

Discharge outcomes

- Patient verbalizes increased self-acceptance.
- Patient states intention to seek further professional assistance.

INTERVENTIONS AND RATIONALES

Initial interventions

- Have the patient create a Family Genogram and personal time line indicating the positive and negative events in his life. *These tools help the patient visualize and understand significant events in his life.*
- Acknowledge the patient's apprehensions about openly discussing sexual concerns *to establish rapport, decrease his feelings of anxiety, and foster trust.*
- Be careful to demonstrate a nonjudgmental attitude at all times. Under no circumstances say anything

that would make the patient feel ashamed. *It is the patient's needs and feelings, not your opinions, that matter.*

Interim interventions

- Ask the patient what he perceives as distressing about his sexual behavior or fantasies *to gain a clear understanding of the factors responsible for psychological distress.*
- Once a trusting relationship has been established, ask direct questions about the patient's sexual behavior and fantasies. Discuss his knowledge about sexuality and dispel myths or misinformation as needed *to enhance his understanding of sexual functioning and sexual response patterns.*
- Encourage the patient to identify and discuss beliefs and values regarding sex. Discuss the effects of childhood experiences, religious beliefs, and his parents' attitudes toward sex and sexual behavior *to assist him in making connections between childhood experiences and adult sexual behavior.*
- Discuss current interpersonal relationships *to assist the patient in making connections between his emotional needs and his sexual behavior and also to help him understand how his behavior affects others.*
- Encourage the patient to identify feelings, such as pleasure, reduced anxiety, increased control, or shame associated with sexual behavior and fantasies, *to provide insight for developing appropriate interventions.*
- Help the patient understand that expressing feelings of anger, hostility, sadness, and fear are not wrong *to facilitate the expression of emotions.*
- Help the patient distinguish between practices that are distressing because

they do not conform to social norms or personal values from those that may place him or others in serious emotional, medical, or legal jeopardy *to reinforce the need to stop behaviors that could harm him or others.*
- Assist the patient in establishing short-term goals for practicing new behaviors or accepting those behaviors that he finds distressing but wants to continue *to provide some resolution for emotional distress.*

Discharge interventions
- Provide the patient with information about community resources, social services, individual and group therapy, support groups (such as Sex and Love Addicts Anonymous), sex therapy, or other sources of support and assistance *to diminish his feelings of helplessness and hopelessness and to help him make decisions regarding his sexual behavior.*
- Emphasize the need for long-term treatment and for persistence in pursuit of his goals. *Deeply rooted emotional and sexual problems may take a long time to heal.*

EVALUATION STATEMENTS

Patient:
- acknowledges personal sexual concerns.
- expresses feelings about sexual behavior or fantasies.
- verbalizes understanding of how personal background affects sexual behavior and fantasies.
- acknowledges behaviors that are emotionally, legally, or medically dangerous (if necessary).

- verbalizes increased acceptance of self.
- expresses need for further assistance.

DOCUMENTATION

- Diagnostic test results
- Patient statements indicating distress over behavior or fantasies
- Nursing interventions
- Patient responses to nursing interventions
- Patient's description of short-term goals
- Referrals to specialized professionals and programs
- Evaluation statements.

Sleep pattern disturbance

related to psychological or biological factors

DEFINITION

Inability to meet individual need for sleep or rest arising from such internal factors as anxiety, depression, stress, illness, drug therapy, or biorhythm disturbance

ASSESSMENT

Cultural status
- *Demographics:* age, sex, level of education, nationality, race, ethnic group
- *History:* beliefs, values, and attitudes about health and illness; health customs, practices, and rituals
- *Diagnostic test:* Cultural Assessment Guide

Neurologic status

- *Mental status:* appearance and attitude, level of consciousness, motor activity, thought and speech, mood and affect, perceptions, orientation, memory, general information, calculations, capacity to read and write, visual-spatial ability, attention span, abstraction, judgment and insight
- *Motor system:* muscle tone, strength, and symmetry; gait; cerebellar function
- *Cranial nerve function*
- *Sensory system:* cortical function (position sense, stereognosis, two-point discrimination, and extinction), dermatome, peripheral sensory system (pain, position, and vibration), paresthesia
- *Reflexes:* deep tendon (biceps, triceps, brachioradialis, quadriceps, achilles), superficial (abdominal, cremasteric, plantar), pathological (palmar grasp, Babinski's, Moro's, tonic neck)
- *Pupillary response*

Nutritional status

- *History:* eating habits, dietary restrictions, nutritional deficiencies, obesity

Psychological status

- *Life changes:* recent divorce, illness, job loss, or loss of loved one
- *Psychiatric history:* age at onset, type and severity of symptoms; impact on functioning; type of treatment; patient's response to treatment
- *Signs and symptoms:* changes in appetite, energy level, motivation, personal hygiene, self-image, self-esteem, sexual drive, or competence

- *Diagnostic tests:* Hamilton Rating Scale for Depression, Beck Depression Inventory, Minnesota Multiphasic Personality Inventory

Sleep pattern status

- *History:* daytime activity, work patterns, time patient normally goes to bed, hours of sleep patient requires to feel rested
- *Medication history:* medications, caffeine, alcohol, amphetamines, benzodiazapines
- *Signs and symptoms:* difficulty falling asleep, nocturnal awakening, early morning awakening, hypersomnia, insomnia, sleep pattern reversal
- *Diagnostic test:* sleep electroencephalography

DEFINING CHARACTERISTICS

- Awakening earlier or later than desired
- Changes in behavior or performance, including disorientation, increased irritability, lethargy, listlessness, restlessness
- Difficulty falling asleep, interrupted sleep
- Evidence of internal factors that prevent or disrupt sleep
- Extreme mood changes
- Fatigue
- History of psychiatric illness
- Misuse of drugs and alcohol
- Obesity, poor nutrition, lack of exercise
- Signs of sleep deprivation, including dark circles under eyes, expressionless face, frequent yawning, mild fleeting nystagmus, ptosis of the eyelid, slight hand tremor, thick speech with mis-

pronunciation and incorrect use of words

ASSOCIATED DISORDERS

Alcohol- or substance-related disorder, anxiety disorders, bipolar disorder, chronic obstructive pulmonary disease, depressive disorder, dementia with depressed mood, pickwickian syndrome, sleep apnea

EXPECTED OUTCOMES

Initial outcomes
- Patient identifies factors that interfere with achieving undisturbed sleep.
- Patient stays out of bed during normal waking hours.
- Patient participates in appropriate unit activities during the day.

Interim outcomes
- Patient identifies measures that help increase amount of sleep.
- Patient adheres to treatment regimen for underlying psychiatric condition.
- Patient reports that he is getting adequate rest.
- Patient sleeps 6 hours each night.

Discharge outcomes
- Patient establishes a bedtime routine that includes relaxation techniques.
- Patient no longer exhibits behavior related to sleep deprivation, such as restlessness, irritability, lethargy, or disorientation.

INTERVENTIONS AND RATIONALES

Initial interventions
- Assess the patient's sleep pattern thoroughly *to identify any underlying physiologic or emotional problem contributing to his sleep pattern disturbance.*
- Ask the patient to describe in specific terms each morning the quality of sleep during the previous night *to provide ongoing assessment.*
- Encourage the patient to discuss concerns that may be preventing sleep. *Active listening helps elicit underlying causes of sleep disturbances.*
- Have the patient keep a sleep diary *so disruptions can be identified and modified.*
- Plan nursing activities to include adequate periods of uninterrupted sleep. *This allows consistent nursing care while affording the patient uninterrupted time for sleep.*
- Create a quiet environment conducive to sleep. For example, provide sleep aids such as pillows or a bath before bedtime, close the curtains, adjust lighting, and close the door. *These measures promote rest and sleep.*
- Plan activities that require the patient to wake at a regular hour and stay out of bed during the day *to reinforce natural circadian rhythms.*
- Closely monitor sleep patterns in a patient with bipolar disorder. *Inadequate sleep can precipitate mania.*

Interim interventions
- As prescribed, administer antidepressant medications to a depressed patient *to control or alleviate factors inhibiting restful sleep.*

- As prescribed, administer sedative-hypnotic agents *to induce sleep* or tranquilizers *to reduce anxiety.*
- Encourage the patient to become involved in an exercise program or other activities during the day. Discuss the relationship of exercise and activity to improved sleep. Discourage excessive napping. *Activity and exercise promote sleep by increasing fatigue and relaxation.*
- Encourage participation in group therapy *to provide an environment where the patient can freely express his feelings.*

Discharge interventions
- Teach the patient relaxation techniques, such as guided imagery, progressive muscle relaxation, and meditation, *to promote rest and sleep.*
- Encourage the patient to maintain regular times to go to sleep and to wake up *to help ensure that progress is maintained once he leaves the hospital.*

EVALUATION STATEMENTS

Patient:
- identifies factors that interfere with achieving undisturbed sleep.
- participates in exercise program or other activity.
- does not exhibit signs and symptoms of sleep deprivation.
- exhibits improved mood, energy, and orientation.
- uses relaxation techniques.

DOCUMENTATION

- Diagnostic test results
- Patient's reports of sleep disturbances

- Patient's description of sleep pattern
- Patient's sleep schedule
- Nursing interventions
- Patient's response to nursing interventions
- Medication record
- Observations of patient moods, behaviors, and physical appearance
- Patient's participation in unit activities and group therapy
- Noted improvement in patient's sleep pattern
- Evaluation statements.

Social interaction impairment

related to codependence

DEFINITION

Social enmeshment or isolation due to attempts to control surroundings or behavior of another person

ASSESSMENT

Cultural status
- *Demographics:* age, sex, level of education, occupation, nationality, race, ethnic group
- *History:* beliefs, values, and attitudes about health and illness; health customs, practices, and rituals
- *Diagnostic test:* Cultural Assessment Guide

Family status
- *Family history:* marital status; sibling birth order; parents' adequacy as role models; extended family and stepfamily; communication patterns;

methods of conflict resolution; discipline methods; sources of emotional, spiritual, physical, and social support; alcohol or drug abuse; physical, emotional, or sexual abuse
- *Socioeconomic factors:* economic status of family; sense of adequacy and self-worth of family members; employment status; attitudes toward work; religious identification; influence of religion on values and daily practices
- *Diagnostic tests:* Family Genogram, Social Readjustment Rating Scale, Family Environment Scale

Neurologic status
- *Mental status:* appearance and attitude, level of consciousness, motor activity, thought and speech, mood and affect, perceptions, orientation, memory, general information, calculations, capacity to read and write, visual-spatial ability, attention span, abstraction, judgment and insight

Psychological status
- *Current illness:* reason for seeking therapy; signs and symptoms; signs of distress; ability to perform activities of daily living; changes in appetite, weight, sleep patterns, or sexual drive
- *History:* past psychiatric therapy or hospitalization; use of alcohol, drugs, or medications
- *Symptoms of codependence:* lack of self-esteem, perception of responsibility for others
- *Childhood development:* developmental milestones; academic performance; behaviors with peers, siblings, parents, extended family; family role; ability to assert needs; personality traits; adaptive and maladaptive be-

haviors; involvement in social groups; feelings of happiness, inclusion, and safety
- *Adolescent development:* academic and social comfort and performance; feeling of being loved by family; relationships with peers, authority figures, parents, extended family; dating history; sexual activities; physical, emotional, or sexual abuse; delinquency
- *Adult development:* satisfaction with life; dating and marital history; patterns of behavior in relationships; academic, military, and occupational history; self-esteem; independence; social interaction; relationships with family, children, in-laws, and neighbors; community standing; employment status and stability; future aspirations
- *Medication history:* anxiolytic agents, antidepressants, antipsychotics, antimanic agents, analgesics, sedative-hypnotics, hormone replacement therapy, other prescribed medications, alcohol, illicit drugs
- *Diagnostic tests:* Minnesota Multiphasic Personality Inventory, Wechsler Adult Intelligence Survey, Myers-Briggs Type Indicator, Fundamental Interpersonal Relations Orientation-Behavior, State-Trait Anxiety Inventory, Beck Depression Inventory, Marital Attitudes Evaluation, Thematic Apperception Test

DEFINING CHARACTERISTICS

- Anxiety, compulsions, denial
- Codependent role models
- Depression or diminished self-esteem
- Enmeshment or isolation
- Family history of physical abuse or alcoholism

- History of physical, emotional, or sexual abuse
- Hypervigilance
- Lack of education and employment skills
- Limited insight
- Perceived responsibility for or need to control others
- Physical fights with partner
- Refusal of help from others
- Rigid family roles
- Substance abuse
- Use of intimate relationship to separate from family of origin

ASSOCIATED DISORDERS

Intermittent explosive disorder, personality disorders (avoidant personality disorder, borderline personality disorder, dependent personality disorder), posttraumatic stress disorder, substance-related disorders

EXPECTED OUTCOMES

Initial outcomes
- Patient acknowledges impairment in social relationships.
- Patient discusses fears of changing codependent behavior.
- Patient discusses need to take greater interest in his own life and activities.
- Patient discusses his level of self-esteem, his emotional history, and his current behavior.
- Patient sets goals for improvement and seeks support and therapy.

Interim outcomes
- Patient recognizes controlling behavior.

- Patient improves ability to recognize problems and use problem-solving skills.
- Patient recognizes lack of assertiveness.
- Patient discusses irrational beliefs.
- Patient receives information about individual, group, and 12-step programs.
- Patient describes aspects of healthy relationships.
- Patient reduces codependent behavior.

Discharge outcomes
- Patient discusses connection between social impairment and codependence.
- Patient demonstrates improved social interactions.
- Patient demonstrates increased assertiveness.
- Patient participates in ongoing therapy or programs.
- Patient identifies characteristics of positive intimate relationship.
- Patient reports improved self-esteem.

INTERVENTIONS AND RATIONALES

Initial interventions
- Assess the patient's history *to diagnose his condition and determine treatment.*
- Help the patient identify behaviors and feelings associated with social relationships *to foster recognition of potential areas for growth.*
- Instruct the patient to examine problems in small units or steps *to avoid becoming overwhelmed.*

- Help the patient recognize his lack of assertiveness *to increase his self-awareness and sense of responsibility for his own behavior.*
- Reassure the patient that his fears will be addressed gradually *to lessen his anxiety and maintain motivation.*
- Discuss the quality of the patient's interpersonal relationships and help him express his fear of intimate relationships *to increase his self-awareness and help him establish goals for improving his social life.*
- Help the patient identify personal strengths *to increase his hope of success.*

Interim interventions
- Help the patient identify his unproductive methods of social interactions *to identify areas of growth.*
- Discuss the history of his codependent behavior *to help him understand how repeated codependent behavior patterns have affected his life.*
- Support the patient's efforts to change behavior *to provide encouragement and build trust in the therapeutic relationship.*
- Teach assertiveness skills *to help the patient adapt new behaviors.*
- Explain that new behaviors can produce anxiety, but will become comfortable with experience *to help sustain healthy behavior.*
- Discuss requirements for participating in group therapy *to foster an informed decision and increase the patient's responsibility for himself.*
- Discuss characteristics of a healthy intimate relationship *to help the patient form realistic expectations of himself and others.*

- Help the patient differentiate between social and intimate relationships *to promote healthy boundaries.*
- Ask the patient to identify activities that foster self-esteem. Assign homework exercises to help him identify personal strengths and techniques for improving self-esteem *to strengthen his commitment to change.*

Discharge interventions
- Work with the patient to develop a plan for improving his opportunities for social interaction *to provide ongoing therapy.*
- Role-play situations in which the patient is prone to codependent behavior *to allow him to practice alternative methods of responding to others.*
- Role-play situations that encourage the patient to use assertiveness skills *to increase his proficiency in using these skills.*
- Praise the patient for successful behavior changes *to help him assume more responsibility for his behavior.*
- Demonstrate use of relaxation techniques, cognitive reframing, and thought stopping *to increase the patient's control of his own behavior.*
- Encourage participation in a fitness program *to foster self-care.*
- Monitor the patient's initial response to the treatment program *to help ensure ongoing participation.*
- Support the patient's attempts to form intimate relationship *to promote personal growth.*
- Encourage participation in ongoing therapy *to enable the patient to get further reality testing, feedback, and support.*

EVALUATION STATEMENTS

Patient:
- identifies problems in interpersonal relations.
- identifies situations that may increase codependent behavior.
- discusses progress toward goals.
- reports increased comfort with acting assertively.
- reports decreased anxiety related to social interactions.
- demonstrates increased skill in personal interactions.
- identifies qualities of healthy social interactions and interpersonal relationships.
- reports improved self-esteem.

DOCUMENTATION

- Patient's statements indicating dissatisfaction with interpersonal relationships
- Diagnostic test results
- Nursing interventions
- Patient responses to nursing interventions
- Patient's periodic reassessments of problems and goals
- Progress reports of therapy
- Patient's reports of behavior outside therapy
- Completion of homework assignments
- Patient's plans for obtaining ongoing care
- Evaluation statements.

Social isolation

related to dysfunctional interpersonal relations

DEFINITION

Unwanted social isolation that the patient perceives as imposed by others, marked by difficulty in developing satisfying relationships

ASSESSMENT

Cultural status
- *Demographics:* age, sex, level of education, occupation, nationality, race, ethnic group
- *History:* beliefs, values, and attitudes about health and illness; health customs, practices, and rituals
- *Diagnostic test:* Cultural Assessment Guide

Family status
- *Marital status*
- *Family roles:* formal and informal roles, role performance, degree of family agreement on each member's role, interrelationships of roles
- *Physical and emotional needs:* ability of family to meet the patient's physical and emotional needs, disparities between patient's needs and family's willingness or ability to meet them
- *Coping patterns:* major life events and their meanings to each family member; usual coping patterns; evidence of physical, sexual, or emotional abuse
- *Socioeconomic factors:* economic status of family, sense of adequacy and

self-worth of family members, employment status, attitudes toward work, religious identification, influence of religious beliefs on values and daily practices
- *Family communication:* style and quality of communication, methods of conflict resolution

Psychological status
- *History:* developmental milestones, earliest memories, significant losses, relationships with peers, religious or social group involvement, evidence of antisocial behavior, symptoms of depression
- *Diagnostic tests:* Hamilton Rating Scale for Depression, Beck Depression Inventory, Minnesota Multiphasic Personality Inventory

Neurologic status
- *Mental status:* appearance and attitude, level of consciousness, motor activity, thought and speech, mood and affect, perceptions, orientation, memory, general information, calculations, capacity to read and write, visual-spatial ability, attention span, abstraction, judgment and insight

Social status
- *History:* conversational skills, interpersonal skills, size of social network, quality of relationships, degree of trust in others, level of self-esteem, ability to function in social and occupational roles, use of alcohol and drugs to provide recreation and socialization
- *Signs and symptoms:* withdrawal, lack of eye contact, lack of social interaction

- *Diagnostic test:* Social Adjustment Scale

DEFINING CHARACTERISTICS

- Bizarre behavior
- Difficulty with English language or recent move to the United States
- Living alone, with few friends and no nearby family support
- Poor social group involvement
- Recent divorce, death in family, or loss of job

ASSOCIATED DISORDERS

Anxiety disorder, dementia, mental retardation, mood disorder, personality disorders (antisocial, avoidant, borderline, paranoid, schizoid, schizotypal), schizophrenia

EXPECTED OUTCOMES

Initial outcomes
- Patient talks about feelings of isolation.
- Patient identifies behaviors that led to social isolation.

Interim outcomes
- Patient spends specified amount of time with other people.
- Patient appears comfortable interacting with others.

Discharge outcome
- Patient plans continued involvement with social groups, recreational activities, family, and job.

INTERVENTIONS AND RATIONALES

Initial interventions

- Assess the patient's primary spoken language and provide an interpreter if needed *to facilitate communication, to reduce feelings of anxiety, and to ensure effective teaching.*
- Establish a trusting relationship *to allow the patient to express himself.*
- Demonstrate eye contact, appropriate physical boundaries, and other socially appropriate behaviors *to provide a model for the patient to imitate.*
- Help the patient identify causes for his social isolation *to assess his perception of the problem.*
- Help the patient express his social goals *to begin the process of setting realistic goals and moving toward them.*

Interim interventions

- Encourage the patient to participate in unit activities *to enable him to practice newly acquired social skills.*
- Explore possible avenues for recreational, social, and occupational involvement. *This helps form social contacts, decreases depression and dysfunction, and provides alternatives to isolation.*
- Encourage the patient to increase the level of his social contact gradually *to avoid becoming overwhelmed.*

Discharge interventions

- Encourage the patient to describe positive changes in his relationships with others. *Self-evaluation allows the patient to see progress and thus reduces his feelings of rejection.*
- Help the patient locate community resources and support groups *to decrease isolation and provide support.*
- Reinforce efforts by family and friends to strengthen their relationship with the patient. *The patient may benefit most from renewing ties with family and friends.*
- Provide the patient with numbers for suicide prevention and mental health hot lines *so he can reach out in the most frightening times of his transition from isolation.*

EVALUATION STATEMENTS

Patient:

- communicates effectively to staff members.
- identifies goals for increasing level of social activity.
- participates in unit activities.
- plans specific social activities for after his discharge.

DOCUMENTATION

- Diagnostic test results
- Patient's expression of loneliness
- Patient's participation in group activities and social behavior on the unit
- Behavioral changes suggested by staff members that help decrease loneliness
- Resources provided to patient for ongoing care
- Communication with family members and friends and their responses
- Evaluation statements.

Social isolation

related to homelessness

DEFINITION

Lack of connection to others, identification with a community, or access to resources, such as housing, food, and physical care

ASSESSMENT

Cultural status
- *Demographics:* age, sex, level of education, occupation, nationality, race, ethnic group
- *History:* beliefs, values, and attitudes about health and illness

Nutritional status
- *History:* nutritional deficiencies; cachexia; food, drug, or environmental allergies
- *Physical examination:* height, weight, skin color and turgor
- *Laboratory tests:* hemoglobin and hematocrit; cholesterol, triglyceride, serum iron, serum albumin, and electrolyte levels

Psychological status
- *Developmental history:* history of violence, legal difficulties, family history, medication history, circumstances leading to homelessness
- *Current illness:* episodes of mental illness, hospitalizations, drug or alcohol dependency, affective state, orientation, level of cognition and thought, short- and long-term memory

- *Personal resources:* family, friends, church, homeless companions
- *Diagnostic tests:* Folstein Mini-Mental Health Status Examination, Brief Psychiatric Rating Scale, Hamilton Rating Scale for Depression or Zung Self-Rating Depression Scale

Self-care status
- *History:* neurologic, sensory, or psychological impairment; ability to carry out voluntary activities; use of adaptive equipment, devices, or supplies
- *Living conditions:* shelter, safety, adequacy of clothing, access to medical resources
- *Diagnostic test:* Self-Care Assessment Tool

DEFINING CHARACTERISTICS

- Emotional or geographic separation from family
- History of alcohol and drug abuse or use of neuroleptics
- History of violent or criminal behavior
- Male, over age 35, with low level of education and evidence of mental illness

ASSOCIATED DISORDERS

Amnestic or other cognitive disorders, bipolar disorder, delirium, dementia, personality disorders, schizophrenia, substance- or alcohol-related disorder. Also may be associated with untreated physical conditions, such as diabetes mellitus, and skin disorders that are aggravated by the patient's limited access to care.

EXPECTED OUTCOMES

Initial outcomes
- Patient's essential needs for food and safety are met.
- Patient develops sufficient trust to cooperate with assessment.

Interim outcomes
- Patient tolerates being in groups in patient community for increasing periods of time.
- Patient accepts treatment for medical and psychiatric condition.

Discharge outcome
- Patient accepts placement in or some connection to a community agency.

INTERVENTIONS AND RATIONALES

Initial interventions
- Act as a patient advocate *to obtain needed services for the patient.*
- Develop or participate in a community outreach program. *Because of mental illness and alienation from society, homeless patients may be reluctant to enter a hospital or clinic.*
- Demonstrate patience and tolerance as you complete the patient's assessment. If necessary, assess him in several brief sessions, not one thorough session, *to accommodate his intolerance for company. The homeless patient may have had bad experiences with the system in the past; overcoming fears and distrust will take time.*
- Meet basic needs for food, comfort, and sense of safety before pursuing issues related to social isolation *to help*

ensure the patient's well-being and build trust.
- Introduce the patient gradually to the therapeutic community, tolerating absence or withdrawal from groups at first, *to allow the patient time to learn to trust new contacts. The homeless patient may require a great deal of time and patience to overcome a long-standing distrust of others.*

Interim interventions
- Explain all treatment measures to the patient and seek his permission to contact family members or community resources *to maintain trust.*
- Provide positive reinforcement for socially acceptable behaviors, such as efforts to improve hygiene and table manners, *so that others will be more accepting of the patient.*
- Offer encouragement in a manner that shows respect for the patient *so he doesn't feel you are talking down to him.*
- Maintain professional objectivity at all times in your relationship with the patient. Don't turn away from the patient, but also don't become too personally involved. If he makes inappropriate remarks, don't personalize them. *The patient may have deficient social skills and not be ready for an intense interpersonal relationship; your objectivity and patience will enable him to take first steps at relating to others.*
- Encourage the patient to gradually increase his participation in group activities in the hospital or shelter *to foster social skills in a safe environment and enhance connections with others.*
- Involve the patient in meetings with representatives from community agencies, church groups, survival services, and medical staff *to foster his commit-*

ment to the treatment plan and provide an opportunity to test newly acquired social skills.

Discharge interventions
- Keep the patient hospitalized until minimal social function is possible *to help him maintain any established community ties and resources.*
- Work with the treatment team *to develop appropriate referral options and community connections.*

EVALUATION STATEMENTS

Patient:
- exhibits decreased distrust of others.
- participates in group activities to the extent possible.
- seeks out social interaction with trusted treatment team members.
- shows diminished physical and psychiatric symptoms.
- expresses positive attitudes toward discharge plan.
- expresses willingness to maintain community contacts.

DOCUMENTATION

- Diagnostic test results
- Patient's statements indicating his degree of comfort with social contact
- Nursing interventions
- Patient's response to nursing interventions
- Information about the patient's relationship with family, other homeless people, church groups, or other community resources
- Patient's comments about treatment and discharge plans
- Evaluation statements.

Social isolation

related to illness or disability

DEFINITION

Unwanted social isolation resulting from a combination of physical, psychological, social, and environmental factors

ASSESSMENT

Cultural status
- *Demographics:* age, sex, marital status, level of education, nationality, race, ethnic group, religion, area of residence (rural, suburban or urban), type of residence (house, apartment, high-rise, with or without handicap access)
- *History:* beliefs, values, and attitudes about health and illness; health customs, practices, and rituals
- *Diagnostic test:* Cultural Assessment Guide

Neurologic status
- *Mental status:* appearance and attitude, affect and mood, thought and speech, orientation, judgment, memory, insight and calculation, levels of consciousness
- *Physical examination:* motor function, sensory function, reflexes

Family status
- *Family roles:* formal and informal roles, role performance, degree of family agreement on each member's role, interrelationships of roles

- *Family communication:* style and quality of communication, methods of conflict resolution
- *Family subsystems:* effect of family alliances on individual members and family as a unit
- *Physical and emotional needs:* family's ability to meet the patient's physical and emotional needs, disparities between patient's needs and family's willingness or ability to meet them
- *Socioeconomic factors:* economic status of family, sense of adequacy and self-worth of family members, employment status, attitudes toward work, religious identification, influence of religious beliefs on values and daily practices
- *Coping patterns:* major life events and their meaning to each family member, usual coping patterns, patient's perception of effectiveness of coping patterns
- *Family health history:* psychiatric illness, stress-related illness, medical illness, suicide, substance abuse, mental retardation; history of violence, physical, emotional, or sexual abuse
- *Diagnostic tests:* Family Environment Scale, Family Adjustment Device, Family Genogram

Psychological status

- *Impact of current illness:* changes in personal hygiene, self-image, or self-esteem; impact on daily functioning; use of alcohol or drugs to cope
- *Psychiatric history:* presence of psychiatric disorder, age at onset, type and severity of symptoms, impact on daily functioning, type of treatment, patient's response to treatment
- *Developmental history:* higher education, occupation and job changes,

dating and marital history, hobbies and recreational activities, spirituality, feelings related to illness and disability
- *Laboratory tests:* urinalysis, hemoglobin and hematocrit, electrolyte and blood glucose levels, thyroid function tests, blood and urine drug toxicology screening
- *Diagnostic tests:* Brief Psychiatric Rating Scale, Hamilton Rating Scale for Depression

Self-care status

- *History:* presence of neurologic, sensory, motor, or psychologic impairment; ability to carry out voluntary activities; ability to perform activities of daily living; use of adaptive equipment, devices, or supplies
- *Physical examination:* gait, fine motor dexterity, activity tolerance, safety of environment
- *Diagnostic tests:* Functional Ability Scale, Self-Care Assessment Tool

Sensory status

- *History:* neurologic or musculoskeletal disease or injury; visual or hearing loss; use of glasses, hearing aids, crutches, or walker; tobacco, alcohol, or illicit drug use; medications
- *Signs and symptoms:* visual hallucinations, blurred vision, ptosis, auditory hallucinations, cerumen, tinnitus, vertigo, pain
- *Physical examination:* vision, hearing, tactile sense
- *Diagnostic tests:* Snellen eye chart, hearing acuity test

Social status

- *History:* conversational skills, interpersonal skills, size of social network, quality of relationships, degree of

trust in others, level of self-esteem, ability to function in social roles
- *Factors interfering with social activity:* physical or psychological impairment, access to and from home, safety of neighborhood, access to public transportation and telephone
- *Signs and symptoms:* withdrawal, lack of eye contact, inability to socialize due to environmental obstacles
- *Diagnostic test:* Social Adjustment Scale

DEFINING CHARACTERISTICS

- Discomfort in social situations
- Expression of feeling of rejection
- Inability to tell others of need for social interaction
- Ineffective social skills and insecurity in public
- Lack of a significant purpose in life
- Lack of supportive family or friends
- Limited mobility or institutionalization
- Living alone
- Physical or mental handicap or onset of illness
- Sad, dull affect; withdrawn; uncommunicative

ASSOCIATED DISORDERS AND TREATMENTS

Acquired immunodeficiency syndrome, arthritis, cancer, cerebrovascular accident, depressive disorder, head or neck surgery, hearing loss, hepatitis, human immunodeficiency virus (HIV) encephalopathy, HIV infection, incontinence, Kaposi's sarcoma, mood disorders, organic brain syndrome, osteoporosis, Parkinson's disease, personality disorders, *Pneumocystis car-*

inii pneumonia, schizophrenia, spinal cord injuries, tuberculosis, vision loss

EXPECTED OUTCOMES

Initial outcomes
- Patient admits that his social relationships are inadequate.
- Patient describes his disease and how it contributes to social isolation.
- Patient expresses grief over loss of social independence caused by the limitations of his disease.

Interim outcomes
- Patient asks for help in increasing social activity.
- Patient interacts with family members, spouse, partner, or members of the health care team.
- Patient gradually increases his level of participation in social activities.

Discharge outcomes
- Patient makes use of hospital or community support groups and other social resources.
- Patient reports an improvement in social relationships and decreased feelings of social isolation.

INTERVENTIONS AND RATIONALES

Initial interventions
- Spend sufficient time with the patient to allow him to express concern over the effect of his illness on his social life (10 minutes each shift, for example) *to foster trust.*
- Help the patient identify factors that contribute to social isolation *to identify his needs and match them to available resources.*

- Ask about physical limitations (secondary to illness), emotional barriers, and environmental factors such as lack of transportation *to help him focus on specific issues instead of general complaints.*
- Encourage the patient to express feelings associated with increased dependence on others *to help relieve his anger.*

Interim interventions
- Involve the patient and the family (if appropriate) in planning his care *to individualize care and reduce feelings of dependency and helplessness.*
- Encourage the patient to communicate his needs assertively to others. *By being assertive, the patient assumes responsibility for getting his needs met in an honest manner, without anger or guilt that frequently accompanies feelings of helplessness.*
- Encourage social interaction between the patient and others. Begin by encouraging short visits with people he feels will not reject him *to foster feelings of acceptance and support.*
- As the patient's comfort level and social skills improve, encourage him to participate in group activities. *Gradually increasing activities helps to reduce the patient's feeling of being overwhelmed.*
- Help the patient identify social activities he can initiate independently, such as calling friends on the phone or writing letters, *to foster feelings of control and contact with others.*
- Help the patient accept the fact that other people may view him differently because of his illness and explore ways of coping with their reactions. *The stigma associated with illness is a reality*

and the patient must learn to cope with it.

Discharge interventions
- Provide positive feedback for effective social interaction *to help the patient recognize his own progress and enhance his self-esteem.*
- Offer referrals to support groups *to help the patient achieve increased social independence.*
- Contact and make referrals to appropriate social service agencies *to provide continuity of care.*

EVALUATION STATEMENTS

Patient:
- describes factors contributing to social isolation.
- seeks assistance to increase social contacts.
- interacts with family, friends, and caregivers.
- accepts assistance with increasing social contacts.
- reports an increase in social contacts.
- describes decreased feelings of social isolation and fear of rejection.

DOCUMENTATION

- Diagnostic test results and laboratory findings
- Patient statements indicating dissatisfaction with social relationships
- Observations of patient's social skills
- Identified causes of patient's social isolation
- Nursing interventions to encourage social interaction
- Patient's response to nursing interventions

- Appropriate resources identified for patient
- Referrals to social service agencies
- Evaluation statements.

Spiritual distress

related to diagnosis of terminal illness

DEFINITION

Feelings of alienation from God, due to the patient's inability to reconcile his fatal illness with his religious or spiritual convictions

ASSESSMENT

Cultural status
- *Demographics:* age, sex, level of education, occupation, nationality, race, ethnic group
- *History:* beliefs, values, and attitudes about dying; health customs, practices, and rituals
- *Diagnostic test:* Cultural Assessment Guide

Family status
- *Marital status*
- *Family roles:* formal and informal roles, role performance, degree of family agreement on each members' role, interrelationships of roles, changes the patient perceives his death will make in family functioning
- *Family rules:* rules that foster stability, maladaptive rules, methods of modifying family rules

- *Family communication:* style and quality of communication, methods of conflict resolution
- *Physical and emotional needs:* family's ability to meet the patient's physical and emotional needs
- *Family goals and values:* extent to which family permits pursuit of individual goals and values; importance of religious identification to family members; extent to which religion defines values systems, norms, and practices
- *Coping patterns:* major life events and their meaning to each family member, usual coping patterns, family's perception of effectiveness of coping patterns

Psychological status
- *Current illness:* changes in appetite, energy level, motivation, personal hygiene, self-image, self-esteem, sleep pattern, sexual drive
- *Medical condition:* apparent symptoms, diagnosis, prognosis, chronology of illness; changes to the patient's usual lifestyle and his ability to pursue life goals; meaning attached to medical condition
- *Life changes:* recent divorce, job loss, onset or exacerbation of medical condition, feelings of responsibility for his condition, manifestations of the disease and the degree to which they impair functioning
- *Diagnostic tests:* Brief Psychiatric Rating Scale, Mini–Mental Status Examination

Social status
- *Signs and symptoms:* withdrawal, lack of eye contact, intrusiveness, inappropriate responses, decreased self-

esteem, diminished ability to function in social and occupational roles
- *Diagnostic test:* Social Adjustment Scale

Spiritual status
- *History:* religious affiliation, current perception of faith and religious practices, spiritual beliefs linked to current distress, change in usual spiritual practices, relationship between spiritual beliefs and everyday living (life-affirming and life-denying influences), unmet spiritual needs (meaning and purpose, love and relatedness, forgiveness)
- *Signs and symptoms:* crying, fanaticism, despair, withdrawal
- *Diagnostic tests:* Spiritual and Religious Concerns Questionnaire, Spiritual Well-Being Scale, Meaning in Suffering Test

DEFINING CHARACTERISTICS

- Anger toward God, church, or religious representatives in response to diagnosis of terminal illness and its manifestations
- Bargaining with God as a stage of anticipatory grieving
- Belief that spirituality or religion plays major role in giving life meaning and purpose
- Changes in sleep patterns or spiritual practices
- Expressions of need for meaning and purpose, love and belonging, healing and reconciliation
- Failure of religious beliefs to serve as effective means of coping

ASSOCIATED DISORDERS

Any newly diagnosed terminal illness, such as acquired immunodeficiency syndrome, amyotrophic lateral sclerosis, cancer, end-stage cardiac, renal, or pulmonary disease

EXPECTED OUTCOMES

Initial outcome
- Patient identifies the spiritual or religious beliefs that precipitated feelings of distress about his condition.

Interim outcomes
- Patient explores spiritual or religious beliefs with a trusted religious advisor.
- Patient makes a conscious decision to affirm, modify, or reject these beliefs.
- Patient identifies the positive and negative aspects of using faith to give meaning to the experience of illness.
- Patient evaluates the extent to which faith will help him cope with illness.

Discharge outcome
- Patient identifies a trusted spiritual or religious advisor, or if unavailable, appropriate resources, to help with his continued exploration of how faith can provide meaning for the experience of illness.

INTERVENTIONS AND RATIONALES

Initial interventions
- Actively listen to the patient's thoughts on spiritual matters. *Acknowledging spiritual issues validates their importance.*

- Help the patient identify the conflict between spiritual or religious beliefs and the diagnosis of terminal illness. For example, the patient may say, "If God knows me and wants the best for me, then He wouldn't let me have a terminal illness." *Values and beliefs that helped in the past may no longer be useful to the patient as he confronts terminal illness.*

Interim interventions
- Ask the patient if he wishes to discuss spiritual concerns with a chosen religious authority *to allow access to expert spiritual care resources.*
- If the patient chooses to consult a trusted religious advisor, arrange a meeting and explain to both parties the importance of clarifying spiritual or religious beliefs *to help the patient affirm, modify, or reject his beliefs.*
- Help the patient identify positive and negative ways in which faith can be used to give meaning to the experience of terminal illness *to help him evaluate the extent to which beliefs help or hinder his ability to cope.*
- Describe the stages of grieving and the emotions and behaviors characteristic of each stage *to help the patient realize that his experiences are normal.*
- Help the patient develop a plan that uses faith to enhance his ability to cope with terminal illness. For example, suggest spiritual readings, attending his place of worship, visiting church members, or other activities. *Planning engages the patient in accepting the diagnosis and is essential for coping with the long-term effects of his illness.*
- Give the patient permission to express his anger toward God. Use active listening to provide an opportunity for him to vent his feelings, or encourage him to punch a pillow or use another safe physical outlet *to relieve tension.*

Discharge intervention
- Encourage the patient to continue to pursue a meaningful dialogue with his chosen spiritual advisor. If his personal spiritual advisor is not available, recommend community-based spiritual resources *to foster the patient's continued exploration of how faith provides meaning for the experience of illness.*

EVALUATION STATEMENTS

Patient:
- identifies the conflict between spiritual or religious beliefs and the diagnosis of terminal illness.
- decides to affirm, modify, or reject religious beliefs.
- identifies positive and negative ways faith can be used to give meaning to the experience of illness.
- evaluates the extent to which faith helps him cope with illness.
- contacts a trusted spiritual or religious leader to help him explore how to use faith to facilitate coping.

DOCUMENTATION

- Diagnostic test results
- Patient's behaviors and reports that signal spiritual distress
- Nursing interventions to help the patient identify the causes of his spiritual distress
- Patient response to visits by a spiritual or religious leader

- Nursing interventions to encourage the patient's positive use of spiritual or religious beliefs
- Patient response to nursing interventions
- Referral to spiritual resources in the community
- Evaluation statements.

Spiritual distress

related to perceived separation from a religious source of hope, strength, and meaning

DEFINITION

Perceived loss of spiritual source of hope or alienation from religious beliefs

ASSESSMENT

Cultural status
- *Demographics* age, sex, level of education, occupation, nationality, ethnic group
- *History:* beliefs, values, and attitudes about health and illness; health customs, practices, and rituals

Psychological status
- *Developmental history:* recent life changes, psychiatric history, substance abuse
- *Signs and symptoms:* changes in appetite, energy level, motivation, personal hygiene, self-image, self-esteem, sleep pattern, sexual drive

Spiritual status
- *History:* religious affiliation; current religious practices and beliefs; beliefs about purpose of life; perception of meaning in suffering; perception of relations between self, others, nature, and God; support network; effects of religious belief on management of stress and maintenance of self-esteem
- *Medical history:* illnesses that cause a change in body image, chronic illness, terminal illness
- *Signs and symptoms:* crying, fanaticism, despair, withdrawal
- *Diagnostic tests:* Spiritual and Religious Concerns Questionnaire, Spiritual Well-Being Scale

DEFINING CHARACTERISTICS

- Anger over current dilemma directed at God or clergy
- Desire for spiritual assistance
- Failure to obtain sufficient support, hope, and meaning from religious values
- Inability to obtain relief from stress and suffering through practice of religious routines
- Low self-esteem, anxiety, depression, impaired cognitive functioning
- Perception that current illness has no meaning

ASSOCIATED CONDITIONS

This diagnosis may be seen in any hospitalized or home care patient, depending on the individual and the circumstances.

EXPECTED OUTCOMES

Initial outcomes
- Patient discusses feelings related to loss of a source of spiritual strength.

- Patient identifies issues that led to spiritual distress.

Interim outcomes
- Patient identifies activities that increase sense of spiritual hope, strength, and meaning.
- Patient practices spiritual activities.

Discharge outcomes
- Patient expresses increased feelings of hope and strength.
- Patient describes plans to maintain contact with spiritual source of hope and strength after discharge.

INTERVENTIONS AND RATIONALES

Initial interventions
- Actively listen to the patient's thoughts on spiritual matters. *Acknowledging spiritual issues validates their importance.*
- Explore the patient's feelings about loss of spiritual hope and strength. Listen for statements, such as, "I have been abandoned by everyone, even God" or, "Why would God allow this to happen to me?" *Listening conveys interest and respect and allows the patient to clarify his spiritual beliefs.*
- Convey a nonjudgmental attitude toward the patient's feelings and beliefs. To convey this attitude, you must be comfortable with your own beliefs. *Acceptance by others promotes self-acceptance and helps the patient explore spiritual questions.*
- Provide comfort as the patient begins to express strong emotions. Stay with him. If the patient finds touching acceptable, pat his hand or hug him.

Therapeutic touch conveys support and strengthens the therapeutic relationship.

Interim interventions
- Assist the patient in identifying factors that interfere with his usual spiritual beliefs and practices. *Identification of the problem is the first step in resolution.*
- Brainstorm with the patient to find possible solutions to his spiritual crisis, such as acquiring religious literature, visiting with clergy, making special dietary accommodations, or scheduling time for religious activities. *Involvement of the patient in finding solutions maintains his sense of responsibility for his own spiritual well-being.*
- Provide verbal reinforcement for the patient's efforts to resolve spiritual crisis. *Reinforced behaviors are more likely to be repeated.*

Discharge interventions
- Encourage the patient to discuss plans for maintaining spiritual practices after discharge, such as setting aside time each day for prayer or meditation. *Because the hospital stay is short-term, behavioral changes must be reinforced to prevent recurrence.*
- Assist the patient in identifying community groups that could provide spiritual support *to prevent development of future crises.*

EVALUATION STATEMENTS

Patient:
- expresses feelings of distress related to his perception of the absence of hope or meaning in current illness.
- lists the events that led to his spiritual crisis.

- discusses usual religious practices that contribute to spiritual well-being.
- requests assistance from clergy.
- expresses feelings of spiritual comfort.
- discusses plans for continuing contact with sources of spiritual comfort after discharge.

DOCUMENTATION

- Diagnostic test results
- Patient's reports of spiritual distress
- Observations of the patient's physical, mental, and emotional status
- Nursing interventions
- Patient's response to nursing interventions
- Evaluation statements.

Thermoregulation, ineffective

related to neuroleptic malignant syndrome

DEFINITION

Ineffective regulation of hypothalamic control of autonomic nervous system caused by use of neuroleptic medications, resulting in severe fluctuations of body temperature

ASSESSMENT

Cardiovascular status
- *Physical examination:* temperature, pulse, respirations, blood pressure
- *Signs and symptoms:* tachycardia, hypertension

- *Laboratory tests:* serum creatinine, phosphokinase, and electrolyte levels

Genitourinary status
- *Signs and symptoms:* incontinence
- *Laboratory tests:* blood urea nitrogen, urinalysis

Integumentary status
- *Skin characteristics:* color, elasticity, texture, turgor
- *Medications:* neuroleptics
- *Signs and symptoms:* diaphoresis

Musculoskeletal status
- *Physical examination:* range of motion of all joints, coordination and gait, muscle strength, functional mobility
- *Signs and symptoms:* rigidity, akinesia, dysarthria, pain or tenderness on movement

Neurologic status
- *Mental status:* appearance, level of consciousness, motor activity, thought and speech, orientation, memory, attention span
- *Motor system:* muscle tone and strength, gait
- *Sensory system:* pupillary response, cortical function, peripheral system
- *Reflexes:* deep tendon, superficial
- *Prior medical conditions:* previous incidence of neuroleptic malignant syndrome (NMS), schizophrenia, amnestic or other cognitive disorders, delirium, dementia, mood disorders
- *Medications:* neuroleptics, lithium, selected antidepressants, anesthetic agents, antiparkinsonian agents
- *Signs and symptoms:* hyperthermia, psychomotor agitation, alterations in

consciousness, dysphagia, apprehension, mutism, exhaustion
- *Laboratory test:* drug toxicology screen

Respiratory status
- *Physical examination:* skin color; nail and lip color; respiratory rate, depth, and pattern; percussion and auscultation of lung fields
- *Signs and symptoms:* tachypnea
- *Laboratory tests:* arterial blood gas levels; hemoglobin and hematocrit

Psychological status
- *Psychiatric history:* age at onset of illness; type and severity of symptoms; type of treatment; patient's response to treatment; family history of schizophrenia, bipolar disorder, or NMS

RISK FACTORS

- Changes in neuroleptic medication, including adjustment of dosage, change to different medication, combination with lithium or another neuroleptic, or withdrawal of dopaminergic medications
- Diaphoresis
- Fluctuations in blood pressure
- Hyperpyrexia
- Insufficient antiparkinsonian medication
- Metabolic acidosis or hypoxia
- Mild to severe hydration
- Preexisting infections
- Psychomotor agitation
- Rapid deterioration of mental status
- Rapid neuroleptization (series of high-dose neuroleptics in quick succession)
- Severe parkinsonian muscular rigidity
- Tachycardia or tachypnea

- Urinary incontinence
- Use of various psychotropic or non-psychiatric medications

ASSOCIATED DISORDERS AND TREATMENTS

Chemical toxicity (pharmacological reaction); delirium, dementia, and amnestic and other cognitive disorders; mood disorders; schizophrenia; use of psychotropic drugs

EXPECTED OUTCOMES

Initial outcomes
- Patient stops taking neuroleptic medications contributing to disorder.
- Patient maintains normal body temperature, heart rate, and blood pressure.
- Patient begins to decrease psychomotor hyperactivity.
- Patient exhibits improved neurological function.
- Patient undergoes medical care to reduce symptoms of exhaustion and dehydration.
- Patient responds to fluid replacement and treatment of cardiac, respiratory, renal, neurologic, or other complications.

Interim outcomes
- Patient does not experience adverse effects in response to medication administration.
- Members of the treatment team review the patient's medication and make recommendations for future pharmacologic interventions.

Discharge outcomes

- Patient is free of psychomotor agitation.
- Patient and family members express understanding of the need for follow-up care.
- Patient and family members identify the signs and symptoms of NMS.
- Patient returns to baseline physiologic parameters without any permanent damage.
- Patient expresses understanding of his medication's indications, dosage, adverse effects, and precautions, and the need for follow-up monitoring.

INTERVENTIONS AND RATIONALES

Initial interventions

- Discontinue neuroleptic medications immediately *because they are the causative agents of NMS.*
- If the patient's condition deteriorates, transfer him to the medical intensive care unit. *The patient's life may be at risk if he develops cardiac arrhythmias, infarction, or failure; respiratory, renal or neurologic complications; hypoxia; hyperthermia; organic amnestic syndromes; peripheral neuropathy; or hematological complications.*
- Monitor vital signs and intake and output every 4 hours *to determine the effectiveness of therapy.*
- For the first week of treatment, assess the patient's neurological status every 4 hours. *Rapid deterioration of mental status is an important indicator of the severity of the syndrome.*
- Request orders to administer appropriate medications or dialysis *to alleviate symptoms, as needed.*

- Force fluids *to counteract the effects of dehydration and hyperthermia.*
- Consult a dietitian for special diet. *The patient may be too active to sit for meals and may require finger foods.*
- Request anticonstipation medications as necessary, *since this limited diet can affect bowel movements.*
- Try to limit the patient's psychomotor agitation by involving him in quiet activities, scheduling rest and sleep periods, using a quiet room, or engaging him in discussion. *The least restrictive methods of controlling psychomotor agitation should be tried first.* Assess the effectiveness of your interventions.
- As a last resort, consider use of physical restraint to limit psychomotor hyperactivity. *Restraint may allow the patient to experience a period of rest. However, if the patient fights restraint, it may be counterproductive.*

Interim interventions

- Continue to monitor the patient throughout his hospital stay and outpatient follow-up *to detect subtle changes in his health status.*
- Although sedatives may be needed, be mindful that the patient's agitation may be an adverse effect of medications already being administered. *The patient can get trapped in a cycle: Medications help cause NMS, but are also needed to treat the condition.*
- Review the patient's past medication history *to make recommendations regarding future pharmacologic interventions.* Involve all team members in assessment of the patient's medication regimen and be prepared to serve as a consultant to other health care professionals. *NMS may be self-limiting once the medication regimen is adjusted.*

Discharge interventions
- Teach the patient and family members about signs and symptoms of NMS and its relationship to neuroleptic therapy *to allow them to take an active role in health maintenance.*
- Teach the patient and family members about follow-up care and the likelihood of recurrence *to encourage compliance with the medical regimen. Family members may need to obtain medical attention for the patient if he is physically or psychologically unable to do so.*
- Explain to the patient and family members how to recognize signs of psychomotor agitation that may require immediate treatment *to foster compliance and help lessen the stigma associated with psychomotor agitation.*
- Explain to the patient that the treatment team is using the most recent research findings to prescribe medications that have the least probability of causing adverse effects and future episodes of NMS. *The patient may be afraid to comply with the medication program following NMS.*
- Work with the outpatient case managers to develop a discharge plan for the patient. He will require ongoing monitoring of his physical status and medications *because one episode of NMS increases the risk of further episodes. A comprehensive discharge plan decreases the likelihood of further serious complications.*

EVALUATION STATEMENTS

Patient:
- shows no evidence of permanent medical complications.
- tolerates tapering of medications to lowest therapeutic dosage.
- maintains normal body temperature, heart rate, and blood pressure.
- maintains hydration, bowel and bladder habits, and skin integrity.
- understands the rationale for physical restraints.
- expresses understanding of the physiology of NMS
- agrees that the adjusted medication regimen is acceptable.
- agrees to adhere to continued treatment.

DOCUMENTATION

- Results of physical examination, laboratory findings, and neurologic assessment
- Patient's intake and output
- Nursing interventions
- Patient's response to nursing interventions
- Results of ongoing monitoring of patient's condition
- Patient's response to new medication regimen
- Patient's perception of problem
- Evaluation statements.

Thought process alteration
related to delusional thinking

DEFINITION

Inability to process thoughts accurately and correctly because of a fixed, false belief that cannot be corrected by logic

ASSESSMENT

Cultural status

- *Demographics:* age, sex, level of education, occupation, nationality, ethnic group
- *History:* beliefs, values, and attitudes about health and illness; health customs, practices, and rituals

Neurologic status

- *Physical examination:* motor activity, cranial nerve function, cerebellar function, sensory system
- *Mental status:* appearance and attitude, level of consciousness, thought and speech, mood and affect, perceptions, judgment, insight, orientation, memory, abstraction, calculations, concentration
- *Medications:* neuroleptics, barbiturates, antimanic agents, antidepressants, narcotics, alcohol, illicit drugs
- *Signs and symptoms:* headache, incoordination, falls, pain, tremors
- *Laboratory tests:* drug toxicology screening, thyroid function tests, serotonin levels, human immunodeficiency virus testing
- *Diagnostic tests:* computed tomography, lumbar puncture, magnetic resonance imaging, electroencephalography, Mini–Mental Status Examination

Psychological status

- *History:* reactions to illness, recent losses, personality traits, number and quality of significant relationships, family history of mental illness, level of emotional functioning
- *Reason for hospitalization:* patient's perception of problem, recent stressors, changes in somatic functioning

- *Signs and symptoms:* behavioral indications of suspicion or mistrust; denial, projection, or rationalization; accusatory statements; statements that are grandiose, contradictory, illogical, or irrelevant; depressive symptoms; hostility
- *Diagnostic tests:* Brief Psychiatric Rating Scale, Hamilton Rating Scale for Depression, Minnesota Multiphasic Personality Inventory

Social status

- *History:* conversational skills, interpersonal skills, size of social network, degree of trust in others, level of self-esteem, ability to function in social and occupational roles
- *Signs and symptoms:* withdrawal, lack of eye contact, intrusiveness, inappropriate responses, social isolation, aggressiveness

DEFINING CHARACTERISTICS

- Behavior based on delusional beliefs
- Behavioral manifestations of anxiety
- Delusions (erotomanic, grandiose, jealous, persecutory, somatic, unspecified)
- Disorientation to time, place, person, circumstances, and events
- Exaggeration
- Impaired ability to reason, think abstractly, or conceptualize
- Inability to distinguish delusion from reality
- Inappropriate interpretation of environment
- Incorporation of mental health professionals, family, or other patients into delusional belief system
- Misinterpretation of words and actions of others

- Thoughts and beliefs not based in reality and not consensually validated

ASSOCIATED DISORDERS

Acquired immunodeficiency syndrome dementia complex, Alzheimer's disease, brain tumor, delusional disorders, dementia, mood disorders, personality disorders, psychotic disorder, psychotic disorders with delusions or hallucinations, schizophrenia, substance- or alcohol-related disorder or withdrawal

EXPECTED OUTCOMES

Initial outcomes
- Patient does not harm self or others.
- Patient complies with medical regimen.
- Patient is oriented to himself and his environment.
- Patient identifies internal and external factors that trigger delusional episodes.

Interim outcomes
- Patient engages in activities to decrease delusions.
- Patient focuses on feelings underlying delusional beliefs.
- Patient takes steps to foster development of social skills.

Discharge outcomes
- Patient considers and develops accurate, reality-based alternatives to meet his needs.
- Patient and family make plans for continued care after discharge.

INTERVENTIONS AND RATIONALES

Initial interventions
- Provide the patient with an area of decreased stimulation such as a quiet room *to enhance safety.*
- Arrange structured visits with the patient and listen actively to him *to project a nonjudgmental attitude.*
- Address the patient by name. Tell him your name *to foster the patient's awareness of himself and his environment.*
- Give short, simple explanations to the patient each time you do something *to avoid confusion.*
- Discuss the importance of adhering to a treatment plan designed to correct any biochemical imbalances *to help decrease his anxiety.*
- Do not argue, reason with, or challenge a patient with delusions; instead, provide comfort and support. *Attempts to correct delusional beliefs will increase his anxiety.*

Interim interventions
- Explore events that trigger delusions. Discuss anxiety associated with triggering events. *Exploring these topics will help you understand the dynamics of the patient's delusional system.*
- Without arguing or agreeing, acknowledge the plausible elements of the delusion. *Delusions usually have some basis in reality. By conveying acceptance of delusions but not belief in them, you can better help the patient.*
- Once the dynamics of the delusions are understood, discourage repetitious talk about delusions and refocus the conversation on the patient's underlying feelings. *As the patient begins to*

learn to cope with his feelings, delusions will become less necessary.

- Teach the patient distraction techniques *to reduce anxiety and fear.*
- Encourage the patient to participate in one-to-one conversation and group activities. Set limits on inappropriate behaviors *to promote development of social skills in a safe atmosphere.*
- Use role modeling to show the patient how to handle social situations that produce anxiety *to promote social development.*

Discharge interventions
- Help the patient find other means of meeting emotional needs. *Delusions usually decrease when needs are met in other ways.*
- Educate the patient and family or companion about signs and symptoms of illness and the effects of medication. *Collaboration with family members promotes continuity of care.*
- Refer the family or companion to appropriate resources to plan for the patient's care after discharge. *This helps provide a comprehensive approach to postdischarge care.*

EVALUATION STATEMENTS

Patient:
- does not harm self or others.
- describes two factors that increase delusions.
- adheres to treatment plan.
- practices at least one distraction technique daily.
- demonstrates increased social skills.
- discusses a reality-based interpretation of events that is validated by another person.

DOCUMENTATION

- Diagnostic test results
- Patient's description of delusion
- Nursing interventions that focus on reality orientation and patient education and patient's response
- Evaluation statements.

Thought process alteration

related to neuropsychiatric manifestations of AIDS

DEFINITION

Inability to process thoughts accurately and correctly because of neurologic effects of acquired immunodeficiency syndrome (AIDS)

ASSESSMENT

Cultural status
- *Demographics:* age, sex, level of education, occupation, nationality, ethnic group
- *History:* beliefs, values, and attitudes about health and illness; health customs, practices, and rituals

Neurologic status
- *Mental status:* abstract thinking; insight regarding present situation; judgment; long- and short-term memory; cognition; orientation to person, place, and time
- *Physical examination:* level of consciousness, sensory ability, fine and gross motor functioning

- *Previous medical conditions:* history of neurologic disorder, head injury, or psychiatric illness

Self-care status
- *History:* eating and drinking, bathing and hygiene, dressing and grooming, toileting, sleep and rest, safety practices

Family status
- *History:* composition of nuclear and extended family, level of communication with family members, degree of separation from family, family's tolerance of patient's choices and decisions, reaction of the family to the patient's AIDS diagnosis

Psychological status
- *Signs and symptoms:* changes in appetite, energy level, motivation, personal hygiene, self-image, self-esteem, sleep pattern, sexual drive, or competence
- *Alcohol or drug abuse:* type of substance, effects on mood and behavior, evidence of abuse or withdrawal, impact on functioning
- *Life changes:* recent divorce, job loss, loss of loved ones
- *Psychiatric history:* age at onset, type and severity of symptoms, impact on functioning, type of treatment, patient's response to treatment

DEFINING CHARACTERISTICS

- Altered attention span; disorientation to time, place, person, events, circumstances
- Clinical evidence of impaired neurologic or psychiatric functioning
- Confabulation

- Human immunodeficiency virus (HIV) positive test result
- Impaired ability to conceptualize, calculate, make decisions, reason, problem-solve, follow directions
- Inappropriate social behaviors
- Memory deficit

ASSOCIATED DISORDERS

AIDS, AIDS dementia complex, HIV infection, HIV encephalopathy, Kaposi's sarcoma, *Pneumocystis carinii* pneumonia

EXPECTED OUTCOMES

Initial outcomes
- Patient maintains orientation to person, place, and time.
- Patient does not sustain injury.

Interim outcomes
- Patient continues to perform activities of daily living (ADLs) to the greatest extent possible.
- Patient demonstrates techniques for coping with memory loss.
- Patient makes necessary decisions as part of planning for progression of illness.
- Family members or companion expresses understanding of care required by patient.

Discharge outcomes
- Family members or companion demonstrates appropriate coping skills as the patient's condition deteriorates.
- Family members or companion identifies available health resources.

INTERVENTIONS AND RATIONALES

Initial interventions

- Observe the patient's thought processes during every shift. Document and report any changes. *Changes may indicate progressive improvement or a decline in the underlying condition.*
- Implement appropriate safety measures to protect the patient from injury. *He may be unable to provide for his own safety needs.*
- Call the patient by name and tell him your name. Provide background information (place, time, date) frequently throughout the day *to provide reality orientation.* Use a reality orientation board *to visually reinforce reality orientation.*

Interim interventions

- Monitor the patient's neurologic signs and level of pain *to assess progression of AIDS.*
- Offer short, simple explanations to the patient each time you carry out any medical regimen *to avoid confusion.*
- Label the patient's personal possessions and photos, keeping them in the same place as much as possible, *to reduce confusion and create a secure environment.*
- Encourage the patient to develop a consistent routine for performing ADLs *to enhance his self-esteem and increase his self-awareness and awareness of environment.*
- Teach the patient ways to cope with memory loss, for example, using a beeper to remind him when to eat or take medications, using a pillbox organized by days of the week, keeping lists in notebooks or a pocket calendar, or having family members or friends remind him of important tasks. *Reminders help to limit the amount of information the patient must maintain in his memory.*
- Assist the patient in making necessary decisions as neuropsychiatric complications progress. These decisions may include assigning durable power of attorney, writing a will, writing a living will, giving up driving a car, stopping work, and making provisions for child care. Help the patient cope with the emotional consequences of decisions *to promote his acceptance of changes brought on by his illness.*
- Encourage family members to discuss familiar occurrences with the patient *to promote a sense of security and comfort.*
- Encourage the patient to voice feelings and concerns about his loss of memory *to reduce anxiety and promote acceptance of his need for additional supervision and care.*
- Help family members or the patient's companion develop the necessary coping skills to deal with the patient *to help ensure their continued involvement in his care.* Teach them what to expect as dementia progresses. The patient may experience increasing memory loss, difficulty concentrating, and increasing apathy marked by a dull affect. Explain to them that when the patient becomes apathetic, it does not mean he is depressed or unhappy, only disconnected *to provide reassurance.* Tell them that the patient will need increased assistance with eating, drinking, dressing, and maintaining hygiene.

Discharge interventions

- Instruct family members or companion on ways to maintain a safe home environment for the patient *to prevent injury.*
- Teach family members or companion to speak to the patient slowly in simple sentences with only a single thought expressed in each sentence *to promote communication and decrease frustration.* Because the patient may have trouble with generalizations, they should make their statements as specific as possible. For example, instead of saying, "We'll go out this afternoon," they should say, "I'll come to your house today at 2:30. Then I'll drive you to the museum."
- Demonstrate reorientation techniques to family members or companion and provide time for supervised return demonstrations. *Informed caregivers will be better prepared to cope with the patient with altered thought processes.*
- Refer the patient, family members, and his companion to community resources *for comprehensive patient care following discharge.*

EVALUATION STATEMENTS

Patient:
- remains free of injury.
- maintains awareness of need for assistance.
- remains oriented to person, place, and time.
- performs ADLs with assistance to the extent possible.
- demonstrates increased skill in coping with memory loss.
- makes necessary decisions to cope with physiologic changes.

Family member or companion:
- identifies partial or complete confusion as part of patient's changing physiologic state.
- reports being able to communicate effectively with patient.
- contacts appropriate resource to arrange home care.

DOCUMENTATION

- Patient's behavior indicating altered thought processes
- Patient's level of pain and measures taken to relieve it
- Nursing interventions performed to facilitate orientation and maintain safety
- Patient's response to nursing interventions
- Family members' or companion's ability to cope with changes in the patient's condition
- Referrals made to professional agencies
- Evaluation statements.

Thought process alteration

related to physiological causes

DEFINITION

Inability to process thoughts accurately and correctly because of physiological causes

ASSESSMENT

Cultural status
- *Demographics:* age, sex, level of education, marital status, nationality

- *History:* beliefs, attitudes, and values about health and illness; health customs, practices, and rituals

Neurologic status
- *Mental status:* appearance and attitude, level of consciousness, motor activity, thought and speech, mood and affect, perceptions, orientation, memory, abstraction, judgment and insight, general information, visual-spatial ability
- *Prior medical conditions:* head injury, brain tumor, Parkinson's disease, multiple sclerosis, dementia, schizophrenia, drug and alcohol abuse, temporal lobe epilepsy
- *Medications:* antianxiety agents, antimanic agents, antidepressants, neuroleptics, antiparkinsonian agents, barbiturates, sedative-hypnotics, antihistamines, amphetamines
- *Signs and symptoms:* lethargy, restlessness, stupor, seizures
- *Diagnostic tests:* Folstein Mini-Mental Status Health Examination, computed tomography scan, magnetic resonance imaging

Psychological status
- *Signs and symptoms:* changes in appetite, energy level, personal hygiene, sleep patterns

Sensory status
- *History:* visual acuity; auditory acuity; use of hearing aid or glasses
- *Prior medical conditions:* hearing loss, neurologic injury, alcohol or drug abuse, psychiatric disorders
- *Physical examination:* visual, auditory, olfactory, gustatory, and tactile examination

- *Signs and symptoms:* visual or auditory hallucinations
- *Diagnostic tests:* Snellen eye chart, Weber test, hearing acuity

Sleep pattern status
- *Medications:* sleeping aids, caffeine, amphetamines
- *Signs and symptoms:* sleep pattern disturbances

Family status
- *Family communication:* style and quality of communication, methods of resolving conflict

DEFINING CHARACTERISTICS

- Altered attention span
- Altered sleep patterns
- Changes in remote, recent, or immediate memory
- Cognitive dissonance
- Confabulation
- Decreased ability to grasp ideas
- Disorientation in time, place, person, circumstances, or events
- Distractibility
- Impaired ability to reason, abstract, solve problems, make decisions, conceptualize, or interpret the environment
- Inappropriate affect
- Inappropriate social behavior
- Verbal report of limitations on usual thought processes

ASSOCIATED DISORDERS

Cerebrovascular accident, brain tumor, dementia, diabetic ketoacidosis, drug or alcohol withdrawal or intoxication, head trauma, hypoxemia or hypercapnia (secondary to acute respiratory failure), malnutrition, sensory deprivation (from isolation, prolonged bed rest, traction), septicemia

EXPECTED OUTCOMES

Initial outcome
- Patient expresses awareness of the need for assistance.

Interim outcomes
- Patient performs activities of daily living (ADLs) with assistance.
- Patient's laboratory values stay within normal range.
- Patient receives treatment for physiologic causes of thought process alteration.
- Family members identify signs and symptoms of partial or complete confusion.

Discharge outcome
- Family members make arrangements for home care.

INTERVENTIONS AND RATIONALES

Initial interventions
- Establish a therapeutic one-to-one relationship with the patient *to build trust.* To the extent possible, consistently assign the same staff members to provide care *to keep confusion to a minimum.*
- Explain the situation slowly and carefully to the patient and make him aware of his need for assistance *to keep him as oriented as possible.*

Interim interventions
- Make sure the patient is receiving appropriate care for any underlying

physiological disorder *to ensure his well-being and optimal recovery.*
- Address the patient by name and tell him your name *to foster his awareness of self and environment.*
- Give short, simple explanations to the patient each time you perform a procedure or task *to decrease confusion.*
- Schedule nursing care to provide quiet times for the patient *to help avoid sensory overload.*
- Mention time, place, and date frequently throughout the day. Have a clock and a calendar where the patient can easily see them; refer to these aids when orienting him *to foster awareness of self and environment.*
- Keep the patient's things in the same places as much as possible. *A consistent, stable environment reduces confusion and frustration and aids completion of ADLs.*
- Use appropriate safety measures *to protect the patient from injury.* Avoid physical restraints *to avoid agitating the patient.*
- Ask family members to bring labeled family photos, and other favorite articles *to create a more secure environment for the patient.*
- Plan the patient's routine and be as consistent as possible in following it. *A consistent daily plan aids task completion and reduces confusion.*
- Speak slowly and clearly, and allow ample time for the patient to respond *to reduce his frustration and promote task completion.*
- Encourage the patient to perform ADLs, dividing tasks into small, critical units. Be patient and specific in providing instructions. Allow time for the patient to perform each task. *These measures enhance his self-esteem and*

help prevent complications related to inactivity.

- Encourage family members to share stories and discuss familiar people and events with the patient. *Sharing stories and familiar subjects promotes a sense of continuity, aids memory, and creates a sense of security and comfort. Note that if the patient's short-term memory is impaired, his remote memory may still be intact.*
- Support family members' attempts to interact with the patient *to provide positive reinforcement.*
- Allow time before and after visits for family members to express their feelings *to help them cope with the patient's illness. Listening to their opinions may also help you assess and monitor the patient's condition.*

Discharge intervention

- Refer family members to appropriate health care professionals and community resources to plan for patient care after discharge, *to ensure a comprehensive approach to postdischarge care.*

EVALUATION STATEMENTS

Patient:
- remains free from injury.
- expresses awareness of need for assistance.
- is oriented to person, place, and time, as revealed by neurologic assessment.
- performs ADLs with assistance.
- receives treatment for the physiologic causes of thought process alteration.
   The family:
- obtains referrals to appropriate resources for home care.

- receives information about the patient's level of confusion obtained during the assessment of his changing mental state.

DOCUMENTATION

- Patient's verbal responses
- Observations of patient's behavior
- Interventions that focus on helping patient maintain reality orientation
- Responses of patient to nursing interventions
- Evaluation statements.

Verbal communication impairment

related to psychological or neurologic impairment

DEFINITION

Decreased ability to speak, understand, or use words appropriately

ASSESSMENT

Cultural status

- *Demographics:* age, sex, level of education, occupation, nationality, ethnic group
- *History:* beliefs, values, and attitudes about health and illness; health customs, practices, and rituals

Neurologic status

- *Mental status:* appearance and attitude, level of consciousness, motor activity, thought and speech, mood and affect, perceptions, orientation, memory, general information, calculations,

capacity to read and write, visual-spatial ability, attention span, abstraction, judgment and insight
- *Medication history:* neuroleptics, anxiolytic agents, antidepressants, barbiturates, pain medications, alcohol, recreational drugs
- *Motor system:* muscle tone, strength, symmetry, and gait; cerebellar function
- *Cranial nerve function*
- *Characteristics of speech:* coherence of topics; logic and relevance of responses; volume; voice tone and modulation; presence of speech defects, such as stuttering, excessively fast or slow speech, sudden interruptions, slurred speech, or overproductive or underproductive speech
- *Signs and symptoms:* dysarthria, garbled speech, echolalia, aphasia, dysphasia
- *Laboratory tests:* electrolyte levels, drug toxicology screening, hemoglobin and hematocrit, blood glucose level, thyroid and liver function tests
- *Diagnostic tests:* computed tomography, magnetic resonance imaging, positron emission tomography, cerebral arteriography, digital subtraction angiography, electroencephalography, Glasgow Coma Scale, Folstein Mini-Mental Health Status Examination

Psychological status
- *Alcohol or drug abuse:* type of substance, effects on mood and behavior, evidence of abuse or withdrawal, impact on functioning
- *Life changes:* recent divorce, job loss, loss of loved ones
- *Psychiatric history:* onset, type, and severity of symptoms; impact on functioning; type of treatment; response to treatment

- *Signs and symptoms:* changes in appetite, energy level, motivation, personal hygiene, self-image, self-esteem, sleep pattern, sexual drive, or competence

DEFINING CHARACTERISTICS

- Aphasia
- Blocking, losing train of thought
- Circumstantiality
- Difficulty with phonation
- Disorientation
- Echolalia
- Flight of ideas
- Inability to identify objects
- Inability to modulate speech, pronounce words, or speak in sentences
- Looseness of association
- Mutism
- Neologisms
- Perseveration
- Pressured speech
- Stuttering or slurring
- Verbigeration

ASSOCIATED DISORDERS

Acquired immunodeficiency syndrome, anxiety disorders, brain tumor, cerebrovascular accident, dementia, head injury, mood disorders, multiple sclerosis, Parkinson's disease, schizophrenia, substance-related disorders, temporal lobe epilepsy, transient ischemic attacks

EXPECTED OUTCOMES

Initial outcomes
- Patient communicates needs and desires to family, friends, or staff.
- Staff meets patient's needs.
- Patient incurs no injury or harm.

Interim outcome

▪ Patient establishes an effective and satisfying method for communicating with others.

Discharge outcome

▪ Patient begins to make plans to use self-help groups, speech therapist, and other resources to improve psychological or neurologic status.

INTERVENTIONS AND RATIONALES

Initial interventions

▪ Observe the patient closely to anticipate his needs; for example, restlessness may indicate a need to urinate. *Nonverbal cues give meaning to actions.*
▪ Minimize environmental stimuli and maintain a quiet, nonthreatening environment *to reduce anxiety.*
▪ Introduce yourself and explain procedures in consistent, simple terms *to foster communication.*
▪ Provide the patient with simple methods to communicate needs that will be recognized by day, evening, and night nurses *to maintain safety and to ensure that his basic needs are met.*
▪ Encourage communication attempts and allow the patient time to respond verbally or in writing *to decrease frustration.* Provide him with words only if he experiences extreme frustration.
▪ Help the patient establish a daily schedule *to help caregivers anticipate his needs and to minimize frustration, fear, and feelings of dependence.*
▪ Maintain a safe environment by using bed side rails, soft restraints or a Posey vest, and other safety measures, according to established policies, *to protect the patient.*

Interim interventions

▪ Assess the patient's communication status daily and record. Match communication needs to interventions: for disorientation, use reality orientation techniques; for alcohol withdrawal syndrome, reassure the patient, don't reinforce the presence of hallucinations, and provide a quiet environment. *Interventions must be tailored to the patient's situation.*
▪ Encourage the patient with dysarthria to speak slowly and to concentrate on forming words and syllables. Encourage him to reduce his speaking rate and increase his volume of speech without shouting *to facilitate clearer communication and to reduce feelings of frustration.*
▪ Provide the patient with aphasia with assistive devices (pad and pencil, alphabet list, flash cards, lapboard with letters, or pictures that convey entire concepts) and mechanical communication devices such as touch-talker computers (for long-term disabilities), establish a set of gestures that have assigned meaning, and document interventions *to provide continuity of care and reduce frustration.*
▪ Encourage the patient with verbal apraxia to repeat himself and persist in efforts to communicate when a word is misarticulated *to promote skill and mastery.*
▪ Encourage the patient with global speech and language loss to use gestures, mime, and pointing *to reduce his frustration.*
▪ For the patient with comprehension deficits, speak slowly, remain within his visual field, and provide as many cues as possible *to maximize comprehension.*

- For the patient with impaired communication secondary to schizophrenia, admit when language is not comprehensible *to promote trust and to provide an opportunity for reality testing.* Administer medications as prescribed *to control symptoms.*
- For the patient with impaired communication secondary to mania, create a calm environment *to prevent overstimulation.* Admit when communication is too fast-paced to be comprehensible. Do not repeatedly identify communication barriers *to avoid frustrating the patient.* Administer medications as prescribed *to control symptoms.*
- Determine the patient's past interests and habits from family members or a friend and discuss them with the patient *to stimulate nonthreatening two-way conversation.*
- Honestly admit when communication is not comprehensible *to foster trust and reduce the patient's feelings of isolation and hopelessness.*

Discharge interventions
- Provide medication teaching to the patient and his family members *to encourage adherence to the regimen.*
- Refer the patient to a psychiatric liaison nurse, social services, and appropriate self-help groups. *Resolution of communication problems may require long-term follow-up.*
- Provide a referral to a speech therapist *to ensure continuity of care.*

EVALUATION STATEMENTS

Patient:
- consistently communicates needs to staff, family, or friends.

- has basic needs met and does not show signs of neglect, such as weight loss, dehydration, or constipation.
- does not show evidence of falls, such as bruises, contusions, or cuts.
- states name, place, and time.
- expresses intent to attend self-help groups.
- identifies resources appropriate to coping with underlying psychological or neurologic problem.
  Family members:
- use appropriate methods to communicate with patient.

DOCUMENTATION

- Diagnostic test results
- Patient's expressions of concern regarding level of communication
- Observations of patient's needs, communication attempts, orientation, and safety measures
- Factors contributing to poor communication and plans to improve psychological or neurologic status
- Nursing interventions carried out to promote communication
- Patient's response to nursing interventions
- Evaluation statements.

Violence, high risk for: Directed at others

related to psychological disturbance

DEFINITION

Presence of risk factors for violence directed at others

ASSESSMENT

Cultural status

- *Demographics:* age, sex, level of education, occupation, nationality
- *History:* beliefs, values, and attitudes about mental illness

Neurologic status

- *Mental status:* appearance and attitude, thought and speech, mood and affect, perceptions, orientation, attention span, abstraction, judgment and insight
- *Physical examination:* motor and sensory function, reflexes
- *Diagnostic tests:* electroencephalography (EEG), magnetic resonance imaging (MRI)
- *Laboratory tests:* serotonin levels, drug toxicology screening

Psychological status

- *History:* use of phencyclidine, alcohol, or other substances; past episodes of violence; family history of violence; incarceration
- *Prior medical conditions:* past psychiatric episodes or hospitalization; alcohol or drug abuse
- *Medication history:* antipsychotics
- *Signs and symptoms:* agitation, irritability, suspiciousness, anger, rage, hostility, cursing, verbal threats, obscene gestures, throwing objects, pacing
- *Diagnostic tests:* Minnesota Multiphasic Personality Inventory, Thematic Apperception Test, Wechsler Adult Intelligence Survey

Social status

- *History:* interpersonal skills, degree of trust in others, level of self-esteem, ability to function in social and occupational roles, criminal activity
- *Signs and symptoms:* withdrawal, lack of eye contact, aggressiveness

Family status

- *Family communication:* style and quality of communication, methods of conflict resolution
- *Family needs:* ability of family to meet patient's physical, social, and emotional needs; disparities between patient's needs and family's ability to meet them
- *Economic factors:* economic status of patient and family; methods of coping with financial stress
- *Coping patterns:* major life events, usual coping patterns, ability of family to cope with violent outbursts
- *Evidence of abuse:* history of physical, emotional, or sexual abuse
- *Family health history:* bipolar disorders, depressive disorder, suicide, schizophrenia, mental retardation, substance-related disorder, stress-related illness, medical illness

RISK FACTORS

- Abnormal EEG results, serotonin levels, MRI, or positive drug toxicology screen
- Aggressive behavior, such as shouting, threatening talk, shaking fists, display of weapons, chair swinging, pounding fists, slamming doors
- Disturbed mood or affect
- Drug or alcohol abuse
- Inability of family to meet physical, social, or emotional needs
- Lack of self-esteem
- Poor family communication and inadequate conflict resolution

- Poor judgment and insight
- Poor orientation to person, place, and time
- Sleep deprivation

ASSOCIATED DISORDERS AND TREATMENTS

Brief psychotic disorder, delirium, delusional disorder, dementia, intermittent explosive disorder, mood disorders, obsessive-compulsive disorder, panic disorder, paranoid type schizophrenia, personality disorders, posttraumatic stress disorder, use of antipsychotic drugs

EXPECTED OUTCOMES

Initial outcome
- Patient gains control over angry impulses through verbalizing his feelings, venting frustration through nondestructive channels, taking time-out, and medications.

Interim outcome
- Patient discusses source of angry feelings and appropriate ways to handle frustration.

Discharge outcomes
- Patient seeks immediate help when beginning to feel out of control.
- Patient makes a commitment to long-term psychological treatment.

INTERVENTIONS AND RATIONALES

Initial interventions
- Inform the patient that you will help him control his behavior *to promote feelings of safety.*

- Provide the patient with the option of seclusion or restraints *to help him gain control of his behavior.*
- Set limits on aggressive behavior and communicate your expectations to the patient *to prevent injury to himself and others.*
- Encourage the patient to discuss his angry feelings. *Discussion may reduce his need to act on his angry thoughts.*
- Make sure the patient understands his medication program and takes his medication as ordered. *Medication can calm the patient, leading to better behavior and greater cooperation.*

Interim interventions
- Work with the patient to identify sources of anger *to help him learn to react nonviolently to problems.*
- Help the patient to identify the consequences of anger to develop awareness of his effect on others.
- Inform the patient of his responsibility for controlling his behavior. Emphasize that he is capable of recognizing feelings and choosing the methods to deal with them. *Through education, the patient can learn that he has choices for responding to anger.*
- Involve the patient in a strenuous exercise program *to decrease the physical energy that accompanies aggression.*

Discharge interventions
- Reward the patient whenever he deals with anger without resorting to violence. *Positive reinforcement helps him continue appropriate behavior.*
- Assess the patient's readiness for group therapy and provide appropriate referrals *to help him learn new ways to deal with people.*

- Refer the patient to an appropriate outpatient mental health clinic *so he can continue to receive therapy.*

EVALUATION STATEMENTS

Patient:
- controls angry impulses and stops violent behavior.
- learns appropriate ways to vent frustration and channel angry impulses.
- follows his medication regimen.
- agrees to seek help when beginning to feel out of control.

DOCUMENTATION

- Patient's behaviors that indicate difficulty controlling aggression
- Use of seclusion or restraint
- Nursing interventions performed to ensure the safety of other patients and staff
- Nursing interventions performed to make patient aware of effects of his behavior on others and options for controlling violent behavior
- Patient's response to nursing interventions
- Referrals to specialized professionals and agencies
- Evaluation statements.

Violence, high risk for: Self-directed

related to suicidal ideation

DEFINITION

The presence of risk factors for suicide

ASSESSMENT

Cultural status
- *Demographics:* age, sex, level of education, occupation, nationality, ethnic group
- *History:* presence or absence of supportive community, degree of social isolation

Neurological status
- *Mental status:* general appearance, attitude, affect and mood, thought and speech, orientation, judgment, memory, insight and calculation
- *Diagnostic test:* Folstein Mini-Mental Health Status Examination

Psychological status
- *History:* mood; alcohol and drug abuse; recent losses and life changes; level of self-esteem; changes in appetite, energy level, sleep pattern, libido, self-care
- *Suicide risk:* thought, plan, means and intent, lethality, previous history
- *Social relationships:* available support systems, quality of relationships
- *Signs and symptoms:* expression of suicidal thoughts, depression, withdrawal, poor eye contact, inappropriate behavior, aggressiveness
- *Diagnostic tests:* Hamilton Rating Scale for Depression, Beck Depression Inventory

Self-care status
- *History:* eating and drinking, bathing and hygiene, dressing and grooming, toileting, sleep and rest, safety practices

RISK FACTORS

- Direct or indirect statements indicating desire to commit suicide
- Disturbed mood and effect; poor judgment and insight
- Fear of own impulsivity
- History of alcohol or drug abuse
- History of multiple suicide attempts
- Multiple losses, such as loss of support of family or friends, deterioration in health status, loss of ability to perform self-care, loss of self-esteem, loss of sense of hope, or loss of control over life circumstances
- Possession of destructive implements (gun, knife, razor blade, scissors)
- Putting affairs in order—writing will, giving away possessions
- Severe depressive disorder manifested by feelings of helplessness, loneliness, hopelessness

ASSOCIATED DISORDERS

Acquired immunodeficiency syndrome, degenerative diseases, dementia, major depressive disorder, personality disorders, schizophrenia, substance-related disorders, terminal illness

EXPECTED OUTCOMES

Initial outcome
- Patient does not harm himself in hospital.

Interim outcomes
- Patient discusses sadness, despair, and other feelings.
- Patient enters into a written contract that specifies he will not harm himself.

- Patient reports decreased desire to kill himself.

Discharge outcomes
- Patient identifies need for continued support and help.
- Patient requests information on support groups and other sources of help.

INTERVENTIONS AND RATIONALES

Initial intervention
- Initiate appropriate safety protocols, such as observing the patient one-on-one, secluding or restraining him to help control his behavior, removing from his environment anything that could be used to inflict self-injury (razor blades, belts, glass objects, pills). *These measures help ensure the patient's safety.*

Interim interventions
- Ask the patient directly: "Have you thought about killing yourself?" If so, "What do you plan to do?" *Suicide risk increases if the patient has a plan and is capable of acting upon it.*
- Make a short-term written contract with the patient that he will not harm himself during a specific time period. Continue negotiating until there is no evidence of suicidal ideation. *A contract gets the subject out in the open, places some responsibility for safety on the patient, and conveys acceptance of him as a worthwhile person.*
- Support the patient, but do not give false reassurance that everything will work out. Let him know that, while no easy answer exists, help is available and you will help him find alternative solutions *to ease despair.*

- Supervise administration of prescribed medications. Be aware of drug actions and adverse effects and make sure that the patient doesn't hoard medications *to ensure he won't harm himself, even inadvertently.*
- Ask the patient to contact staff for help if he's feeling highly anxious or overwhelmed *to help ensure his safety.*
- Do not agree to keep information about suicidal thoughts confidential *to preserve an honest relationship.*
- Assist the patient in identifying sources of depression and hopelessness *to help him deal with these feelings without resorting to a suicide attempt.* Use a warm, caring, nonjudgmental manner *to show unconditional positive regard.* Listen carefully to the patient and don't challenge him *to assure him of undivided attention, concern, and support.* Place limits on excessive talk about suicide. Tell the patient you'll discuss feelings but not details of previous suicide attempts *to help him focus on his feelings.*
- Help the patient identify positive qualities in himself. Decrease environmental stimuli when necessary and provide a safe outlet for releasing emotions and anger. Review situations that cause stress for the patient and help him develop plans for dealing with them. *These measures will help the patient cope better with depression.*
- Encourage family members to talk with one another and develop improved coping strategies *to foster enhanced family functioning.*

Discharge interventions
- Make appropriate referrals to mental health professionals *to help the patient work through suicidal feelings.*

- Help the patient set a goal for obtaining long-term psychiatric care. *Ambivalence about psychiatric care or refusal to consult with a therapist usually indicates lack of insight and use of denial.*
- Provide the patient with telephone numbers and information about crisis centers, hot lines, counselors, and other emergency services *to help ensure his safety following discharge from the hospital.*

EVALUATION STATEMENTS

Patient:
- does not harm himself while in hospital.
- enters into contract stating that he will not attempt suicide and will contact staff if he's feeling anxious.
- expresses feelings of depression and anxiety.
- identifies sources of depression and anxiety.
- identifies positive qualities in himself.
- expresses need for ongoing treatment and support.

DOCUMENTATION

- Patient's comments indicating suicidal ideation
- Contracts signed by patient
- Observations of patient's behaviors and interactions with others
- Safety measures and nursing interventions
- Patient's responses to interventions
- Evaluation statements.

PART TWO

CHILD AND ADOLESCENT MENTAL HEALTH

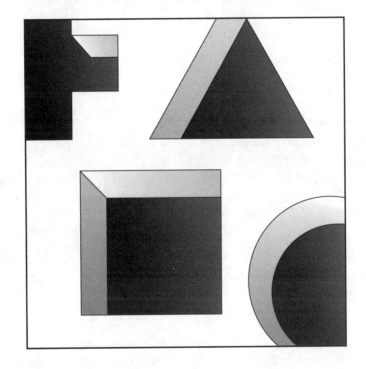

Anxiety

related to separation from parents and unfamiliarity with caregivers

DEFINITION

Feelings of threat or danger caused by separation from parents and lack of familiarity with the health care environment

ASSESSMENT

Family status
- *Demographic and cultural factors:* age and sex of all family members, level of education, developmental stage of siblings, nationality, religious affiliation, ethnicity, attitudes and beliefs about health care
- *Family development:* family roles, dynamics, problem-solving strategies, methods of communicating affection and emotional support, socioeconomic status

Psychological status
- *Childhood development:* use of emotional supports (blanket or pillow, stuffed animal, pictures), eating, sleeping, and toileting patterns
- *Current illness:* changes in self-image, self-esteem, sleep pattern, or level of competence
- *Health history:* psychiatric illness and treatment, substance use, prescribed psychiatric medications

Neurologic status
- *Mental status:* appearance, attitude, mood and affect, thought and speech, ability to understand, attention span, abstract thinking, insight, judgment, orientation, perceptions
- *Physical examination:* reflexes, motor function, sensory function

DEFINING CHARACTERISTICS

- Autonomic hyperactivity (abdominal distress, clammy skin, difficulty swallowing, dry mouth, feeling dizzy or light-headed, feeling flushed or chilled, frequent urination, shortness of breath)
- Developmental immaturity or regressive behavior
- Fear
- Hyperactivity
- Low self-esteem
- Motor tension (achiness, restlessness, trembling, twitching, muscle tension)
- Sleep disturbances

ASSOCIATED DISORDERS AND TREATMENTS

This diagnosis may accompany any hospitalization that separates the child and parents, such as for diagnostic tests, surgery, or traumatic injury.

EXPECTED OUTCOMES

Initial outcomes
- Child remains safe during hospitalization.
- Child receives age-appropriate explanations of routines and procedures.

Interim outcomes
- Child interacts calmly with members of the hospital staff.

- Child expresses feelings of fear and anxiety.
- Child uses appropriate emotional supports to reduce anxiety.
- Child does not experience symptoms of extreme anxiety.

Discharge outcomes
- Child expresses reduced feelings of fear and anxiety.
- Child exhibits few or no signs and symptoms of anxiety.
- Child resumes appropriate developmental tasks.

INTERVENTIONS AND RATIONALES

Initial interventions
- Assign one nurse to care for the child. *This provides the child and family with a sense of security, which promotes trust and reduces tension.*
- Provide the child with age-appropriate explanations of routines and procedures *to promote trust and reduce confusion and fear.*

Interim interventions
- Use age-appropriate props, such as puppets and toys, during teaching sessions *to adjust teaching to the child's developmental needs.*
- Talk with the child about his feelings. *Quiet talks help reduce anxiety and improve self-esteem.*
- Talk with the child about the health care regimen; ask for his impressions from time to time *to help the child feel involved in making decisions about his care, which can reduce anxiety.*
- Allow the child extra visiting periods with his parents and family. *Spending time with parents and siblings reduces anxiety.*
- Provide the parents with regular progress reports *to foster awareness, build trust, and allay fears.*

Discharge intervention
- Explain to the parents that their child will need to express feelings and question the need for hospitalization from time to time. *Guidance concerning possible reactions will prepare the family to meet the child's emotional needs after discharge.*

EVALUATION STATEMENTS

Child:
- remains safe during hospitalization.
- cries less and is less withdrawn.
- expresses or uses appropriate props to express feelings of fear or anxiety.
- interacts calmly with members of the hospital staff.
- participates in constructive age-appropriate diversions while hospitalized.
- uses appropriate emotional supports to reduce anxiety.
- does not experience symptoms of extreme anxiety.
- expresses reduced feelings of fear and anxiety.

DOCUMENTATION

- Child's expressions of fear, loneliness, or anxiety
- Behaviors indicating anxiety
- Nursing interventions performed to ensure the child's safety and reduce his anxiety
- Teaching topics covered and props used, if any

- Child's responses to nursing interventions
- Referrals to specialized professionals, agencies, and community services
- Evaluation statements.

Body image disturbance

related to an eating disorder

DEFINITION

Inaccurate self-perception leading to an eating disorder in an attempt to conform to an idealized body image

ASSESSMENT

Family status
- *Demographics:* age, sex, level of education (for all family members); parents' occupations
- *Cultural influences:* ethnicity, nationality, religious affiliation; values and beliefs regarding parenting, child rearing, and health care; rituals pertaining to food and mealtimes

Cardiovascular status
- *History:* use of tobacco or caffeine
- *Physical examination:* skin color and temperature, vital signs, carotid and apical pulses, heart sounds
- *Signs and symptoms:* chest pain, fatigue, palpitations, syncope, orthopnea, dyspnea, headache, shortness of breath, heart murmur
- *Diagnostic test:* electrocardiography

Gastrointestinal status
- *History:* food intake patterns, dieting history, bowel patterns

- *Medications:* laxatives, diuretics, diet pills, oral contraceptives
- *Physical examination:* vital signs, weight, height, stool characteristics, bowel sounds, integrity of oral mucosa, rectal and abdominal examination
- *Signs and symptoms:* nausea, vomiting, weight loss, change in appetite, constipation, diarrhea, mouth sores, tooth enamel erosion
- *Laboratory tests:* complete blood count (CBC), electrolyte levels, hemoculture

Nutritional status

- *History:* exercise pattern, attitude toward food, use of multivitamins
- *Physical examination:* percentage of body fat; basal energy expenditure; skin turgor, temperature, and color; characteristics of skin, nails, and hair; reflexes; muscle strength; inspection of hands
- *Signs and symptoms:* change in body weight, structure, or function; reduced fat distribution; pallor; irritability; cravings; binging and purging; amenorrhea or menstrual irregularity; periods of fatigue and hyperactivity; cold intolerance; fainting; decreased reflexes; weakness; bite marks on knuckles
- *Laboratory tests:* urinalysis; liver and thyroid function tests; levels of follicle-stimulating hormone, serum iron, serum albumin, total protein, and serum transferrin; total lymphocyte count; nitrogen balance; creatinine-height index
- *Diagnostic tests:* upper GI series

Integumentary status
- *Physical examination:* skin characteristics, excoriated areas, edema, pressure ulcers

Neurologic status
- *Mental status:* abstract thinking; insight about present situation; judgment; long- and short-term memory; cognition; orientation to person, place, and time
- *Physical examination:* level of consciousness, sensory ability, fine and gross motor functioning

Psychological status
- *History:* appetite; energy level; dieting; previous eating disorders; feelings about control over self and life situation; recent emotional crisis; ability to cope with stress; sleep pattern changes; work and study habits; history of physical, sexual, or emotional abuse
- *Body image:* past, current, and desired body image; perception of ideal body form; feelings about weight gain
- *Development:* birth order, number of siblings, family structure and roles, academic performance, relationships with peers, social group involvement, recreational activities and hobbies, coping mechanisms, self-perception, family's methods of resolving conflict
- *Medications:* antidepressants, alcohol or drug use, antipsychotic drugs
- *Diagnostic tests:* Brief Psychiatric Rating Scale, Hamilton Rating Scale for Depression, Eating Attitudes Test, Compulsive Eating Scale, Concern Over Weight and Dieting Scale, Yale-Brown Obsessive Compulsive Eating Disorder Scale

Parental status
- *History:* attitudes toward discipline, expectations for child, stability of parental relationship, understanding of adolescent's illness

Social status
- *History:* conversational and interpersonal skills, quality of relationships, dating history

DEFINING CHARACTERISTICS
- Abnormal electrolyte levels, ECG, urinalysis, or CBC results; low body weight
- Absence of three consecutive menstrual cycles
- Binge eating (minimum of two episodes weekly for at least three months), binging and purging
- Cold intolerance
- Constipation
- Decreased blood pressure, pulse, and temperature; decreased reflexes; fainting
- Denial of eating disorder
- Distorted body image
- Excessive, vigorous exercise
- Fear of weight gain, refusal to maintain more than minimal body weight
- Feeling of lack of control over eating behavior
- Food obsession, including hoarding food
- Irritability and perfectionism
- Physical signs of an eating disorder, such as dry, brittle hair or nails, lanugo hair, muscle weakness, tooth enamel erosion
- Pica
- Ritualized eating or exercise patterns; fasting
- Sleep pattern disturbance

- Social withdrawal and isolation
- Use of laxatives, diuretics, or diet pills
- Wearing of large, concealing clothing

ASSOCIATED DISORDERS

Amenorrhea, anemia, anorexia nervosa, arrhythmia, bulimia nervosa, dehydration, depressive disorder, diarrhea, electrolyte imbalance, esophagitis, growth disturbance, hemorrhoids, malabsorption syndrome, malnutrition, nutrient deficiency

EXPECTED OUTCOMES

Initial outcomes
- Adolescent adheres to treatment regimen.
- Adolescent acknowledges self-destructive eating and exercise patterns.
- Adolescent seeks help in overcoming eating disorder.

Interim outcomes
- Adolescent expresses feelings associated with food, exercise, weight loss, and medical condition.
- Adolescent participates in decisions about care and treatment.
- Adolescent helps develop written contract that establishes target weight gain.
- Adolescent expresses insight about eating patterns and self-destructive behaviors.
- Adolescent describes how arbitrary social standards of beauty have affected her self-perception.

Discharge outcomes
- Adolescent participates in eating disorder support group.

- Adolescent's parents participate in group therapy.
- Adolescent demonstrates new coping behaviors.
- Adolescent expresses positive feelings about self.
- Adolescent expresses satisfaction with parents' involvement in care.

INTERVENTIONS AND RATIONALES

Initial interventions
- Document vital signs and hydration status *to assess cardiovascular functioning and nutritional intake. This information is also required for decisions on enteral feedings.*
- Monitor the patient's eating patterns, fluid and electrolyte status, and daily weight *to ensure her well-being.*
- Observe the adolescent during mealtimes and in the bathroom *to make sure she is not hoarding food, discarding food, or purging.*
- Discuss the patient's medical condition and reasons for diet changes with her and her parents *to help ensure compliance.*
- Convey a favorable, caring attitude *to foster a positive relationship.* Take steps to ensure continuity of care during hospitalization *to foster trust and establish a therapeutic relationship.*
- Encourage the patient to participate in self-care and maintain interest in treatment decisions *to foster a sense of control in restoring health.*
- Tell the patient that you accept her as a person and provide reassurance that she can overcome her problems *to validate self-perception and enhance confidence.*

Interim interventions

- Encourage the patient to express thoughts and concerns about diagnosis and treatment, eating, exercise, and self-image *to prevent misconceptions and allow the patient to express feelings.*
- Ask the adolescent to help develop and sign a written contract with mutually agreed upon goals for weight gain *to give her control over her care and help her develop realistic expectations.*
- Implement behavior modification strategies consistently *to enable the patient to predict consequences of behavior.* Reinforce appropriate behaviors *to encourage the patient to comply with therapy and to participate in care.*
- Confront the patient directly with your concerns and tell her you expect her to do the same *to establish the precedent that manipulative behavior is not acceptable.*
- Avoid using coercive techniques to make the patient participate in care or adhere to rules. *Use of coercion may encourage the patient to view manipulative behavior as acceptable.*
- Without conveying distrust, monitor for signs that the adolescent isn't adhering to treatment *to assess self-destructive behavior.*
- Discuss the patient's progress with her *to increase awareness of achievements and to promote continued effort.*
- Discuss the adolescent's perception of her appearance. Help her understand how arbitrary social standards for beauty have affected her self-perception. Point out that she does not have to accept society's equation of thinness with beauty. Explain that she has a right to think of herself as beautiful regardless of how she compares with others *to build self-esteem.*

- Encourage participation in constructive activities *to divert the patient's need for control away from body image and eating.*

Discharge interventions

- Encourage the adolescent to participate in group therapy with peers with eating disorders *to foster insight and group support.*
- Encourage the parents to demonstrate emotional support for the patient *to strengthen the family support system.* Discuss with the parents their expectations for their daughter and how these expectations may be affecting her *to enhance their awareness.*
- Encourage the parents to join a support group for parents of children with eating disorders *to provide a forum for expressing feelings and obtaining support from individuals who can understand their concerns.*
- Remind the adolescent and her family of interventions to assist her in dealing with thoughts and feelings, such as role playing, therapeutic listening, and keeping a journal *to provide ongoing opportunities to deal with feelings.*
- Teach the parents the signs of relapse into self-destructive behaviors *to help them obtain early assistance and to enhance their confidence in their ability to protect their child from harm.*

EVALUATION STATEMENTS

Adolescent:
- completes treatment regimen.
- acknowledges self-destructive eating and exercise patterns.
- achieves and maintains body weight within 10% of ideal weight.

- discusses feelings about diagnosis of body image disturbance, seeks help, and participates in care decisions.
- participates in group therapy.
- makes healthy choices regarding meals and exercise and demonstrates new coping behaviors.
- expresses positive feelings about herself and insight about self-destructive behaviors.
- expresses need for further treatment and seeks help when feeling out of control.

Parents:
- provide emotional support.
- participate in group therapy.

Adolescent and parents:
- demonstrate effective coping and conflict resolution methods.

DOCUMENTATION

- Daily weight
- Diagnostic test results
- Food consumed at each meal and exercise patterns
- Adolescent's description of self
- Rituals involving food or exercise
- Adolescent's participation in and response to support group
- Evidence of self-destructive or manipulative behavior
- Nursing interventions to teach behavior modification techniques
- Adolescent's response to therapy and nursing interventions
- Statements indicating change in adolescent's self-perception
- Adolescent's interactions with parents and peers
- Evaluation statements.

Decisional conflict

related to sexual activity

DEFINITION

Uncertainty about whether to engage in sexual activity

ASSESSMENT

Family status
- *Demographics:* age, sex, level of education of all family members; socioeconomic status
- *Cultural influences:* ethnicity, religious affiliation, beliefs and attitudes regarding health practices and sexual activity
- *Relationships:* family alliances, evidence of conflict

Neurologic status
- *Mental status:* appearance and attitude, level of consciousness, motor activity, thought and speech, mood and affect, perceptions, orientation, memory, general information, capacity to read and write, attention span, abstraction, judgment and insight

Sexuality status
- *History:* contraceptive practices; drug and alcohol use; attitudes toward sex; sexual orientation, practices, experimentation; traumatic sexual experiences
- *Sexually transmitted diseases:* gonorrhea, syphilis, acquired immunodeficiency syndrome, chlamydial or herpesvirus infection

Social status

- *History:* learning ability, obstacles to learning, decision-making abilities (especially with regard to sexual relationships), support systems (family, friends, partner, teachers)

Psychological status

- *History:* level of functioning, coping mechanisms, support systems, self-image, self-esteem, attitude toward physical appearance
- *Developmental stage:* physical maturity, cognition, beliefs, values, ethics

DEFINING CHARACTERISTICS

- Adolescent reports feeling pressure to have sex
- Adolescent uses sex to bolster weak self-esteem or receive peer approval
- Lack of knowledge or indifference about possible consequences of sexual activity
- Signs of anxiety, distress, fear, uncertainty (expressed or behavioral)
- Vacillating decisions about sexual behavior

ASSOCIATED DISORDERS

Anorexia nervosa, anxiety disorders, bulimia nervosa, depressive disorders, obesity, personality disorders, pregnancy, sexually transmitted diseases, substance-related disorders

EXPECTED OUTCOMES

Initial outcome

- Adolescent expresses feelings about sexuality and sexual activity.

Interim outcomes

- Adolescent identifies desirable and undesirable consequences of sexual activity.
- Adolescent discusses conflicts between personal values and social pressures to be sexually active.
- Adolescent describes family conflicts and explores their potential effects on sexual conduct.

Discharge outcomes

- Adolescent accepts help from parents, family, friends, and health professionals.
- Adolescent reports confidence in choosing sexual behavior that's consistent with personal values.

INTERVENTIONS AND RATIONALES

Initial intervention

- Visit the adolescent frequently *to promote a therapeutic relationship.* Encourage her to express feelings about social and sexual life *to improve recognition of feelings and foster open discussion.*

Interim interventions

- Assess the adolescent's knowledge of sex and sexuality. Discuss sexual behavior and its potential consequences. Teach her about safer sex practices and birth control. Mention abstinence as an option. *Correct information about sexual practices reduces the adolescent's confusion over whether to be sexually active.*
- Listen attentively and remain nonjudgmental as the adolescent describes personal fears, values, and desires.

Nonjudgmental, active listening demonstrates your unconditional positive regard for the patient.
- Provide guidance as the adolescent explores options for sexual activity *to promote trust in her ability to make choices.*
- Discuss issues surrounding peer pressure. Ask the adolescent if she feels strong social pressure to be sexually active. In what other ways do her peers exert an influence on her? Explore ways of coping with peer pressure. *Peer pressure is a reality that each adolescent must learn to deal with.*
- Discuss family conflicts. Ask the adolescent if she feels troubled family relationships are pushing her to become sexually active. *Adolescents may seek in sexual relationships the love they are unable to obtain from family members.*

Discharge interventions
- Respect the adolescent's right to make choices based upon her personal values, desires, religious beliefs, cultural norms, and sexual preference *to foster autonomy and self-confidence.*
- Help the adolescent identify a support network (friends, family, community services, church or synagogue groups) and encourage her to use this network to aid in decision making. *An effective support system provides an emotional underpinning and helps the adolescent make decisions and resolve conflicts.*

EVALUATION STATEMENTS

Adolescent:
- describes feelings related to sexuality and sexual activity.

- describes conflicts between her personal values and social pressure to become sexually active.
- discusses possible influences, including peer pressure and conflicts with her family, on her decision to be sexually active.
- expresses increased understanding of her options regarding sexual activity and their potential consequences
- identifies a support network and uses it to aid decision making.
- reports feeling more comfortable with her ability to make decisions about sexuality and sexual activity.

DOCUMENTATION

- Statements indicating conflict over the decision to be sexually active
- Adolescent's cognitive, emotional, and behavioral levels of function
- Adolescent's knowledge of birth control and safer sex practices
- Nursing interventions to help adolescent make choices regarding whether to be sexually active
- Adolescent's responses to interventions
- Evaluation statements.

Decisional conflict
related to substance use

DEFINITION

State of uncertainty about whether to use recreational drugs

ASSESSMENT

Family status

- *Demographics:* family compositions; level of education of family members; parents' occupation; adolescent's grade level; urban, suburban, or rural residency
- *Family roles:* degree of family agreement on roles, interrelationship of various roles
- *Family rules:* rules that foster stability, maladaptive rules, willingness of parents to modify rules, consequences when rules are broken
- *Family communication:* style and quality of communication, methods of conflict resolution
- *Family subsystems:* family alliances and their effects on family stability
- *Physical and emotional needs:* ability of family to meet adolescent's physical and emotional needs, disparities between adolescent's needs and family's ability to meet them
- *Family goals and values:* extent to which family permits adolescent to pursue individual goals and values
- *Socioeconomic factors:* economic status of family, effect of financial pressures on adolescent's sense of adequacy and self-worth
- *Coping patterns:* usual coping patterns, family member's perception of effectiveness of coping patterns
- *Evidence of abuse:* physical and behavioral indicators
- *Diagnostic test:* Family Genogram

Psychological status

- *History:* birth order; appetite, energy, and motivation levels; personal hygiene; self-image; self-esteem; sleep patterns; alcohol or drug abuse; reaction to puberty; relationships with peers and authority figures; scholastic performance
- *Recent events:* divorce of parents, illness, job loss, loss of loved one, recent move or change in school
- *Social interaction:* interpersonal skills, social network, ability to function at school and work, level of trust in others, ability to seek assistance, aggressive behaviors

Neurologic status

- *Mental status:* appearance and attitude, level of consciousness, motor activity, thought and speech, mood and affect, perceptions, orientation, memory, general information, ability to read and write, judgment and insight
- *Laboratory tests:* drug toxicology screening; thyroid and liver function tests; serotonin, electrolyte, hemoglobin, and blood glucose levels; human immunodeficiency virus testing; urinalysis

DEFINING CHARACTERISTICS

- Evidence of experimentation with drugs
- Expressed feelings of indestructibility
- Expressions of distress and tension related to uncertainty about drug use
- Expressions of fear related to consequences of drug use
- Indifference toward risks associated with substance abuse
- Need for peer approval and conformity

ASSOCIATED DISORDERS

This diagnosis commonly accompanies any diagnosis related to substance abuse or psychiatric illness and may coincide with many other diagnoses.

EXPECTED OUTCOMES

Initial outcome
■ Adolescent discusses conflict over drug use.

Interim outcomes
■ Adolescent describes conflict between personal values and options and external value systems (parental, societal, peer, and legal).
■ Adolescent identifies perceived desirable and undesirable consequences of drug use.
■ Adolescent accepts assistance from parents, other family members, friends, and health care provider.

Discharge outcomes
■ Adolescent reports increased comfort with making choices that are consistent with personal values.
■ Adolescent discusses options for obtaining long-term counseling.

INTERVENTIONS AND RATIONALES

Initial interventions
■ Visit the adolescent frequently. Schedule a specific amount of non-care-related time each day for visits *to promote trust and provide a time when the adolescent can discuss his feelings confidentially.*
■ Make the adolescent aware that you are willing to discuss all topics, including substance use. Reassure him that all information will be kept confidential *to encourage honest discussion of concerns.*

Interim interventions
■ Encourage adolescent to explore feelings related to drug use, school, family, friends, and other vital topics. Remain nonjudgmental *to demonstrate your regard of him as a worthwhile person with valid values and beliefs.*
■ Ask the adolescent to describe his family and home life *to assess for family conflict that may be creating emotional distress.* Provide referrals for family counseling if needed.
■ Ask the adolescent if he experiences peer pressure to use drugs. Explore ways of coping with peer pressure. *Peer pressure is a reality that all adolescents must learn to cope with.*
■ Discuss self-esteem and explore ways of building self-esteem *to strengthen the adolescent's ability to deal with peer pressure.*
■ Help the adolescent explore alternative recreational activities, such as sports, art, music, community service, or participation in church or synagogue groups *to help him develop alternatives to substance use.*
■ Teach the adolescent about the health and legal consequences of substance use and abuse. *Accurate information will help the adolescent make informed and rational decisions.*
■ Encourage the adolescent to identify and use support systems, such as family, friends, clinics, a school nurse, or another health care provider. *A support network and emotional support are important tools in resolving emotional conflicts.*

Discharge intervention

- Refer the adolescent for long-term counseling, if necessary. *Long-standing emotional conflicts may require more in-depth intervention.*

EVALUATION STATEMENTS

Adolescent:
- discusses conflict over whether to use drugs.
- identifies health and legal consequences of drug use.
- discusses peer pressure, family conflict, or other factors that may be influencing him to use drugs.
- identifies available sources of emotional support and requests help, if needed.
- reports increased self-esteem and ability to deal with peer pressure.

DOCUMENTATION

- Evidence of drug use
- Adolescent's stated feelings about drug use
- Adolescent's level of functioning (cognitive, emotional, behavioral)
- Nursing interventions to help the adolescent make choices regarding drug use
- Adolescent's responses to interventions
- Evaluation statements.

Growth and development alteration

related to cognitive difficulties

DEFINITION

Delay or disruption in a child's acquisition of self-care skills related to a congenital or acquired deficit in intellectual functioning

ASSESSMENT

Family status

- *Demographics:* age, sex, and developmental stage of all children; age, occupation, marital status, level of education, and socioeconomic status of parents
- *Cultural influences:* nationality, ethnicity, religious affiliation; beliefs, attitudes, and values about health and illness; health customs, practices, and rituals
- *Parent's child-rearing skills:* ability to meet children's physical and emotional needs, disciplinary history and current disciplinary style, knowledge of normal childhood patterns of growth and development
- *Parents' reaction to child's illness:* past methods of coping with crises; stability of parental relationship; reaction to having a child with a cognitive deficit; stage of grieving over the loss of normalcy of their child; understanding of their child's cognitive deficits, developmental delays, and prognosis; expectations for their child's growth and development; level of con-

cern regarding delays in their child's acquisition of self-care skills
- *Diagnostic test:* Family Genogram

Neurologic status
- *Health history:* child's exposure to environmental toxins, family safety practices
- *Medication history:* anticonvulsants, psychotropics, neuroleptics, antidepressants, stimulants, or amphetamines
- *Mental status:* environmental awareness, speech and language development, articulation, attention span
- *Motor development:* muscle tone, strength, and symmetry; hand and leg dominance; sitting balance; gait; cerebellar function
- *Cranial nerve function*
- *Sensory function:* cortical, visual, and auditory function; peripheral sensory function (pain, position, vibration)
- *Reflexes:* deep tendon, primitive, superficial, pathological
- *Signs and symptoms:* self-care deficits, muscle tone abnormalities, abnormal movements, tremors, seizure activity, aura, myoclonus, sensory deficits, postictal state
- *Laboratory tests:* anticonvulsant, ammonia, carnitine, and electrolyte levels; thyroid function test; amino acid screen; viral titers
- *Diagnostic tests:* computed tomography, magnetic resonance imaging, positron emission tomography, electromyography, closed circuit television electroencephalography, visual and auditory evoked potential studies, Connors Parent-Teacher Rating Scales

Psychological status
- *Childhood development:* significant events (prenatal, perinatal, postnatal), difficulties with attachment or feeding in infancy, usual sleep pattern and difficulties, number of siblings and child's birth order, composition of extended family, developmental milestones, temperament (infancy, childhood), personality traits, learning style (visual, auditory, haptic), attention span, school history, recreational activities, quality of relationships (peer, parental, sibling)
- *Signs and symptoms:* behavioral disorders (self-stimulatory, self-injurious, autism-like, or antisocial behaviors), hyperactivity, poor attention span, tantrums, aggression, depressive disorders, change in eating habits
- *Diagnostic tests:* Bayley Scales of Infant Development, Stanford Binet Intelligence Scale, Wechsler Intelligence Scales for Children (WISC-III), Wechsler Preschool and Primary Scale of Intelligence (WPPSI-R)

Self-care status
- *History:* ability, willingness, and prerequisite skills necessary to perform self-care tasks; competency in feeding, toileting, dressing; use of adaptive equipment, utensils, or supplies; parent-child interaction during self-help activities; behaviors that interfere with task completion
- *Signs and symptoms:* delays in learning self-care or adaptive activities; neurologic, musculoskeletal, sensory, or psychological impairment
- *Diagnostic tests:* Washington Guide to Promoting Development in the Young Child, American Association on Mental Retardation Adaptive Be-

havior Scales, Vineland Social Maturity Scale

DEFINING CHARACTERISTICS

- Delay in acquiring self-care skills
- Delay in normal childhood development

ASSOCIATED DISORDERS

Attention-deficit and hyperactivity disorder, brain tumor, chromosomal abnormalities, cognitive deficits, complications or trauma (prenatal, perinatal, postnatal), cortical dysfunction related to environmental causes (for example, lead poisoning, chemical toxicity, intrauterine viral infection), head injury, hydrocephalus with shunting, motor deficits, movement disorders, seizure disorder, single-gene defects, sporadic syndromes associated with cognitive deficits, tardive dyskinesia

EXPECTED OUTCOMES

Initial outcomes

- Parents express feelings, such as anger, guilt, frustration, and disappointment, associated with teaching their child.
- Parents identify their child's strengths and needs.
- Parents recognize and identify personal strengths and abilities to help nurture their child and promote his development.

Interim outcomes

- Parents describe and demonstrate proper techniques for teaching a child with cognitive impairment.

- Parents participate in planning and implementing a program to improve their child's self-help skills.
- Parents report increased feelings of self-esteem regarding their roles as teachers and nurturers.
- Child demonstrates improved attention to tasks and fewer digressions (tantrums, distraction, manipulative behavior) during teaching sessions.
- Child makes systematic, steady progress toward acquiring self-help skills.

Discharge outcomes

- Parents agree to continue their child's developmental program at home.
- Parents identify and use a support system that includes professional assistance when needed.
- Child performs self-care tasks to the best of his ability.
- Child demonstrates or expresses improved self-esteem related to increased independence.
- Parents report a decrease in their child's social isolation related to improved social skills.

INTERVENTIONS AND RATIONALES

Initial interventions

- Follow the medical regimen *to help the child recover from his current illness or injury and promote safety.*
- Provide the parents with a nonjudgmental and supportive atmosphere *to encourage an open expression of feelings, such as anger, frustration, and disappointment, they may have experienced while raising their child.*
- Provide the parents with positive feedback about their actions to pro-

mote optimal child development *to ease any feelings of inadequacy or guilt.*
▪ Help the parents identify personal strengths as well as the strengths and needs of their child *to promote understanding, improve their self-esteem, and encourage an ongoing commitment to providing their child with necessary teaching and assistance.*
▪ Involve the parents (and child when appropriate) in planning, documenting, and implementing teaching sessions *to foster compliance and improve the quality of interaction between the child and his parents.*

Interim interventions
▪ Teach the parents the principles of behavior modification and demonstrate applicable techniques. *Consistent use of behavior modification will help the child develop and refine desirable self-care skills.* Tell them to:
– provide prompt positive reinforcement when their child performs a desired behavior.
– ignore undesirable behavior.
– provide continual reinforcement when seeking to establish a desired behavior and follow up with intermittent reinforcement *to help make sure the behavior will continue.*
– reward small successes *to help their child build upon simple behavioral improvements before mastering complex behaviors.*
▪ Record the child's progress on a chart or graph prominently displayed in the child's room *to provide the child and parents with positive reinforcement.*
▪ Teach the parents how to record data on their child's progress chart. *The chart reinforces both the parents' teach-*ing efforts and their child's efforts to master desired behaviors.*

Discharge interventions
▪ Provide the parents with a written copy of the teaching plan *to encourage consistent implementation of the plan at home, thus promoting continuity of care.*
▪ Encourage the parents to describe the teaching plan to the child's teachers, grandparents, sitters, and other companions *to ensure consistent implementation.*
▪ Provide the parents with referrals to appropriate community services or counseling professionals. If necessary, call or visit the family regularly *to monitor its progress, help update goals, provide emotional support, and encourage it to continue the program.*

EVALUATION STATEMENTS

Child:
▪ expresses his feelings about behavioral problems and parental responses related to his disorder.
▪ expresses and exhibits a desire to learn self-care skills.
▪ demonstrates regular, systematic progress in acquiring self-care skills.
▪ expresses and demonstrates improved self-esteem and self-concept as he makes progress.
  Parents:
▪ express feelings, such as anger, frustration, depression, guilt, or inadequacy, associated with their child's disorder and their role as parents.
▪ accurately describe personal strengths and the strengths and needs of their child.

- describe ways to incorporate their child's strengths into an effective teaching program for him.
- describe and demonstrate behavior modification techniques appropriate for their child's teaching program.
- maintain a written record of their child's progress.
- express positive feelings about their child and his progress.
- promote socialization outside the home for their child.
- describe an effective support system comprised of family, friends, community resources, trained professionals, and parent support groups.

DOCUMENTATION

- Diagnostic test results
- Feelings expressed by family members regarding the child's developmental delays and cognitive impairment
- Feelings expressed by the child about his behavioral problems and his parents' response to his disability
- Observations of parent-child interactions
- Nursing interventions to promote the acquisition of self-care skills
- Copy of teaching plan developed with the parents
- Copy of graph indicating progress toward specific behavioral goals
- Responses of the child and his parents to nursing interventions
- Parents' compliance with behavior modification plan
- Referrals to community resources, home care services, trained professionals, or parent support groups
- Evaluation statements.

Growth and development alteration

related to illness or physical disability

DEFINITION

Delay or disruption in a child's performance of normal developmental tasks due to chronic illness or congenital or acquired physical disability

ASSESSMENT

Family status
- *Demographics:* age, sex, and level of education of all family members; parents' marital status; developmental stage of siblings; family developmental stage
- *Cultural influences:* nationality, ethnicity, religious affiliation; beliefs, attitudes, and values about health and illness; health customs, practices, and rituals
- *Family development:* informal and formal family roles, rules and expectations, attitudes regarding independence, quality of sibling and parent-child relationships, reaction of siblings to child's disability, family goals and aspirations
- *Parents' child-rearing skills:* ability of parents to meet the physical and emotional needs of their children; history and current style of discipline; knowledge of normal patterns of childhood growth and development; strategies for preventing trauma, poisoning, or exposure to environmental toxins and ensuring infant and child safety

- *Parents' coping strategies:* usual coping methods and their effectiveness, prior experience coping with crises, stability of parents' relationship, presence of support system, history of substance abuse
- *Parents' reaction to child's illness:* emotions associated with having a physically disabled child; current stage in the process of grieving the loss of a "normal" child; expectations for their child's growth and development; level of concern regarding their child's delayed development; level of knowledge concerning child's disability, developmental delays, and prognosis
- *Diagnostic tests:* Family Genogram, Cultural Assessment Guide, Comprehensive Parent-Child Screening Profile, Caldwell Home Inventory

Cardiovascular status

- *Health history:* strep infection, rheumatic fever, kidney disease, chromosomal abnormalities, recurrent respiratory infection, congenital cardiovascular or cardiopulmonary disease
- *Physical examination:* activity level, breath sounds, motor skills, skin color and temperature, vital signs, precordial inspection (heart size, rate, and rhythm; heart sounds), physical development
- *Signs and symptoms:* weak cry (infant), squatting, poor activity tolerance, poor eating habits, tachycardia, syncope, vein distention, edema, nail clubbing, cyanosis, diaphoresis, breathing difficulties (adventitious breath sounds), chest deformity
- *Laboratory test:* lipid profile
- *Diagnostic tests:* electrocardiography, echocardiography, cardiac catheterization

Musculoskeletal status

- *Health history:* neuromuscular deficits, skeletal deformities, trauma, congenital limb deformities, prior musculoskeletal surgery; prescribed anti-inflammatory agents or muscle relaxants
- *Physical examination:* range of motion (all joints); joint and muscle symmetry; joint deformities; contractures; muscle size, strength, and tone; coordination; gait; functional mobility and use of mobility aides (wheelchair, braces, crutches, cane, walker); motor-skill milestones
- *Signs and symptoms:* limited range of motion, subluxation, dislocation, contracture, muscle atrophy, poor muscle strength, scoliosis, abnormal muscle tone
- *Diagnostic tests:* electromyography, Milani-Comparetti Motor Screening Test, Bayley Scales of Infant Development (motor skills)

Neurologic status

- *Health history:* mother's exposure to environmental teratogens during pregnancy; complications or trauma (prenatal, perinatal, postnatal); Apgar scores; motor, cognitive, or attention deficits; head or spinal cord injury; neural tube defects; difficulty feeding or swallowing
- *Medication history:* anticonvulsants, antidepressants, stimulants
- *Mental status:* awareness, language development, articulation, attention span
- *Motor status:* motor skills, gait, cerebellar functions, hand dominance
- *Cranial nerve function*
- *Reflexes:* deep tendon reflexes; infantile, superficial, and pathological reflexes

- *Signs and symptoms:* delayed motor skills, gait disturbance, hypotonia or hypertonia, spasticity, athetoid movements, dystonia, perseverance of primitive reflexes, hyperreflexia, seizures, aura, myoclonus, sensory deficits, tremors, postictal state
- *Laboratory tests:* levels of anticonvulsant medications, ammonia, carnitine and electrolytes; thyroid function test, amino acid assay, viral titers
- *Diagnostic tests:* computed tomography, magnetic resonance imaging, positron emission tomography, closed circuit television electroencephalography, visual and auditory evoked potentials, Connors Parent-Teacher Rating Scales, Primitive Reflex Profile

Psychological status
- *Childhood development:* significant events (prenatal, perinatal, postnatal), difficulties with attachment or feeding in infancy, usual patterns of sleep and nutrition, number of siblings and child's birth order, composition of extended family, developmental milestones, personality and temperament (infancy and childhood), learning style (visual, auditory, haptic) and adjustment to school, learning disabilities, socialization skills, quality of relationships (peer, parental, sibling), hobbies, recreational activities
- *Signs and symptoms:* antisocial behavior (tantrums, aggression, self-injury, autism-like behavior, depression, substance use or abuse), hyperactivity, poor attention span, change in eating habits
- *Diagnostic tests:* Bayley Scales of Infant Development, Stanford Binet Intelligence Scale, Wechsler Intelligence Scales for Children (WISC-III),

Wechsler Preschool and Primary Scale of Intelligence (WPPSI-R)

Self-care status
- *History:* ability, willingness, and prerequisite skills necessary to perform self-care tasks; competency in feeding, toileting, dressing; use of adaptive equipment, utensils, or supplies; parent-child interaction during self-help activities; behaviors that interfere with task completion
- *Signs and symptoms:* delays in learning self-care or adaptive activities; neurologic, musculoskeletal, sensory, or psychological impairment
- *Diagnostic tests:* Washington Guide to Promoting Development in the Young Child, American Association on Mental Retardation Adaptive Behavior Scales, Vineland Social Maturity Scale

Sensory status
- *Visual examination:* position, size, and symmetry of the child's eyes; congenital eye malformations; visual field; extraocular movements; corneal opacities; visual tracking and acuity; pupillary reaction; tearing; diplopia; strabismus; nystagmus; ptosis
- *Auditory examination:* position, size, and symmetry of the child's ears; congenital ear malformations; condition of auditory canal and tympanic membrane; cerumen impaction; otic drainage; auditory tracking
- *Olfactory examination:* congenital nasal deformities; sense of taste; condition of nasal mucosa, turbinate, septum
- *Gustatory examination:* congenital oral defects; appetite, taste; weight

change; bruxism; condition of the gums, dentition, and buccal cavity
- *Tactile examination:* awareness of position in space; sensitivity to touch, temperature, pressure, and pain
- *Diagnostic tests:* audiometry, tympanometry, optokinetic response test, "E" chart, Allen Kindergarten Eye Chart, Test of Sensory Integration Functions in Infants, Sensory Integration and Praxis Test

DEFINING CHARACTERISTICS

- Delayed ability to perform age-appropriate developmental tasks
- Delayed pattern of growth and development
- Inability to perform age-appropriate self-care skills

ASSOCIATED DISORDERS AND TREATMENTS

Brain tumor; cardiovascular or cardiopulmonary disease or defect (congenital or acquired); cerebral thrombosis; craniostenosis; failure to thrive; head or spinal cord trauma; hydrocephalus or shunting; intraventricular hemorrhage; kidney disease; movement disorders; musculoskeletal, orthopedic, or neuromuscular disorder; neural tube defects; neuropathies; physical abuse; seizure disorders

EXPECTED OUTCOMES

Initial outcomes
- Child achieves optimal health and remains free from injury.
- Parents begin the process of grieving the loss of a normal childhood for their child.

- Parents identify their child's unique strengths and express positive feelings about him.
- Parents and child demonstrate appropriate attachment behaviors.
- Parents identify personal strengths and abilities that will help them nurture their child and promote optimal development.
- Parents accurately describe the nature of their child's disability and his prognosis.

Interim outcomes
- Parents engage their child in age-appropriate recreational and social activities.
- Child makes steady, systematic progress in developmental growth and in acquiring self-care skills.
- Parents identify and use adaptive coping strategies.
- Child participates in activities appropriate for his age and developmental stage.
- Child expresses an age-appropriate understanding of the nature of his disability and is able to communicate this understanding to peers and other social contacts.

Discharge outcomes
- Child demonstrates improved developmental skills enabling integration into his family, school, and community.
- Child achieves and maintains an optimal level of developmental functioning and self-care ability.
- Parents identify and use community services, educational systems, and support groups to help them adapt to the child's disorder and meet the needs of all family members.

INTERVENTIONS AND RATIONALES

Initial interventions

- Follow the medical regimen *to ensure optimal health for the child and promote safety.*
- Provide the parents with a nonjudgmental and supportive atmosphere *to validate the grieving process; encourage expressions of anger, frustration, disappointment, or guilt; and promote a trusting therapeutic relationship.*
- Praise the parents for their attempts to promote optimal child development *to ease any feelings of inadequacy or guilt.*
- Help the parents identify personal strengths as well as the strengths and needs of their child *to promote their understanding and self-esteem and enhance their attachment to him.*
- Involve the parents in planning, documenting, and implementing teaching sessions for their child *to foster compliance and improve the quality of interaction between the child and his parents.*
- Provide clear, honest answers to the parents' questions about their child's disability. Provide information in easily understandable increments to avoid overwhelming them. *This helps them build knowledge about their child's disorder, which promotes acceptance and encourages compliance with the teaching regimen.*

Interim interventions

- Teach the parents about developmental, recreational, and social tasks that are appropriate for their child's developmental stage *to promote understanding and enhance their abilities to*

help their child meet developmental *goals.*
- Teach the parents techniques for promoting their child's progress in acquiring self-care skills. Record the child's progress on a chart or graph prominently displayed in the child's room *to provide both the child and his parents with positive reinforcement.*
- Explain the importance of scheduling time for personal relaxation and recreation *to reduce tension.*
- Discuss the possibility of engaging a home health care agency to help the parents care for their child *to effectively meet all of the child's health care needs.*
- Teach the parents ways to integrate their child into normal family and social activities *to promote attachment to their child and reduce fears of social isolation caused by the child's disability.*
- Help the child develop a simple, honest explanation of his disability for peers and other social contacts *to promote his self-esteem and reduce any sense of social isolation.*

Discharge interventions

- Provide the parents with a written copy of the teaching plan *to encourage consistent implementation of the plan at home.*
- Show the parents how to record data on their child's progress chart. *At home, the chart reinforces both the parents' teaching efforts and their child's efforts to master desired behaviors.*
- Encourage the parents to share their teaching plan with teachers, grandparents, sitters, and other important people in the child's life *to ensure consistent implementation.*

- Provide the parents with referrals to appropriate community services (financial, educational, technical), counseling professionals, or parenting support groups. If appropriate, call or visit the family regularly. *Having a comprehensive support network helps allay anxieties and fears about integrating the child into normal home and community life. Calling or visiting lets you monitor their progress, help update goals, provide emotional support, and encourage the family to continue with the program.*

EVALUATION STATEMENTS

Parents:
- openly express feelings of shock, denial, disbelief, or anger related to their child's disability.
- identify personal strengths and the strengths and needs of their child.
- develop a support system composed of family, friends, and trained professionals to help them meet the needs of their child and family.
- seek opportunities to interact with their child and participate in his care.
- express their desire to understand the nature of their child's disability and his prognosis.
- express positive feelings about their child.
- describe normal child development and activities that will optimize their child's development.
- identify and use community resources to help them care for their disabled child.
- pursue their child's rights concerning access to education and health care.

Child:
- achieves optimal health status and is free from injury.
- demonstrates steady, systematic growth in development and in acquiring age-appropriate self-care skills.
- participates in age-appropriate ways in teaching sessions, family get-togethers, and social activities.
- comfortably describes the nature of his disability to others.
- demonstrates self-care skills that are consistent with his age and developmental level.

DOCUMENTATION

- Diagnostic test results
- Parents' expressed feelings about their child's disability and its impact on the family
- Observations of parent-child interaction
- Frequency and reasons for child's health care visits
- Parents' knowledge about their child's disability and prognosis
- Child's current growth and developmental level
- Teaching topics for parents and child
- Family actions to promote the child's growth and development and to integrate him into family and community life
- Referrals provided to home health agencies, community services, medical supply companies, teaching centers, counselors, parenting support groups
- Evaluation statements.

Hopelessness

related to mood disturbance

DEFINITION

Lack of hope caused by unsettled emotions

ASSESSMENT

Family status
- *Demographics:* family composition; level of education of family members; parents' occupations; child's grade level; urban, suburban, or rural residency
- *Physical and emotional needs:* ability of family to meet child's physical and emotional needs
- *Coping patterns:* family members' sense of self-worth and adequacy, family members' perception of effectiveness of coping patterns
- *Evidence of abuse:* physical and behavioral indicators
- *Family health history:* history of mood disorders
- *Diagnostic test:* Family Genogram

Parental status
- *History:* knowledge of normal growth and development in children, usual coping mechanisms, disciplinary measures, stability of parental relationship, parent's understanding of child's illness, available support systems

Psychological status
- *Current illness:* changes in appetite, energy level, motivation, personal hy-

giene, self-image, sleep pattern; evidence of alcohol or drug abuse
- *Life changes:* recent move, parental divorce, loss of loved one or pet
- *Psychiatric history:* type and severity of symptoms, impact on functioning, child's response to treatment
- *Childhood development:* birth order, number of siblings, developmental milestones, earliest and continuous memories, academic performance, relationship with peers, involvement with social groups
- *Diagnostic tests:* Hopelessness Scale for Children, Children Depression Inventory

Self-care status
- *History:* ability to carry out activities of daily living, amount of needed assistance

Sleep pattern status
- *History:* usual hours of sleep, helpful techniques used to fall asleep
- *Signs and symptoms:* difficulty falling asleep, nocturnal or early morning awakening, hypersomnia, insomnia, nightmares or night terrors
- *Diagnostic tests:* sleep electroencephalography (EEG), sleep-deprived EEG

Social status
- *History:* quality of relationships, degree of trust in others, level of self-esteem, ability to function in social and academic roles
- *Signs and symptoms:* withdrawal, lack of eye contact, aggressiveness

DEFINING CHARACTERISTICS

- Decreased affect and verbalization

- Decreased appetite
- Decreased initiative and involvement in school or play
- Increased sleep or sleep pattern disturbances
- Nonverbal cues, such as minimal eye contact, shrugging in response to questions, turning away from speaker
- Problems in peer and family relationships
- Verbal cues, including frequent sighing and hopeless responses, such as "I can't" or "What's the use?"

ASSOCIATED DISORDERS

Adjustment disorders, anxiety disorder, conduct disorder, mood disorders, posttraumatic stress disorder, reactive attachment disorder of infancy or early childhood, separation anxiety disorder

EXPECTED OUTCOMES

Initial outcome
- Child does not harm himself while in hospital.

Interim outcomes
- Child completes activities of daily living with assistance.
- Child participates in therapeutic play with dolls or other toys.
- Child identifies feelings and seeks help when they are overwhelming.
- Child accepts praise from others.

Discharge outcomes
- Child discusses ways to deal with stress at home or school and with feelings of hopelessness.
- Child makes positive statements about himself and others.

- Child and family members make plans to continue treatment.

INTERVENTIONS AND RATIONALES

Initial interventions
- Provide a safe and secure environment *to establish a therapeutic relationship and maintain the patient's safety.*
- Make a short-term contract with the child that he will not harm himself during a specific time period *to help him accept responsibility for his safety.*
- Encourage the child to discuss any thoughts of harming himself. *This will emphasize that you care, reinforce feelings of safety, and encourage responsibility.*

Interim interventions
- Monitor the child's affect and behavior *to ensure safety.*
- Provide structured playing time by using puppets, dolls, and games *to provide an opportunity for the child to express his feelings. Playing is a form of communication for children. It decreases anxieties and facilitates discussion.*
- Encourage the child to attend group therapy *to help him learn ways to cope with feelings and promote peer interaction.*
- Provide the child with a "Positives Book," a small notebook where he can write down things that happen throughout the day that make him feel good about himself *to encourage him to focus on his strengths and to enhance his self-esteem.*
- Encourage the child to participate in self-care to the extent possible. Praise even small accomplishments. *These*

*measures enhance self-esteem and re-
duce feelings of helplessness.*
- Ask the child to identify friends and
enjoyable diversions. Encourage him
to make contact with friends and participate in recreational activities. *A
lack of friends or pleasurable diversions
increases the severity of hopelessness.*
- Ask family members or friends to
bring the child personal belongings
from home; for example, photographs, a stuffed animal, or a pillow.
*Bringing familiar items to the child's
hospital room may reduce stress.*
- Offer the child praise for participating
in therapeutic activities, completing daily activities, and making positive statements *to enhance his self-esteem.*
- Educate his parents and teachers
about interventions that increase the
child's self-esteem *so that he continues
to receive support after discharge.*

Discharge outcomes
- Assist child in identifying ways to
deal with stress at home and school,
such as talking to a teacher or counsel-
or when feeling hopeless. *A support
network will ensure feelings of safety.*
- Teach the child, caregivers, and teachers about his medication regimen, including purpose, schedule, and potential adverse effects *to aide compliance.*
- Emphasize the need for follow-up
appointments with the child and his
caregivers *to ensure continuing care.*

EVALUATION STATEMENTS

Child:
- remains free from injury.
- names specific feelings, such as anger, sadness, guilt, nervousness, and
loneliness.

- seeks out staff when upset and participates in group therapy.
- demonstrates less agitation when
given positive feedback.
- expresses positive themes during
play.
- participates in self-care to extent
possible.
- states positive characteristics about
self and others.
   Caregivers, family members, and
child:
- express willingness to continue treatment.
   Teachers and school administrators:
- express willingness to adapt to special needs of the child.

DOCUMENTATION

- Child's ability to commit himself to
maintaining safety and adherence to
behavioral contracts
- Child's affect and behavior
- Nursing interventions that stabilize
mood and maintain safety
- Response to prescribed medications
and frequency of medications
- Themes expressed by child during
play therapy
- Referrals to community agencies
- Evaluation statements.

Incontinence, functional

related to developmental lags

DEFINITION

*Involuntary passage of urine or stool
related to inability to function at age-
appropriate stage*

ASSESSMENT

Family status
- *Demographics:* family composition, level of education of family members, parents' occupations, child's grade level
- *Communication patterns:* methods of conflict resolution, ability to discuss feelings
- *Coping patterns:* usual coping patterns, family member's perception of effectiveness of coping patterns

Gastrointestinal status
- *History:* bowel patterns, dietary intake, behavior modification to decrease episodes of encopresis
- *Signs and symptoms:* encopresis, nausea, vomiting, constipation

Genitourinary status
- *History:* urinary pattern; frequency and time of incontinence; urgency; hesitancy; use of devices to decrease nocturnal enuresis, such as bell and pad; behavior modification; history of urinary tract infections
- *Medications:* tricyclic antidepressants, nasal spray
- *Laboratory tests:* urinalysis, urine culture, sensitivity testing

Parental status
- *History:* disciplinary methods, parents' understanding of child's problems with incontinence

Psychological status
- *Current problems:* impact on functioning; recent life changes, such as recent move, separation, change in school; coping mechanisms; ability to talk about thoughts and feelings

DEFINING CHARACTERISTICS

- History of frequent urinary tract infections
- History or presence of fecal impaction
- Incontinence
- Presence of psychological risk factors for incontinence, such as inability to express thoughts or feelings, inadequate coping skills, inconsistent discipline, parental discord, recent life changes, or an unstable environment
- Voiding that occurs in socially unacceptable situations

ASSOCIATED DISORDERS

Adjustment disorder, anxiety disorders, autism, disruptive behavior disorder, encopresis, enuresis, pervasive developmental disorder

EXPECTED OUTCOMES

Initial outcome
- Child and family members express feelings related to incontinence.

Interim outcomes
- Child cooperates with interventions to decrease enuresis or encopresis.
- Child demonstrates increased awareness of the need to void or move bowels.
- Child uses play or other means to communicate feelings.

Discharge outcomes
- Family members and teachers exhibit nonjudgmental attitude toward child.
- Child and family members plan to continue interventions at home.

INTERVENTIONS AND RATIONALES

Initial intervention

- Obtain a history of incontinent episodes from parents. Discuss parents' and child's frustrations and concerns *to develop a foundation for nursing interventions.*

Interim interventions

- Implement behavior interventions, such as decreasing fluids in the evenings, waking the child 30 minutes before usual enuresis time, and establishing a time after meals and before bed for the child to sit on the toilet *to encourage routine physiologic function.*
- Provide rewards for compliance with the behavior modification program *to foster a sense of control.*
- Educate the child and family members about psychological factors contributing to incontinence, such as stress, changes at home, inability to release disturbing thoughts and feelings. *A child may communicate troubled feelings through an inability to control bowel and bladder functions.*
- Use toys, puppets, or drawings to help the child identify feelings, such as anger, anxiety, sadness, and happiness. *This helps him understand feelings and cope with stress.*

Discharge outcomes

- Emphasize to family members and teachers the need to display a nonjudgmental attitude toward the child *to prevent damage to his self-esteem.*
- Teach family members about interventions to help decrease incontinence *to ensure continuation of treatment.*

- Educate the child and family members about prescribed medications *to help ensure compliance.*

EVALUATION STATEMENTS

Child:
- participates in behavioral modification program.
- learns to communicate disturbing thoughts and feelings.
- exhibits a decrease in incontinence.
  Child and family members:
- express a desire to continue treatment following discharge.

DOCUMENTATION

- Frequency and time of incontinent episodes
- Daily nursing interventions and child's response
- Patient and family teaching
- Evaluation statements.

Injury, high risk for

related to impulsive or antisocial behavior

DEFINITION

High risk of injury resulting from an inability or refusal to consider the consequences of impulsive antisocial behaviors

ASSESSMENT

Family status
- *Demographics:* family composition; level of education of family members;

parents' occupations; child's grade level; urban, suburban, or rural residency
- *Family roles:* degree of family agreement on roles
- *Family rules:* maladaptive rules, flexibility regarding rules, consequences when rules are broken
- *Family communication:* style and quality of communication, methods of conflict resolution
- *Family subsystems:* alliances between family members, effect of alliances on family stability
- *Physical and emotional needs:* ability of family to meet child's physical and emotional needs, disparities between child's needs and family's willingness or ability to meet them
- *Cultural factors:* identification with racial, cultural, or ethnic group; religious identification; influence of religious beliefs on values and practices
- *Coping patterns:* effectiveness of coping patterns
- *Evidence of abuse or family violence:* physical and behavioral indicators, history of incarceration of family members
- *Family health history:* bipolar disorder, depressive disorder, suicide, substance-related disorder, learning disorders, attention-deficit disorder
- *Diagnostic test:* Family Genogram

Neurologic status
- *Physical examination:* cerebellar function, cranial nerve function, fine and gross motor functioning, pupillary response, sensory ability
- *Mental status:* appearance and attitude, level of consciousness, motor activity, thought and speech, mood and affect, cognition, long- and short-term memory, general information, at-

tention span, abstract thinking, judgment and insight, orientation to person, place, and time
- *Signs and symptoms:* headaches, seizures, poor coordination, vocal or motor tics
- *Laboratory tests:* drug toxicology screening, thyroid function test, metabolic screening, electrolyte levels
- *Diagnostic tests:* electroencephalography (EEG), sleep-deprived EEG, magnetic resonance imaging

Parental status
- *History:* knowledge of normal growth and development, feelings about discipline, stability of parent's relationship, involvement with social service agencies, parent's understanding of child's illness

Psychological status
- *Current problems:* changes in self-image or self-esteem; aggressive behaviors; attempts to set fires; suicidal ideation or attempts; alcohol or drug abuse; sleep pattern disturbances; recent divorce, move, or change in school; loss of loved one or pet; losses through separation, divorce, foster placement, or death
- *Psychiatric history:* age at onset of disorder, past psychiatric hospitalizations, type of treatment, medication regimen, response to treatment and medication
- *Childhood development:* age at which development milestones were achieved, maladaptive behaviors, academic performance, relationships with peers, social group involvement, hobbies, life events in childhood, evidence of antisocial behavior

- *Laboratory tests:* urinalysis, human immunodeficiency virus testing
- *Diagnostic tests:* Rorschach test, Thematic Apperception Test, Children's Apperception Test, Roberts Apperception Test for Children, Revised Children Manifest Anxiety Scale, Children Depression Inventory, Children's Perceived Self-Control Scale

Social status
- *History:* interpersonal skills, size of social network, quality of relationships, degree of trust in others, level of self-esteem, ability to function in social and academic roles

RISK FACTORS

- Alcohol or drug abuse by parents or child
- History of harming self, others, or animals
- History of physical or sexual abuse
- Inability of parents to understand child's illness or meet his needs
- Inability to control aggression, trust others, or cope with problems
- Inconsistent parental discipline or poor parental relationships
- Lack of parental support
- Lack of social network
- Poor communication between family members and difficulty resolving conflicts
- Poor self-esteem

ASSOCIATED DISORDERS

Attention-deficit and hyperactivity disorder, brain tumor, conduct disorder, genetic anomalies, head injury, mood disorders, oppositional defiant disorder, pervasive developmental disorders, posttraumatic stress disorder, psychotic disorders, seizure disorder, Tourette's disorder

EXPECTED OUTCOMES

Initial outcomes
- Child refrains from harming himself or others by accepting redirection, time-outs, seclusion, and medications.
- Child expresses understanding of safety rules.

Interim outcomes
- Child redirects energies to constructive activities.
- Child expresses feelings in socially appropriate manners.
- Child takes time-outs or leaves room when beginning to feel out of control.
- Child uses play or other means to communicate feelings.
- Child participates in therapeutic group activities and outings.
- Child stops to consider consequences of behavior.

Discharge outcomes
- Family participates in appropriate educational sessions.
- Child and family members plan to continue treatment.
- Parents establish a plan for crisis situations.

INTERVENTIONS AND RATIONALES

Initial interventions
- Provide a private room to reduce external stimuli and remove any dangerous articles *to keep the child and those around him safe.*

- Approach the child calmly. Communicate that you accept him but not his destructive behaviors *to avoid damaging his sense of self-worth.*
- Inform the child that the environment is safe and that you will keep him safe from harming himself or others *to decrease his anxiety.*
- Establish boundaries around the patient's behavior by setting firm, consistent limits and making expectations clear. *Structure and consistency will improve communication and reduce anxiety.*

Interim interventions
- Refrain from arguing with the child and avoid power struggles *to maintain a therapeutic relationship.*
- Educate the patient about socially inappropriate behaviors and redirect his energy to constructive activities. *Redirection will help the child improve his peer and family relationships.*
- Point out antisocial or impulsive behaviors to the child and immediately inquire about his feelings *to correlate feelings and behaviors.*
- Use toys, puppets, or drawings to help the patient identify feelings, such as anger, anxiety, sadness, and happiness. *This helps the child to understand his feelings.*
- Through role playing and metaphoric play with toys, teach the child that certain feelings trigger impulsive behaviors *to help him understand and control his actions.*
- Involve the child in therapeutic group activities *to enhance social skills and peer relationships.*
- Reward the child for refraining from antisocial or impulsive behaviors *to en-*hance his self-esteem and reduce the risk of injury.*
- Discuss home and school situations with the child and teach him to stop, think, feel, and act *to help him deal with stress.*

Discharge interventions
- Educate the family, patient, school counselors, and teachers about prescribed medications *to maintain compliance with the medication regimen.*
- Discuss with the family, teacher, and outpatient clinician interventions to enhance socially appropriate behaviors *to promote continuation of newly learned behaviors.*
- Review follow-up appointments and emergency numbers *to reinforce the importance of continued care in an outpatient setting.*
- Teach parents to adopt behavioral modification techniques in the home *to continue interventions.*

EVALUATION STATEMENTS

Child:
- doesn't attempt to harm himself or others.
- complies with interventions such as time-outs and redirection to constructive activities.
- exhibits fewer socially inappropriate behaviors.
- states consequences of impulsive behaviors.
- identifies such feelings as anger, sadness, boredom, or loneliness.
- talks about why he feels upset.
- takes time-outs or leaves the room when he begins to feel out of control.
- participates in therapeutic group activities and outings.

Family members:
- attend family therapy and educational groups.
- express the need for ongoing treatment.
- cooperate with community agencies, the school system, and the inpatient team in planning ongoing treatment.

DOCUMENTATION

- Diagnostic test results
- Nursing interventions to ensure safety of patient, other children, and staff
- Behaviors that lead to time-out or seclusion, frequency of time-outs and seclusion
- Effectiveness of nursing interventions to redirect the child's energies to constructive activities
- Specialized behavioral modification plans and their effectiveness
- Effectiveness of medications used to assist patient in gaining control
- Child's and family members' responses to education and discharge planning
- Evaluation statements.

Knowledge deficit

related to lack of information about safer sex practices

DEFINITION

Inadequate understanding of safer sexual practices that puts the adolescent and partner at risk for infection by sexually transmitted diseases

ASSESSMENT

Family status
- *Demographics:* age, sex, level of education of all family members; socioeconomic status
- *Cultural influences:* ethnicity, religious affiliation, beliefs and attitudes regarding health practices and sexual activity

Neurologic status
- *Mental status:* appearance and attitude, level of consciousness, motor activity, thought and speech, mood and affect, perceptions, orientation, memory, general information, capacity to read and write, attention span, abstraction, judgment and insight

Sexuality status
- *History:* contraceptive practices; drug and alcohol use; attitudes toward sex; sexual orientation; sexual practices; history of gonorrhea, syphilis, acquired immunodeficiency syndrome (AIDS), chlamydia, herpes, or venereal disease

Social status
- *History:* developmental stage, learning ability, obstacles to learning, decision-making abilities (especially with regard to sexual relationships), support systems (family, friends, partner, teachers)

DEFINING CHARACTERISTICS

- Expressed, implied, or observed lack of knowledge concerning sexual practices and relative risks
- Poor negotiating skills, especially within sexual relationships

- Sexual behavior that increases the adolescent's or partner's risk of infection by sexually transmitted diseases
- Substance use or abuse or any other behavior that impairs decision-making abilities regarding sexual activity

ASSOCIATED DISORDERS

AIDS, chancroid, chlamydial infection, genital herpes, genital warts, gonorrhea, human immunodeficiency virus (HIV) infection, syphilis, trichomoniasis

EXPECTED OUTCOMES

Initial outcome
- Adolescent describes his current sexual practices and his understanding of associated risks.

Interim outcomes
- Adolescent describes safer sexual practices.
- Adolescent exhibits improved interpersonal negotiation skills.
- Adolescent describes proper use of a condom or rubber dam.
- Adolescent states his intention to use safer sexual practices and negotiate appropriate boundaries in sexual relationships.

Discharge outcomes
- Adolescent describes feelings about safer sex practices.
- Adolescent obtains appropriate referrals to community resources.

INTERVENTIONS AND RATIONALES

Initial intervention
- Using a nonjudgmental approach, assess the adolescent's sexual practices and awareness of risks associated with various sexual behaviors *to target your teaching plan.*

Interim interventions
- Describe the relative risk associated with specific sexual activities:
– high-risk practices, such as vaginal or anal intercourse without a condom, unprotected oral sex, manual anal intercourse, oral-anal contact, blood contact, and ingesting urine or semen.
– moderate-risk practices, such as french kissing, anal or vaginal intercourse using nonoxynol 9 and a latex condom, fellatio interruptus using nonoxynol 9 and a latex condom, cunnilingus using a rubber dam, and urine contact.
– low-risk practices, such as mutual masturbation, wearing a latex glove when exploring rectum or vagina, closed-mouth kissing, massage, hugging, body-to-body rubbing. *Knowledge of risks will empower the adolescent to make appropriate choices about sexual behavior.*
- Explain that absolutely safe behaviors include abstinence, solitary masturbation, fantasy, voyeurism, or a mutually monogamous relationship with a noninfected partner *to reinforce that all other sexual practices carry varying degrees of risk.*
- As appropriate, discuss populations at high risk for sexually transmitted diseases. For example, if you suspect that the adolescent or the adolescent's

partner is an I.V. drug abuser, discuss the high risk of HIV transmission for members of this population group. *Adolescents who are members of high-risk groups or whose partners are members of high-risk groups need to be especially vigilant about practicing safer sex to avoid disease transmission through repeated exposure.*
- Provide the adolescent with basic information about how to effect change. Discuss the need to acknowledge that one's own behavior may create risk, make a commitment to change, and involve one's sexual partner or partners in the process. *Discussing how to effect change may empower the adolescent to modify his risk profile.*
- Discuss the steps the adolescent needs to take to ensure safer sex. For example, before becoming aroused, the adolescent should discuss the boundaries of a sexual relationship with a potential partner. *Planning in advance for sexual activity will further empower the adolescent to decrease risky behavior.*
- Support the adolescent's efforts to be assertive in setting sexual practice boundaries *to increase his self-confidence and decrease his perception of powerlessness.*
- Instruct the adolescent in proper use of a condom and rubber dam *to reduce the risk of infection.* Describe the proper use of a condom or dam during sexual activity:
– Fully unroll a condom over the erect penis while pinching the end of the condom to provide a reservoir for semen. Hold the condom at the base of the penis when withdrawing.
– Place the dam over the entire vulva or rectum holding two edges of the dam with his hands. Use separate dams when practicing both oral-vaginal and oral-anal sex. Keep the condom or dam in a readily accessible place.
– Always use a new condom or dam for each act of intercourse.
– Never use petroleum-based lubricants with condoms or rubber dams. *Petroleum-based lubricants greatly increase the risk of breaks or leaks in the protective materials.*

Discharge interventions
- Ask the adolescent how he feels about the information you provide on safer sex practices and listen openly to his response. *Getting adolescent feedback will help you evaluate the learning process.*
- Provide the adolescent with names and telephone numbers of resource people or organizations, such as a community AIDS task force, *to provide continuity of care and follow-up after discharge.*

EVALUATION STATEMENTS
Adolescent:
- describes high-, moderate-, and low-risk sexual practices.
- demonstrates improved negotiating skills.
- describes safer sexual practices.
- reports an intention to use safer sexual practices and negotiate appropriate boundaries in sexual relationships.
- describes available community resources for further information and counseling.

DOCUMENTATION

- Adolescent's knowledge about sexual practices and their relative health risks and about sexually transmitted diseases
- Statements reflecting the adolescent's concern about risks that may be incurred by current sexual practices
- Patient teaching provided
- Adolescent's response to teaching, including statements about changes in sexual practices
- Evaluation statements.

Parental role conflict

related to child's hospitalization

DEFINITION

State in which one or both parents experience role confusion and conflict in response to hospitalization of their child

ASSESSMENT

Family status
- *Demographics:* age, sex, and developmental stages of children; age, level of education, occupation, and marital status of parents
- *Cultural influences:* nationality, ethnicity, religious affiliation; values and beliefs regarding parenting, child development, and illness; health practices, rituals, and customs
- *Family development:* severity of the child's condition, number and ages of siblings, developmental stage of the family, conflict between family's life-

style and child's needs, authority within family, level of financial security
- *Parenting skills:* age and maturity, employment skills, knowledge of normal childhood growth and development, level of knowledge regarding the child's condition and prognosis, expectations for the child, ability to meet physical and emotional needs of all children
- *Parent-child interaction:* eye contact, attitude, facial expressions (smiling, frowning), verbal expressions of support, touching, response to child's appearance (bandages, deformities, hospital equipment), quality of parent-child interaction prior to hospitalization
- *Parents' adaptation to child's illness:* severity of child's illness and reason for hospitalization, child's developmental and health care needs, stability of marriage and quality of communication between parents, methods of resolving conflicts, usual coping strategies and their perceived effectiveness, history of using alcohol or drugs (prescribed, OTC, illicit) as a coping mechanism, prior responses to crises, level of community involvement, support systems (extended family, friends, community resources), concurrent family problems
- *Diagnostic tests:* Family Genogram, Cultural Assessment Guide

DEFINING CHARACTERISTICS

- Breakdown in marital relationship (reduction in mutual support and poor communication)
- Changes in the usual pattern of parent-child interaction due to hospitalization

- Expressed or demonstrated inability to cope with parental responsibilities at home
- Expressions of anger, apprehension, anxiety, confusion, doubt, fear, financial worry, or guilt related to child's illness or need for hospitalization
- Inability or unwillingness to participate in child's physical or emotional care

ASSOCIATED DISORDERS AND TREATMENTS

This diagnosis may accompany any condition necessitating hospitalization of the child, such as asthma, burns, cancer, failure to thrive, fractures, head injury, or seizure disorders.

EXPECTED OUTCOMES

Initial outcomes
- Child remains safe during hospitalization.
- Parents express their feelings and concerns about their child's illness and need for hospitalization.

Interim outcomes
- Parents identify and use adaptive coping strategies.
- Parents provide daily physical and emotional care for their child.
- Parents demonstrate improved knowledge of their child's illness, prognosis, and developmental needs.
- Parents reestablish usual patterns of interaction (talking, touching, eye contact) with their child.
- Parents report feeling less threatened by their child's illness.

Discharge outcomes
- Parents develop an effective support system of family, friends, and community services.
- Parents report feeling in control of circumstances and capable of meeting the needs of their child.

INTERVENTIONS AND RATIONALES

Initial interventions
- Follow the medical regimen in caring for the child's current illness *to ensure the child's safety and return to optimal health.*
- Discuss the child's illness and prognosis with the parents *to assess their level of understanding and ability to adapt to their child's illness.*
- Explain the hospital environment, including procedures, medical equipment, visitation, and staff responsibilities to the parents. *This reduces anxiety and promotes a trusting therapeutic relationship.*

Interim interventions
- Involve the parents in the child's care. Acknowledge their role as primary caretakers, provide information necessary to help them make informed decisions, and encourage them to provide their child with emotional support during difficult, painful, or complex procedures. *Parents have intuitive insights into the needs of their child and should act as primary caregivers whenever possible. Also, participating in care can reduce feelings of anxiety, guilt, and helplessness.*
- Teach the parents about normal childhood physical and psychological development *to help them identify and*

address developmental delays or changes brought on by the child's illness.
▪ Assess the parents' coping strategies. Be prepared to discuss and demonstrate constructive alternatives to maladaptive behaviors. *Adaptive coping strategies strengthen the family and help the parents cope effectively with unavoidable family crises.*
▪ Help the parents develop realistic short-term family goals *to reduce feelings of frustration and helplessness.*
▪ Encourage the parents to cooperate with each other and to provide mutual support during their child's illness. *This reduces anxiety and confusion in the family, strengthens the marriage, and enhances the child's sense of security.*
▪ Provide the parents with appropriate amenities when care activities keep them on the unit for long periods. For example, arrange a shower or a place to eat, sleep, or just relax. Be available to care for their child if the parents need a respite. *By helping the parents meet personal needs, you empower them to meet their child's health care needs.*

Discharge intervention
▪ Provide the parents with appropriate referrals to support groups, community services, or trained professionals. *Providing appropriate referrals helps ensure emotional support for the parents, stability for the family, and continuity of care for the child.*

EVALUATION STATEMENTS

Parents:
▪ openly express their feelings and concerns regarding their child's illness and need for hospitalization.
▪ provide their child with daily emotional and physical care.
▪ identify and use adaptive coping strategies.
▪ identify areas of marital stress and work cooperatively to improve mutual support during the child's hospitalization.
▪ demonstrate improved knowledge of the developmental needs of their child.
▪ reestablish normal interaction with their child, holding and touching him and expressing their affection and concern.
▪ report regaining a sense of control.
▪ develop and use a support system comprised of family members, friends, community services, support groups, and medical professionals to help them cope with their child's illness.

DOCUMENTATION

▪ Feelings expressed by the parents relating to their child's illness and need for hospitalization
▪ Observed or reported ineffective coping strategies
▪ Initial level of parents' involvement in their child's daily care
▪ Nursing interventions to help parents improve coping skills and to reestablish usual parent-child interaction
▪ Referrals to community services, support groups, and trained professionals

- Child's response to nursing interventions
- Parents' response to nursing interventions
- Indications of improved parent-child interaction and improved coping abilities of parents
- Improvement in child's emotional state
- Evaluation statements.

Parental role conflict

related to home care of a child with special needs

DEFINITION

State in which one or both parents experience role confusion and crisis in response to the special care needs of a child at home

ASSESSMENT

Family status
- *Demographics:* age, sex, level of education, and occupation of parents
- *Cultural influences:* ethnicity, nationality, religious affiliation; values and beliefs regarding parenting, child rearing, and health care
- *Family development:* extent of child's special needs; number and ages of siblings; developmental stage of family; conflict between family's lifestyle and child's needs; authority within family; level of financial security; family's ability to meet physical, emotional, and social needs of child
- *Parenting skills:* age and maturity level, marital status, employment history, stability of parental relationship, knowledge of normal growth and development, understanding of child's condition and prognosis, expectations regarding child, response to identification of child's special needs
- *Coping mechanisms:* involvement in community, usual response to crises, support systems (relatives, friends, visiting nurse, community resources)

DEFINING CHARACTERISTICS
- Delayed growth and development of child
- Expressions of apprehension, fear, or inadequacy regarding caring for the child
- Expressions of feeling overwhelmed by the child's condition and health care needs
- Inability or unwillingness of one or both parents to physically, psychologically, or financially participate in child's physical and emotional care
- Inadequate physical and psychosocial care of child with special needs
- Inappropriate or inconsistent discipline
- Lack of physical contact between parents and child
- Poor understanding of child's condition, prognosis, and care requirements
- Presence of child who is chronically ill or technology-dependent and requires multiple daily home treatments or careful monitoring

ASSOCIATED DISORDERS AND TREATMENTS

This diagnosis may be associated with any condition requiring long-term home care such as acquired immunodeficiency syndrome, cystic fibrosis, disorders requiring parenteral nutrition therapy, Down syndrome and other developmental disabilities, hemophilia, and respiratory disorders requiring mechanical ventilation.

EXPECTED OUTCOMES

Initial outcomes
- Parents seek external support, education, and assistance to better care for their child at home.
- Parents and siblings discuss their feelings about the child's illness and its impact on family life.

Interim outcomes
- Parents demonstrate improved knowledge concerning the child's developmental needs.
- Parents provide appropriate physical, emotional, and developmental care for their child at home.
- Parents seek emotional support and periodic respites to address personal and marital needs.
- Siblings demonstrate age-appropriate skills in providing care for their brother or sister.
- Siblings report improved feelings of self-esteem and control.

Discharge outcomes
- Parents report feelings of increased confidence regarding meeting their child's needs and acknowledge need to avoid overprotective care.
- Child's self-esteem and social interaction improve.

INTERVENTIONS AND RATIONALES

Initial interventions
- Follow the prescribed medical regimen in caring for the child *to ensure his well-being and return to optimal health.*
- Discuss the child's special needs and home care activities with the parents *to assess the quality of home care and the educational needs of the parents.*
- Encourage the parents and other children to discuss their feelings about the child's condition and care. *Commonly, parents and siblings harbor unexpressed feelings of anxiety, inadequacy, anger, or fear about the child's condition and its impact on family life. Bringing these feelings into the open is the first step in finding solutions.*

Interim interventions
- Involve the parents in the child's care. Acknowledge their role as primary caretakers, provide any information needed to help them make informed decisions, and encourage them to provide their child with emotional support during painful procedures. *Parents have intuitive insight into their child's needs and, therefore, are usually the best primary caregivers.*
- Talk with the parents about the importance of arranging time for activities that enhance their relationship. Explain how respite care can help. Provide information about local agencies that provide respite care and other community resources that support home care. *To provide quality home care for their child, parents must arrange time to address personal needs as well.*

- Help the parents develop realistic expectations of their child and formulate achievable short-term goals based on the child's needs and abilities to reduce feelings of frustration and helplessness.
- Assess the parents' ability to address routine health needs of the child, such as regular dental care, immunizations, personal safety issues, and nutrition. Provide teaching as needed. *A chronically ill child needs complete home health care, not just interventions focused on his illness.*
- Assess the needs of the child's siblings. As you talk with them, ask how it feels to have a brother or sister with special needs; ask how their friends react. If appropriate, contact the school nurse for additional information. Encourage the children to help care for their brother or sister in age-appropriate ways. *Being involved in care activities often improves the siblings' sense of self-esteem and control.*

Discharge interventions
- Advocate normal growth and development for the child. Encourage the parents to allow visits by friends and discourage overprotective behavior. *This promotes social acceptance. Family, friends, and others begin to view the child as a unique, worthwhile individual. This, in turn, helps improve the child's self-esteem.*
- Act as a liaison between the family and health care team, equipment vendors, and community agencies, as needed, *to promote an organized approach, reduce stress, and enhance continuity of care.*

EVALUATION STATEMENTS

Parents:
- demonstrate improved knowledge of their child's condition, prognosis, and home care needs.
- use community resources to help them meet their child's physical, psychological, emotional, and educational needs.
- develop and use a support system to meet personal, emotional, and developmental needs.
   Child's siblings:
- voice their acceptance of having a brother or sister with special needs.
- assist with home care of their brother or sister in age-appropriate ways.

DOCUMENTATION

- Feelings expressed by parents regarding home care of their child
- Feelings expressed by siblings about their brother or sister's condition and its impact on their life
- Observations of parents' interaction with their child
- Description of the child's condition and his special needs
- Nursing interventions to resolve parental role conflicts
- Response of parents, child, and siblings to interventions
- Evaluation statements.

Parenting alteration

related to physical or psychological abuse

DEFINITION

Behavior on the part of the parents that threatens the child's physical safety, psychological well-being, or both, and impairs normal childhood growth and development

ASSESSMENT

Family status

▪ *Demographics:* child's age, sex, developmental stage, and level of education; age, level of education, occupation, socioeconomic and marital status of parents

▪ *Cultural influences:* nationality, ethnicity, religious affiliation; beliefs, attitudes, and values regarding family, child rearing, discipline, health, and illness; health customs, practices, and rituals

▪ *Family roles:* formal and informal roles, family hierarchy, interrelationship of roles and degree of role rigidity, family alliances

▪ *Family rules:* rules that foster stability, maladaptive or inconsistently applied rules, methods of modifying family rules

▪ *Family communication:* style and quality of communication, methods of conflict resolution,

▪ *Goals and values:* extent to which family members agree about goals and values and permit individual members to pursue personal goals

▪ *Family coping patterns:* ability to meet children's physical and emotional needs, major life events, usual coping methods and their perceived effectiveness

▪ *Diagnostic tests:* Family Coping Index, Feetham Family Functioning Survey, Family Genogram, Family Ecomap, Cultural Assessment Guide

Child's health status

▪ *Integumentary examination:* skin characteristics, hygiene, presence of scars or lesions

▪ *Musculoskeletal examination:* range of motion of all joints; joint and muscle symmetry; evidence of swelling, masses, or deformity; pain or tenderness on movement; muscle size, strength, and tone; functional mobility

▪ *Nutritional status:* height and weight in relation to norms for child's developmental stage; usual eating, exercise, and sleeping patterns; basal energy expenditure; anthropometric measurements; abdominal examination

▪ *Mental status:* appearance and attitude, level of consciousness, motor activity, mood and affect, perceptions, orientation, memory, calculations, ability to read and write, visual-spatial ability, attention span, abstraction, judgment, insight

▪ *Laboratory tests:* drug toxicology screen, hemoglobin and hematocrit levels

▪ *Diagnostic test:* Folstein Mini-Mental Health Status Examination

Parental status

▪ *Child rearing skills:* level of maturity, temperament, past responses to crises, knowledge of normal childhood

growth and development, expectations regarding children, disciplinary measures (type, frequency, severity), employment skills and opportunities, stability of parents' relationship, available support systems
- *Parent-child interaction:* parents' caretaking behavior during hospitalization; frequency of eye contact with child; smiling, touching, and verbal expressions of affection and support; parents' response to child's appearance, attitude, and expressions
- *Social behavior:* interpersonal skills; level of self-esteem and self-confidence; comfort level in social settings; evidence of maladaptive behaviors, such as aggression, distrust, social withdrawal, or isolation
- *Diagnostic tests:* Caldwell HOME Inventory, Polansky Childhood Level of Living Scale (CAL) or Child Well-Being Scale, Rubin's Interpersonal Problem-Solving Scale, MESSEY Social Skills Assessment Scale, Social Network Map

DEFINING CHARACTERISTICS

- Delay in child's growth and development
- Evidence of physical or psychological trauma
- Expressions of feeling overwhelmed by demands of parenting
- Expressions of resentment, dislike, or disrespect toward child
- Failure to provide for the child's basic needs
- Failure to thrive (infant)
- Family history of child abuse or abandonment

- Inadequate visual, tactile, or auditory stimulation for the child's developmental stage
- Inconsistent or inappropriate discipline
- Lack of emotional attachment to child
- Lack of knowledge regarding normal childhood growth and development
- Missed appointments with health care professionals
- Poor family communication
- Substance abuse or psychiatric disorder (parents)

ASSOCIATED DISORDERS

Battered child syndrome, burns, child abuse, depressive disorder (parent or child), failure to thrive, fractures, head trauma, neglect, neuromuscular or skeletal accidents or trauma, shaken baby syndrome, soft-tissue injuries

EXPECTED OUTCOMES

Initial outcomes
- Child recovers from his injuries and remains safe during hospital stay.
- Child's diagnostic and laboratory tests suggest or confirm suspected child abuse.

Interim outcomes
- Parents acknowledge their need for help in stopping abusive behavior.
- Parents attend counseling or therapy sessions to address abusive behavior.
- Parents describe appropriate ways to express and cope with anger and frustration.

- Parents reestablish physical and emotional ties with their child (eye contact, touching, talking).
- Parents participate in caring for the child and express their affection and concern for him.
- Parents demonstrate an improved understanding of normal childhood growth and development.

Discharge outcomes
- Parents receive emergency phone numbers and make arrangements for ongoing counseling.
- Child receives post-discharge accommodations that ensure his safety.
- Parents identify and use a support system that includes family, friends, community resources, and appropriate health professionals or counselors.
- Child grows and develops at age-appropriate rate.

INTERVENTIONS AND RATIONALES

Initial interventions
- Follow the prescribed medical regimen *to ensure the child's safety and optimal recovery from injuries.*
- If you suspect child abuse, ask the doctor or radiologist to perform a total-body X-ray. If you suspect that the child has been forced to ingest drugs or alcohol, get an order for toxicology studies (urine and blood). If he is badly bruised, get an order for blood coagulation studies *to obtain evidence of abuse and assess the child's needs.*
- If X-rays or other studies suggest the child has been abused, talk to the doctor about confronting the parents. Follow your hospital's protocol for notifying the appropriate state or local agen-

cy responsible for investigating cases of suspected abuse *to protect the child from further harm and fulfill your legal obligations. Nurses in all states are legally required to report cases of child abuse.*
- Separate the parents and ask each individually about the child's injuries and assess their willingness and ability to acknowledge abusive behaviors. *Typically, abusive parents are impatient with staff and respond to questions about the child's injuries with evasive or vague answers. Denial, indignation, and even indifference to events are common responses to evidence of child abuse. Conflicting accounts are also common.*

Interim interventions
- Attempt to provide abusive parents with referrals to psychiatric counseling and support groups, such as a local chapter of Parents Anonymous, a self-help group made up of former child abusers. Arrange psychosocial service consultation. *The abuser will pose a continued threat until he gets help in understanding his abusive behavior and how to change it.*
- Provide the child with a safe, caring environment and visit him frequently. Encourage him to talk about his injuries, feelings, and abusive behavior at home. Act as a role model for the child, demonstrating appropriate adult-child interaction. For example, show the child how to express his feelings, listen carefully to what the child has to say, provide age-appropriate toys and activities that promote development and self-expression, provide a nutritional diet, and show him ways of dealing with feelings that do not involve resorting to violence. *Often,*

abused children are emotionally with-drawn and fearful of hospital staff and procedures. Building a trusting thera-peutic relationship may help the child begin the process of emotional healing.

- If the parents are receptive, involve them in the care of their child, with ad-equate supervision *to help the parents begin to develop an appropriate attach-ment to the child. Strengthening the par-ents' bond with their child may ease their fears and anxiety, help them to cope with guilt and shame, and improve their sense of control and self-esteem.*

- Assess the parents' child rearing skills, knowledge of normal childhood development, and willingness to learn. If parents are receptive, provide teach-ing to address deficits in their knowl-edge of normal developmental tasks, proper child care (bathing, clothing, feeding), nutritional requirements, and routine health care. Encourage questions and provide thorough an-swers. *Commonly, abusive parents were abused themselves during childhood, and thus grew up with poor parental role models and insufficient opportuni-ties to learn normal child rearing prac-tices. Teaching may help them cope with parenting responsibilities.*

- Provide positive reinforcement when the parents demonstrate appro-priate parenting skills *to help them gain confidence in their parenting abili-ties.*

Discharge interventions
- Provide the parents with emergency numbers to contact in times of crisis if they feel they are about to lose their temper *to promote safety and adaptive coping.*

- Arrange appropriate follow-up care including ongoing counseling for par-ents and child *to provide continuity of care.*

- Prepare the child and family for post-discharge accommodations, in-cluding possible foster care *to ensure the child's safety.*

- Help the parents identify a support network, which may include family members, friends, counselors, mem-bers of their church, and members of Parents Anonymous *to provide ongo-ing emotional support, provide con-structive role models, and improve their coping and child rearing skills.*

EVALUATION STATEMENTS

Child:
- remains safe during hospitalization.
- expresses his feelings about abuse in the home.
   Parents:
- acknowledge their abusive behavior and ask for help.
- express and demonstrate their will-ingness to take steps to end abusive be-havior.
- demonstrate physical, verbal, and vi-sual contact with the child that en-hances parent-child attachment.
- describe and demonstrate an im-proved understanding of normal childhood development tasks.
- express positive feelings about their child.
- identify appropriate methods of ex-pressing anger and frustration with their child.
- identify an appropriate support net-work.

DOCUMENTATION

- Parents' expression of feelings about their child
- Physical evidence suggesting child abuse
- Notification of appropriate authorities
- Parents' level of bonding, caretaking, and knowledge
- Nursing interventions to help the child deal with physical and emotional aspects of abuse
- Nursing interventions to help parents stop abusive behaviors
- Response of parents and child to nursing interventions
- Evaluation statements.

Parenting alteration, high risk for

related to lack of resources (money, education, family support, social support)

DEFINITION

Presence of risk factors that interfere with a mother's ability to promote optimum growth and development in an infant or child, such as lack of financial resources, poor education, lack of role models for parenting skills, inadequate social network

ASSESSMENT

Family status
- *Demographics:* child's age, sex, developmental stage; mother's age, occupation, level of education

- *Cultural influences:* nationality, ethnicity, religious affiliation; values, beliefs, and practices regarding child rearing, education, illness, and health care
- *Mother-child attachment:* communication patterns (verbal, physical, eye contact), mother's feelings regarding her role as a parent and the child's appearance and sex, responses to the child's needs
- *Diagnostic tests:* Family Genogram, Cultural Assessment Guide, Caldwell HOME Inventory

Psychological status
- *Mother's history:* developmental stage, available support systems, usual coping mechanisms, role models, relationship with family (especially her own parents), relationship with child's father, level of knowledge regarding child development and parenting, usual recreational activities, financial stressors, previous parenting experience, work demands

Financial status
- *History:* employment history, debt history, motivation to work, skills, level of financial and emotional support provided by extended family, ability to integrate work or school demands with parenting responsibilities

Child's health status
- *History:* routine well-child examinations, immunization dates
- *Physical examination:* height, weight, anthropometric measurements
- *Nutritional status:* daily food intake, basal energy expenditure
- *Integumentary examination:* hygiene, lesions, scars

- *Musculoskeletal examination:* range of motion; evidence of swelling, masses, or deformity; pain or tenderness on movement; history of skeletal injuries

RISK FACTORS

- Adolescent or teenage mother
- Child's father does not accept family responsibilities
- Delay in child's growth and development
- Evidence of poverty
- Expressions of depression, frustration, anger, sadness, or hopelessness by mother
- Expressions of disappointment regarding child's appearance, sex, abilities
- Failure to attend to the child's basic physical and emotional needs
- Failure to keep routine health care appointments
- Failure to provide appropriate visual, tactile, or auditory stimulation
- Frequent accidents
- History of abandonment or abuse
- Inability to afford basic items for child care (clothes, blankets, developmental toys, food, safety items)
- Inadequate mother-child attachment
- Lack of knowledge regarding proper parenting
- Poor or nonexistent role model for parenting skills
- Poor understanding of normal child growth and development and of parenting tasks
- Unrealistic expectations regarding child's behavior

ASSOCIATED DISORDERS

Burns, child abuse or neglect, congenital anomalies, failure to thrive, fractures, head trauma, high-risk pregnancy (teenage, multiple), parent-child relational problem, premature birth, soft-tissue injuries, substance-related disorders

EXPECTED OUTCOMES

Initial outcomes

- Mother expresses feelings, such as anger, anxiety, depression, fear, or sadness related to parenting responsibilities.
- Mother expresses feelings about her child's appearance and abilities.
- Mother asks for financial, emotional, and educational assistance to improve her parenting skills and ability to meet her child's basic needs.

Interim outcomes

- Mother demonstrates appropriate attachment behaviors, such as talking and playing with her child, holding him, and making eye contact.
- Mother demonstrates an improved understanding of child development and her child's developmental tasks.
- Mother describes her child's nutritional requirements and appropriate patterns of eating, sleeping, and recreation.
- Mother identifies and uses coping techniques to reduce anxiety, tension, and stress.
- Mother schedules routine health care examinations of her child at the clinic and arranges transportation.

Discharge outcomes
- Mother reports feeling comfortable asking questions about basic child care practices.
- Mother contacts appropriate social service agencies to arrange financial assistance.
- Mother identifies and uses appropriate sources of support, which may include the child's father, extended family, members of her church, health care professionals, social service agencies, child care facilities, or a support group.

INTERVENTIONS AND RATIONALES

Initial interventions
- Assign one primary nurse to care for the child and mother *to promote a trusting therapeutic relationship.*
- Encourage the mother to express her feelings regarding her child, financial stress, and new role as parent. Listen carefully and avoid expressing judgment. *Discussing feelings in a safe, secure environment helps allay the mother's fear, tension, and anxiety and promotes a trusting therapeutic relationship. Active listening also helps you identify specific difficulties.*
- Explain hospital routines, procedures, and visiting policies. If possible, arrange for her to room with her child or to stay for extended visits. *This enhances mother-child attachment and provides the mother with ample opportunity to observe appropriate parenting behaviors.*
- Assess the amount of developmental stimulation provided by the mother, her knowledge of normal child growth and development and parenting skills, and her willingness to learn. *This information reveals knowledge deficits and provides the basis for planning teaching topics and role modeling.*

Interim interventions
- Involve the mother immediately in caring for her child *to promote attachment.*
- Teach the mother the basics of proper child care. For example, if she has an infant, teach her proper techniques for breast- or bottle-feeding (proper positioning, amount to offer, and frequency of feedings), bathing and safety precautions, and appropriate dressing. *Research shows that the primary source of information about parenting is the mother's own parents. If the mother lacks an effective role model, you may need to supply basic information about parenting.*
- Teach the mother how to detect illness; for example, by taking the infant's temperature, assessing his respiratory status, and watching for such cues as ear pulling, increased crying, or drawing his legs up to his abdomen *to improve her ability to monitor her child's health.*
- When caring for the child in the mother's presence, act as a role model for proper parenting techniques. Demonstrate comfort measures, such as rocking the infant, and show the mother how to hold the infant in an en face position. *This improves her understanding of routine child care practices. She may learn as much or more by watching your actions as she does in teaching sessions.*
- Teach the mother about normal growth and development, and identify

ages at which the child should master developmental tasks, such as rolling over, crawling, and walking. Also discuss problem behaviors associated with specific ages, such as colic, temper tantrums, and sleeping difficulties *to help her understand her child's growth and development.*
- Discuss the need for safety measures, such as blocking stairways and keeping crib rails secured, *to prevent accidents.*
- Explain the child's need for tactile and sensory stimulation. Demonstrate play activities that promote developmental skills. For example, explain that shaking a rattle in front of an infant helps build eye-hand coordination and placing a mobile above the infant promotes visual tracking and trunk and head control. *Teaching should enhance the mother's understanding that sensory experiences promote cognitive development.*
- Praise the mother's progress whenever she demonstrates proper parenting skills. *Positive reinforcement is crucial in helping her develop confidence and self-esteem.*
- Emphasize the importance of bringing the child to the clinic for routine health care examinations even when the child appears healthy. *Routine visits are important for the early detection of developmental delays and for preventive care such as immunizations.*

Discharge interventions
- Encourage the mother to ask questions about infant and child care. Reassure her that other parents also need to ask basic questions. *A mother who lacks effective parenting role models may not know what questions to ask or she may hesitate to ask questions because of embarrassment.*
- Provide the mother with all appropriate referrals—for example, to a doctor, nurse practitioner, social service agency, or parent support group, *to ensure continuity of care.*

EVALUATION STATEMENTS

Child or infant:
- recovers from his current illness or injury and remains safe during hospital stay.
  Mother:
- expresses feelings about parenthood, her child's appearance and behavior, and her financial problems.
- asks for educational and financial assistance in meeting the basic needs of her child.
- demonstrates appropriate mother-child attachment behavior (physical contact, eye contact, and verbalization).
- demonstrates proper bathing, feeding, and dressing techniques.
- describes tasks associated with normal childhood growth and development and accurately assesses her child's developmental status and needs.
- engages in age-appropriate developmental play with her child.
- schedules and keeps appointments for routine examinations of her child at the clinic.
- contacts appropriate social services to arrange financial assistance.

DOCUMENTATION
- Evidence of the child's developmental abilities

- Level of mother-child attachment
- Observations of the mother's level of knowledge of normal child development and child rearing skills
- Observations of behaviors indicating the mother's ignorance or neglect of routine child care
- Requests for financial, educational, or emotional assistance by the mother
- Nursing interventions to enhance the child's growth and development and promote mother-child attachment
- Teaching provided
- Referrals to social services for financial assistance, parent support groups, health care professionals, job-training or placement services, other community services
- Mother's response to nursing interventions
- Evaluation statements.

Posttrauma response

related to incest

DEFINITION

Sustained harm to a child's physical, psychological, and spiritual well-being due to incest

ASSESSMENT

Family status
- *Demographics:* family composition; level of education of family members; parents' occupations; child's grade level; urban, suburban, or rural residency
- *Cultural factors:* nationality, race, ethnic group; customs and rituals, especially pertaining to sexuality and sexual development of children
- *History:* family roles and role performance, degree of family agreement on roles, interrelationships of various roles
- *Family subsystems:* relationships between nuclear and extended family members, relationships between siblings and stepbrothers and stepsisters, function of family alliances, presence of family secrets
- *Family rules:* rules that foster stability, maladaptive rules, methods of rule modification, consequences of breaking rules
- *Developmental stage:* changes in family responsibilities over time, frequency with which family members enter and exit family system, sleeping arrangements within family
- *Physical and emotional needs:* ability of family to meet child's physical and emotional needs, family boundaries, extent to which family permits pursuit of individual goals
- *Socioeconomic factors:* economic status of family, sense of adequacy and self-worth of members, employment and attitudes toward work
- *Coping patterns:* usual coping patterns; family members' perceptions of effectiveness of coping patterns
- *Evidence of abuse:* evidence of physical, sexual, or emotional abuse within family (victims and victimizers), ability of family members to protect children and correctly judge situations as being safe or unsafe
- *Family health history:* alcoholism, substance abuse, incarceration of family members, stress-related illness
- *Diagnostic test:* Family Genogram

Gastrointestinal status
- *Physical examination:* abdominal inspection, palpation, and auscultation; rectal examination
- *Signs and symptoms:* anal tearing; trauma to anal area including lacerations, hematomas, petechiae, edema, contusions, bleeding, pain; prolapse of anal tissue; fissures; changes in skin pigmentation; anal skin tags; hemorrhoids; scar tissue; changes in the tone of the anal sphincter; changes in bowel patterns due to anal trauma

Genitourinary status
- *Physical examination:* pelvic, genital, abdominal, rectal
- *Prior medical conditions:* urinary tract infections, vaginal infections, infections of penis, sexually transmitted disease, vaginal warts, start of menarche
- *Signs and symptoms:* trauma to penis or vaginal area, nonintact hymen, clefts or bumps on hymenal membrane, labial adhesions, alteration or widening of the hymenal edge, distorted shape of hymenal membrane caused by scar tissue and adhesions
- *Laboratory tests:* urinalysis, culture and sensitivity, venereal disease research laboratory tests, human immunodeficiency virus testing, vaginal cultures

Parental status
- *History:* marital relationship; past sexual relationships; ability to control impulses; degree of participation in routine child care activities such as bathing, diapering, and toileting; interactions between mother and child; interactions between father and child; ability of parents to choose appropriate caregivers; usual supervision practices
- *Previous conditions:* substance abuse, cognitive or psychiatric impairment, physical or sexual abuse, family violence, sexual dysfunction, deviant sexual behavior

Psychological status
- *Signs and symptoms:* changes in appetite, personal hygiene, self-image, self-esteem, sleep patterns, school performance; changes in behavior, such as aggression, withdrawal, inability to socialize; changes in mood, such as crying, mood swings, irritability; substance abuse
- *Childhood development:* birth order, number of siblings, developmental milestones, parents' ability to recall developmental milestones; school performance, relationships with peers, social activity, life events in childhood, evidence of antisocial behavior, evidence of inappropriate sexual behavior
- *Diagnostic tests:* Revised Children Manifest Anxiety Scale, Children Depression Inventory, Hopelessness Scale for Children, State-Trait Anger Scale, Behavioral Checklist

Sexuality status
- *History:* sexual activity, age of first sexual encounter, attitudes toward sex, exposure to pornographic material, involvement with prostitution, sexually transmitted disease, menstrual history
- *Signs and symptoms:* decreased or increased libido, frequent masturbation, sexual acting out

Sleep pattern status

- *Signs and symptoms:* nightmares, night terrors, difficulty falling asleep, aggressive outbursts prior to bedtime, nocturnal awakening
- *Medications:* sleeping aids

Social status

- *Signs and symptoms:* withdrawal; lack of eye contact; intrusiveness; inappropriate responses; hypersexual behavior toward other children, adults, animals, or objects; aggressiveness

Spiritual status

- *History:* religious identification; family members' and child's perception about life, death, and suffering; spiritual support network

DEFINING CHARACTERISTICS

Family members:
- deviant, unsafe sexual behaviors
- enmeshment
- family secrets or refusal to deal with family problems
- frequent entering and exiting into and out of family system by variety of individuals
- history of incest or sexual abuse
- hostility toward outsiders
- inability to control impulses
- inability to provide for child's basic physical and emotional needs
- inability to recognize deviant sexual behaviors
- inappropriate or explicit touching of child's genitals during bathing, diapering, or toileting practices
- inappropriate sleeping arrangements
- lack of appropriate boundaries between family members
- overprotective behavior

- patriarchal, rigid, or chaotic family structure
- pornography, substance abuse, history of incarcerations due to illegal sexual acts
- religious practices that condone sexualized behaviors between family members

Child:
- behavioral indicators, including frequent masturbation and placing objects in vaginal or anal areas; increased aggression; increase in sexual acting out
- disclosure of sexual fondling or penetration
- fearfulness, discomfort, or anger during interactions with parents
- frequent nightmares and inability to fall asleep
- parent-child role reversals (parentified child)
- sexually transmitted disease or trauma to genital or anal areas

ASSOCIATED DISORDERS

Anxiety disorders, behavioral disorders, depressive disorders, eating disorders, parent-child relational problem, physical abuse of child, posttraumatic stress disorder, sexual abuse of child, sexually transmitted diseases, thought process disorders

EXPECTED OUTCOMES

Initial outcomes
- Child does not harm self or others.
- Child enters into contract to maintain personal safety with staff members.

Interim outcomes

- Child begins to use words to express his feelings.
- Child participates in one-to-one therapeutic sessions.
- Child accepts positive feedback and makes positive statements about himself.

Discharge outcomes

- Child can describe steps to take to maintain safety.
- Child expresses awareness of placement following discharge (home, foster care, group home, or day treatment program).

INTERVENTIONS AND RATIONALES

Initial interventions

- Monitor physiological parameters and follow the medical regimen to treat physical injuries *to prevent further trauma or injury.*
- Inform the members of the treatment team and appropriate family service agencies that the child may be a victim of incest *to assure the child's safety following discharge and fulfill your legal responsibility.*
- Monitor the child for changes in mood or behavior, statements of intention to harm himself, or impulsive gestures. Ask directly about suicidal ideation. *A child who has recently disclosed sexual trauma has a high suicide risk.*
- Ask the child to agree to verbal and written safety contracts stating that he will not harm himself for a specified period of time. *A safety contract provides the patient with a tangible, concrete reminder of how to cope with crisis.*

- If the child's aggressive or inappropriate sexualized behaviors become disruptive, establish limits and provide him with an environment where stimulation is decreased *to provide safety for the patient and other children.*
- Be aware that aggressive or sexual acting out behaviors may indicate that the child is reexperiencing the traumatic event, but does not yet have the capacity to verbally express fear, anger, or sadness. Help him by providing support and consistent structure *to avoid punishing the child for his feelings and assist him in coming to terms with trauma.*

Interim interventions

- If the child wants to talk about the traumatic event, actively listen to the him *to reassure him that what he tells you is important and that you are concerned for him.*
- Encourage the child to express fear, anger, and guilt, feelings commonly associated with incest. *Talking about feelings can reduce the child's episodes of aggression and sexual acting out.*
- Praise the child for participating in one-to-one therapy sessions or group therapeutic activities *to encourage participation and enhance his sense of self-worth.*
- Recognize the child's accomplishments and praise him at all opportunities *to empower him and enhance his self-esteem, thereby reducing the chance of further victimization.*

Discharge interventions

- Help the child identify adults who can be trusted, such as a school counselor, mother or father, foster parents, clergy person, teacher, or therapist, *to help prevent further episodes of incest following discharge.*

▪ Discuss the child's thoughts and feelings about foster care *to help alleviate his fears and anxiety regarding foster placement.* Explain the child's concerns to the foster parents. Also discuss the child's psychological needs *to prepare them for future interactions with the child.*

▪ Discuss ways to ensure the child's safety following discharge, such as close supervision with unfamiliar adults and identifying potential victimizers, with the child's caregivers *to reduce the potential for further episodes of incest.*

▪ Make appropriate referrals to mental health professionals and social workers and review the discharge plan with the child and appropriate caregivers *to encourage follow-up care.*

EVALUATION STATEMENTS

Child:
▪ makes a contract for safety.
▪ responds to limits in order to decrease stimulation and maintain safety.
▪ calms down if behaviors become unsafe and out of control.
▪ talks to a staff member about thoughts and feelings related to episodes of incest.
▪ accepts positive feedback from staff members.
▪ participates in group activities.
▪ identifies specific people to seek out for help (school counselor, mother or father, clergy person, teacher, therapist).
  Caregivers:
▪ state specific ways to provide safety for the child.

▪ agree to provide follow-up care for child.

DOCUMENTATION

▪ Frequency and time of day of time-outs or seclusion
▪ Written or verbal safety contracts
▪ Exact quotes of child if any disclosures are made regarding incest
▪ Child-protective services and treatment team members who were notified about the disclosure
▪ Nursing interventions to prompt the child's expression of thoughts and feelings
▪ Child's statements indicating anger, fear, guilt, or other response to incest
▪ Education provided to the parents, foster parents, or other appropriate caregivers
▪ Child's behavior during and after visitation by family members
▪ Discharge plans for placement
▪ Evaluation statements.

Role performance alteration
related to a learning disability

DEFINITION

Impaired personal, academic, or social development caused by a learning disability

ASSESSMENT

Family status
▪ *Demographics:* age, sex, grade level, and developmental stage of child; age,

occupation, and marital status of parents
- *Cultural influences:* nationality, ethnicity, and religious affiliation; values, beliefs, and practices regarding child rearing, education, illness, and health care
- *Diagnostic tests:* Family Genogram, Cultural Assessment Guide

Neurologic status
- *Mental status:* thought and speech, mood and affect, perceptions, memory, calculations, ability to read and write, visual-spatial ability, attention span, abstraction, judgment and insight, motor system
- *Sensory status:* visual acuity and fields; auditory perception, memory, and discrimination; sensitivity to touch, pressure, and temperature; kinesthetic perception
- *Physical examination:* fine and gross motor skills, cranial nerve function, peripheral sensory system
- *Signs and symptoms:* lethargy, restlessness, seizures
- *Laboratory tests:* drug toxicology screen, lead screening
- *Diagnostic tests:* electroencephalography, Snellen vision test, audiometry

Psychological status
- *Childhood development:* developmental milestones, major life events, academic performance, language development, relationships with peers, energy level, motivation, self-image, self-esteem, evidence of substance abuse
- *Social development:* social skills (language, conversation, interpersonal and social behavior), size and quality of social network, evidence of disruptive behavior in classroom or social settings (playground, store, get-togethers)
- *Signs and symptoms:* withdrawal, lack of eye contact, inappropriate responses, aggressiveness
- *Diagnostic tests:* Vineland Adaptive Behavior Scale, Bayley Mental and Motor Scales of Development, Wechsler Intelligence Scales for Children, Peabody Picture Vocabulary Test, Pediatric Examination of Educational Readiness, McCarthy Scales of Children's Ability, MESSEY Social Skills Assessment Scale

DEFINING CHARACTERISTICS

- Below-normal reading, writing, or math skills
- Depression
- Inability to recall details of school lessons
- Low self-confidence and self-esteem
- Perceptual deficits
- Poor auditory memory skills
- Poor interpersonal and social skills
- Poor problem-solving skills (cognitive, social)
- Poor self-concept
- Poor spatial orientation, body image, and motor coordination
- Poor visual-spatial skills
- Short attention span

ASSOCIATED DISORDERS AND TREATMENTS

This diagnosis commonly accompanies a diagnosed learning disorder (disorder of written expression, mathematics disorder, reading disorder), and may accompany any neurologic or musculoskeletal developmental disorder or disease, exposure to lead or other environmental toxins, fetal alcohol syndrome, head injury, hearing loss, treatment with anticonvulsants, or vision or ocular disorders.

EXPECTED OUTCOMES

Initial outcomes
- Child expresses his feelings about trouble with school, teachers, peers, or parents.
- Child cooperates with testing to investigate possible learning disorders.

Interim outcomes
- Parents express feelings, such as anger, anxiety, or frustration, regarding their child's developmental delay.
- Parents demonstrate improved understanding of their child's learning disability and associated needs.
- Child demonstrates improved attention to tasks, such as homework, classroom assignments, and household duties.
- Child reports feeling more confident about his ability to perform assigned tasks in allotted time.
- Child identifies his own special talents and abilities.

Discharge outcomes
- Parents obtain referrals for ongoing emotional and educational support for their child.
- Child demonstrates academic, social, and personal development appropriate for his age and development stage.

INTERVENTIONS AND RATIONALES

Initial interventions
- Schedule uninterrupted non-care-related time to talk with the child about his feelings regarding his academic, social, and personal concerns. *Commonly, a learning disabled child is completely bewildered by his difficulty and senses that he is different from other children. This can lead to feelings of confusion, frustration, fear, and guilt. Listening and providing guidance about learning disabilities improves the child's understanding, reduces his anxiety, and helps build a trusting therapeutic relationship.*
- Refer parents and the child to an educational psychologist *to evaluate the child's learning skills and identify specific disabilities.*

Interim interventions
- Provide positive reinforcement when the child exhibits adaptive behaviors *to encourage appropriate behavior.*
- Discuss the child's learning disability with his parents. Assess their level of knowledge about learning disabilities and acceptance. Listen to them without conveying judgment. *Parents need accurate information about the type and severity of their child's learning disability. They may react with guilt, anger, anxiety, or frustration and need to vent these feelings. Talking with the parents helps you identify family problems or parental deficiencies that need to be addressed in teaching sessions.*
- Explain the nature of the disability and its prognosis. *This helps the par-*

ents *adjust their expectations for their child.*

- Teach the parents about normal tasks for their child's development stage. Discuss ways they can help their child meet normal developmental goals *to provide insight into normal child behavior and how their child differs. Getting parents involved improves their sense of control over circumstances and helps reduce anxiety.*
- Tell the parents to discuss the child's disability and recommended interventions with teachers and counselors at his school *to provide an ongoing program for enhancing the child's learning skills and opportunities.*
- Teach the parents to:
– limit distractions when the child is doing homework *to help him remain focused.*
– break large tasks into smaller sequential steps *to make lessons easier to understand and provide more opportunities for positive reinforcement.*
– permit periodic breaks from studying *to provide opportunities for gross motor activity, which helps release energy and reduces feelings of frustration or anxiety.*
– stay nearby *to provide encouragement and positive feedback.*
- Suggest that the parents talk to the child's teacher about using oral rather than written tests. *A verbal quiz may provide a more accurate assessment of the child's learning. For learning disabled children, translating thoughts into words and then writing them down can be complex and frustrating.*
- Recommend that parents provide the child with sensory experiences that enhance learning, such as tracing letters in sand with his finger, *to help improve his perceptual skills.*
- Tell parents to provide the child with frequent and consistent positive feedback and to set time limits on study assignments *to reduce anxiety and frustration, provide structure, and promote self-confidence and self-esteem.*
- Encourage the child to identify and develop his special talents *to boost his self-esteem.*

Discharge intervention
- Provide the family with appropriate referrals to community services, support groups, and educational and psychiatric professionals *to ensure continuity of care.*

EVALUATION STATEMENTS

Child:
- expresses feelings such as anxiety, frustration, and confusion regarding his learning and socialization difficulties.
- identifies personal strengths and coping techniques to help compensate for his disability.
- demonstrates an ability to remain focused during study periods.
- begins to complete assignments accurately and on time.
- reports feeling less frustrated and more confident.
    Parents:
- express feelings of anxiety, concern, guilt, or frustration related to their child's delayed development and academic difficulties.
- demonstrate an understanding of their child's disability and its effect on his development.

- participate in developing and implementing a treatment plan that addresses the child's learning disability.
- provide their child with emotional support and encouragement.
- enlist the help of teachers and health professionals in providing enhanced learning opportunities for their child.
- identify and use a support system that includes community resources and health professionals.

DOCUMENTATION

- Diagnostic test results
- Child's academic status and reported difficulties
- Child's attitude about school and learning, based upon reports from the child, parents, and teachers
- Parents' expression of concern regarding delays in the child's development
- Child's diagnosed learning disability
- Nursing interventions to help family members adapt to the child's disability
- Responses of parents and child to interventions
- Evaluation statements.

Self-esteem disturbance

related to adverse relationship with parents

DEFINITION

Presence of a parent-adolescent conflict that damages the adolescent's self-esteem

ASSESSMENT

Family status
- *Demographics:* family composition; level of education of all family members; parents' occupations; adolescent's grade level; urban, suburban, or rural residency
- *Family roles:* degree of family agreement on roles, interrelationship of various roles
- *Family rules:* rules that foster stability, maladaptive rules, willingness of parents to modify rules, consequences when rules are broken
- *Family communication:* style and quality of communication, methods of conflict resolution
- *Family subsystems:* family alliances and their effects on family stability
- *Family needs:* ability of family to meet adolescent's physical and emotional needs, disparities between adolescent's needs and family's ability to meet them
- *Family goals and values:* extent to which family permits adolescent to pursue individual goals and values
- *Socioeconomic factors:* economic status of family, effect of financial pressures on members' sense of adequacy and self-worth
- *Coping patterns:* usual coping patterns, family members' perceptions of effectiveness of coping patterns
- *Evidence of abuse:* physical and behavioral indicators
- *Diagnostic test:* Family Genogram

Psychological status
- *History:* birth order; changes in appetite, energy level, motivation, personal hygiene, self-image, self-esteem, sleep patterns; alcohol or drug abuse;

reaction to puberty; quality of relationships with authority figures; scholastic performance
- *Recent events:* divorce of parents, illness, job loss, loss of loved one; recent move or change in school
- *Diagnostic tests:* Children Depressive Inventory, Hopelessness Scale for Children, Child Attitude Toward Father and Mother Scales

Parental status
- *History:* knowledge of normal growth and development, attitudes about discipline, ability to agree on disciplining children, stability of parental relationship, understanding of adolescent's self-esteem disturbance, ability to recognize adolescent's achievement of developmental milestones
- *Diagnostic test:* Index of Parental Attitudes

DEFINING CHARACTERISTICS

- Disagreement about family rules between adolescent and parents
- Financial stress or abusive or chaotic family environment
- Frequent fights or arguments between adolescent and parents
- Inability of family members to communicate or to resolve conflicts
- Inability of family members to recognize adolescent's emotional, physical, and social needs or to help him meet them
- Lack of appropriate boundaries between family members
- Lack of flexibility in family rules and rigid consequences when rules are broken

- Parental discord or lack of knowledge of normal growth and development in children

ASSOCIATED DISORDERS

Adolescent antisocial behavior, communication disorders, conduct disorder, learning disabilities, mood disorders, oppositional defiant disorder, parent-child relational problem, posttraumatic stress disorder

EXPECTED OUTCOMES

Initial outcome
- Adolescent and family describe areas of conflict.

Interim outcomes
- Adolescent begins to express feelings.
- Parents encourage and support adolescent's attempts to express feelings.
- Adolescent uses "I" statements to express feelings.
- Adolescent states positive attributes about self.
- Parents state positive attributes about adolescent and family as a whole.

Discharge outcome
- Parents and adolescent make a commitment to continue outpatient family treatment.

INTERVENTIONS AND RATIONALES

Initial interventions
- Provide a safe, structured environment for adolescent and parents *to encourage open discussion of family conflicts.*

- Discuss with the adolescent and parents the schedule, purpose, and goals of individual and family treatment. *Awareness of the reasons and expectations of treatment will enhance cooperation.*

Interim interventions

- Encourage the adolescent to participate in group activities, group therapy, and individual counseling *to provide opportunities to strengthen self-esteem.*
- Encourage the adolescent to use "I" statements to express feelings; for example, "I am mad because of my curfew." *Using "I" statements may help him get in touch with and talk about feelings.*
- Inform the parents that their adolescent is learning how to talk about feelings and using "I" statements. *Because family communication patterns are deeply ingrained, parents may need time to adjust to their child's assertiveness.*
- Assist the parents in understanding the value of talking about feelings *to encourage them to express emotions appropriately and to discourage them from punishing their child for expressing his feelings toward them.*
- Provide the adolescent with a "Positive Book," a small notebook where he can write down things that happen throughout the day that make him feel good about himself *to encourage him to focus on his strengths and to enhance his self-esteem.*
- Teach parents to reward and praise the adolescent for expressing his feelings appropriately *to encourage them to focus on the child's strengths and to strengthen the entire family system.*
- Role-play with the adolescent to explore different ways to respond to specific family conflicts that occur at home *to help him develop problem-solving and negotiating skills.*

Discharge interventions

- Communicate with an outpatient clinician *to plan continued treatment for family.*
- Emphasize to the adolescent and his parents the need for continued support and family therapy after discharge *to enhance compliance.*

EVALUATION STATEMENTS

Adolescent and parents:
- begin to talk about difficulties at home.
- identify how they feel during times of conflict.
- agree to participate in outpatient treatment.

Adolescent:
- begins to express feelings using "I" statements.
- participates in group activities and individual and family therapy.
- uses more positive statements when talking about himself and family.

Parents:
- attend family therapy and educational groups.
- make positive statements about adolescent and the family as a whole.

DOCUMENTATION

- Family conflicts as described by adolescent and parents
- Adolescent's and parents' behavior when interacting with each other
- Nursing interventions to facilitate family communication and expression of feelings

- Frequency of family visits and family therapy appointments
- Adolescent's description of his own strengths
- Referrals for continued treatment following discharge
- Evaluation statements.

Social interaction impairment

related to externalizing behaviors

DEFINITION

Inability to engage in social activity due to counterproductive behaviors, such as temper tantrums, irritability, hostility, biting, bullying, stealing, or aggressive sexual behavior

ASSESSMENT

Family status
- *Demographics:* age, sex, level of education of all family members
- *Family rules:* maladaptive rules, willingness of parents to modify rules, consequences if rules are broken
- *Family communication:* style and quality of communication, methods of conflict resolution
- *Physical and emotional needs:* ability of family to meet child's physical and emotional needs
- *Coping patterns:* usual coping patterns, major life events, family members' perceptions of effectiveness of coping patterns
- *Evidence of abuse or neglect:* physical and behavioral indicators
- *Family health history:* substance-related disorders, violent behaviors, depressive disorders, suicide, learning disabilities, communication disorders
- *Diagnostic test:* Family Genogram

Neurologic status
- *Mental status:* abstract thinking; insight regarding present situation; judgment; long- and short-term memory; cognition; attention span; orientation to person, place, and time
- *Physical examination:* level of consciousness, sensory ability, fine and gross motor functioning
- *Prior medical conditions:* seizure disorder, brain tumor, Tourette's disorder
- *Laboratory tests:* drug toxicology screen, thyroid function test, metabolic screens, electrolyte levels
- *Diagnostic tests:* electroencephalography (EEG), sleep-deprived EEG, magnetic resonance imaging

Parental status
- *History:* knowledge of normal growth and development in children, ability to recognize child's achievement of developmental milestones, understanding of child's illness, available support systems, involvement with social service agencies

Psychological status
- *Childhood development:* developmental milestones, losses through separation or death, maladaptive behaviors, relationship with peers, evidence of antisocial behavior, such as stealing, lying, acts of physical cruelty, truancy, or property destruction
- *Recent events:* loss of pet or loved one, parental divorce or separation, move to foster home, other traumatic events

- *Medications:* neuroleptics, anxiolytics
- *Signs and symptoms:* aggressive behaviors, inappropriate sexual behaviors, changes in self-image or self-esteem
- *Laboratory tests:* urinalysis, human immunodeficiency virus test, drug toxicology screens
- *Diagnostic tests:* Revised Children Manifest Anxiety Scale, Children Depression Inventory, Behavioral Checklist, Wisconsin Card Sort

Social status

- *History:* interpersonal skills, size of social network, degree of trust in others, level of self-esteem
- *Signs and symptoms:* aggression toward self, others, or environment; inability to function in social and academic situations

DEFINING CHARACTERISTICS

- Blaming others for own misbehavior
- Deliberate destruction of another's property
- Frequent temper tantrums or angry outbursts
- Inability to function in social settings
- Presence of risk factors for impaired social development, such as poor self-esteem, family history of mental illness, poor family communication, inability of family to meet child's physical and emotional needs, physical abuse, sexual abuse, or neglect
- Sexual aggression
- Spiteful or vindictive behavior
- Violent behaviors, such as starting fights or physical cruelty to people or animals

ASSOCIATED DISORDERS

Anxiety disorders, attention-deficit hyperactivity disorder, child or adolescent antisocial behavior, communication disorders, conduct disorder, mood disorders, obsessive-compulsive disorder, oppositional defiant disorder, parent-child relational problem, posttraumatic stress disorder, Tourette's disorder

EXPECTED OUTCOMES

Initial outcomes

- Child expresses understanding of connection between behavior and safety.
- Child does not perform physically damaging acts toward self, others, or his environment.

Interim outcomes

- Child channels uncontrollable feelings safely into constructive outlets.
- Child participates in group activities.

Discharge outcomes

- Child begins to express feelings verbally.
- Child initiates appropriate interactions with peers.
- Child and family members plan continued treatment.

INTERVENTIONS AND RATIONALES

Initial interventions

- Convey your acceptance of the child but not his behavior. *Unconditional acceptance increases the child's feelings of self-worth and helps establish a trusting relationship.*

- Talk to the child about the difference between acceptable and unacceptable behavior. In a matter-of-fact manner, describe the consequences of misbehavior and then follow through if it recurs. *Knowledge that unacceptable behavior has specific consequences may discourage such behavior.*
- Provide clear expectations regarding socially appropriate behaviors *to give the child structure and decrease anxiety.*
- Provide consistent limit setting, direction, and redirection toward constructive activities *to decrease aggressive and sexualized behavior.*
- Minimize stimulation by providing the child with a private room and time-out periods. *Overstimulation causes anxiety and can lead to impulsive or socially inappropriate behavior.*

Interim interventions
- Help the child learn to recognize and deal with his uncontrollable feelings before they emerge as unacceptable behaviors. Suggest activities, such as sports or exercise, that can act as an outlet for these feelings. *This will help the child learn constructive alternatives for aggressive and other unacceptable behavior.*
- Encourage participation in group activities, such as therapy and recreational play, *to allow the child to observe how other children interact socially and to practice his own social skills.*
- Monitor the child's ability to regulate aggressive and sexualized behaviors in group settings *to determine types of feelings that cause stress for the child and his ability to cope with group interaction.*
- Instruct the child to remove himself from overstimulating situations. Re-

mind him of this option when he appears to be becoming anxious *to ensure his safety and the safety of other children.*

Discharge interventions
- Educate the child about different types of feelings *to help him express himself verbally rather than through aggressive behavior.* Discuss feelings of anger, sadness, frustration, and fear. *The child will be better able to come to terms with feelings when discussing them in a calm, supportive situation.*
- Role-play and model appropriate social skills for the child using examples of situations that trigger inappropriate behavior *to increase his sense of control and lessen anxiety regarding discharge.*
- Discuss with community agencies and the child's parents the interventions that were most helpful *to ensure continuity of care.*

EVALUATION STATEMENTS

Child:
- follows the unit routine.
- is able to take time-outs or respond to redirection.
- participates in one-on-one and group activities.
- decreases aggressive and sexualized behaviors.
- begins to talk about feelings.
- seeks staff when upset.
- can remove self from overstimulating environment.
- learns to act out uncontrollable feelings safely in private.

DOCUMENTATION

- Specific behaviors that are unsafe or socially inappropriate
- Child's ability to understand directions and express thoughts and feelings
- Level of supervision required to maintain safety
- Nursing interventions that are effective in maintaining safety and enhancing social skills
- Frequency of time-outs and seclusion
- Description of thoughts and feelings that trigger sexualized or aggressive behaviors
- Education of family members and their willingness to seek follow-up care
- Evaluation statements.

Social interaction impairment

related to internalizing behaviors

DEFINITION

Insufficient or ineffective social interaction due to depressed mood, withdrawal, shyness, lack of connection to others, or lack of interest in activities

ASSESSMENT

Family status
- *Demographics:* age, sex, level of education of all family members; parents' marital status
- *Family roles:* formal and informal roles and role performance, degree of

family agreement on roles, interrelationships of various roles
- *Family rules:* rules that foster stability, maladaptive family rules, methods of rule modification, consistency of enforcement
- *Family communication:* style and quality of communication, methods of conflict resolution
- *Developmental stage of family:* problem-solving skills, problems adjusting to change
- *Family subsystems:* conflicts and alliances between family members
- *Sociocultural factors:* economic status of family, members' sense of adequacy and self-worth, members' identity with cultural or ethnic group
- *Coping patterns:* major life events, usual coping patterns, family's perception of effectiveness of coping patterns
- *Evidence of physical or emotional abuse:* physical or behavioral indicators
- *Family health history:* depressive disorder, suicide, autistic disorder, learning disorders, sensory handicaps, physiological illness
- *Diagnostic test:* Family Genogram

Neurologic status
- *Mental status:* motor activity, mood, affect, perceptions, attention span, sensory function
- *Prior medical conditions:* seizure disorders, sensory difficulties (hearing loss, poor eye sight, sensory deprivation), Tourette's disorder, tic disorders
- *Medications:* anticonvulsants, neuroleptics
- *Signs and symptoms:* seizures, tremors, tics, gross or fine motor impairment

- *Laboratory test:* electrolyte levels
- *Diagnostic tests:* magnetic resonance imaging, electroencephalography

Parental status
- *History:* parents' knowledge of normal growth and development in children, ability to recognize child's achievement of developmental milestones, disciplinary measures, stability of parental relationship, understanding of child's illness

Psychological status
- *Childhood development:* developmental milestones, losses through separation or death, ability to attach to caregivers, social group involvement, life events, energy level, motivation, self-image, self-esteem
- *Recent life changes:* divorce of parents, recent move, change in school, loss of loved one or pet
- *Diagnostic tests:* Revised Children Manifest Anxiety Scale, Children Depression Inventory, Behavioral Checklist

Sensory status
- *Assistive devices:* glasses, contact lenses, hearing aids, history of myringotomy tube insertion
- *Physical examination:* visual and auditory examination, tactile examination
- *Prior medical conditions:* eye disorders, hearing loss
- *Signs and symptoms:* inability to respond to stimuli
- *Diagnostic tests:* Snellen eye chart, hearing acuity test

Social status
- *History:* conversational skills, quality of relationships, ability to function at school and play
- *Signs and symptoms:* withdrawal, lack of eye contact, inappropriate responses, self-stimulating behaviors

DEFINING CHARACTERISTICS

- Dysfunctional interaction with family, peers, others
- Inability to function in groups at school or play
- Inability to receive or communicate a sense of belonging, caring, or interest
- Lack of coping skills; low self-esteem
- Lack of knowledge of normal stages of child development (parents)
- Presence of risk factors for psychological disturbances, such as abuse or neglect, excessive or inconsistent punishment, family history of mental illness or neurologic difficulties, lack of nurturing caregiver or social support, maladaptive family alliances or family rules, poor family communication
- Repeated unsuccessful patterns of social interaction
- Visible discomfort in social situations
- Withdrawal, sad affect

ASSOCIATED DISORDERS

Acquired immunodeficiency syndrome, autistic disorder, childhood disintegrative disorder, mood disorders, neurologic impairment, posttraumatic stress disorder, physical disability or deformity, reactive attachment disorders of infancy or early childhood, schizophrenia, sensory disorders, separation anxiety disorder

EXPECTED OUTCOMES

Initial outcome
- Child and family members cooperate with assessment and interventions.

Interim outcomes
- Child begins to communicate needs to staff.
- Child seeks out staff members for social as well as therapeutic interaction.
- Child expresses interest and satisfaction with play activities.
- Child initiates and maintains a satisfactory interpersonal relationship with another patient.
- Child willingly participates in group activities.

Discharge outcomes
- Child and family continue with treatment following discharge.
- Child is referred to specialized outpatient services.

INTERVENTIONS AND RATIONALES

Initial interventions
- Introduce the child to staff and other children in a clear, calm manner *to decrease anxiety and facilitate trust.*
- Explain the reasons for assessment and treatment to the child and family *to enhance compliance with the admission process and establish rapport.*

Interim interventions
- Spend uninterrupted time with the child during each shift to discuss his favorite activities and thoughts and feelings about interacting with others *to convey concern, identify problems, and provide support.*
- Provide the child with dolls or puppets and then observe his interaction with them *to help the child develop social interaction skills.*
- Act as a role model, demonstrating appropriate interpersonal and social skills when interacting with other patients and staff members *to reinforce social skills discussed in teaching sessions.*
- Provide the child with positive reinforcement as he tries to relate to others. When possible, be on hand during social situations. *The presence of an individual that the child trusts helps him feel more secure in social situations.*
- Encourage the child to initiate a relationship with at least one other patient and to interact with this new friend on a regular schedule each day *to promote age-appropriate socialization.*
- Note any abrupt changes in the child's behavior or mood. *Changes in behavior can signify agitation or increased anxiety.*
- Support participation in group activities. Start with small groups or parallel play and progress to social skills training groups. *Group interactions help the child learn socially acceptable behaviors as he receives positive and negative feedback from peers.*

Discharge interventions
- Provide the parents with references to community resources and discuss continued treatment *to ensure compliance with outpatient therapy.*

- Discuss effective interventions with representatives from appropriate community resources *to facilitate continuity of care.*

EVALUATION STATEMENTS

Child and family:
- comply with assessment and treatment.
- commit to continuing therapy after discharge.
  Child:
- establishes eye contact.
- shows increased social skills, as evidenced by eating meals with group and playing and speaking with others.
- maintains safety.
- begins to communicate his needs to staff.

DOCUMENTATION

- Child's ability to seek out staff and parents for soothing and comfort
- Participation in group activities
- Nursing interventions to enhance social interaction and self-esteem and child's response
- Parents' and child's understanding of nursing interventions
- Parents' stated agreement to continue treatment
- Evaluation statements.

Social isolation

related to unacceptable social behavior or inability to develop satisfying relationships

DEFINITION

State of social detachment or aloneness due to inappropriate behavior or to being ostracized by peer group

ASSESSMENT

Family status
- *Demographic and cultural factors:* age and sex of all family members; level of education; developmental stage of siblings; nationality; identification with racial, cultural, or ethnic group; influence of religious beliefs on daily life; attitudes and beliefs about health care
- *Family roles:* degree of family agreement on roles, interrelationships of family roles
- *Family subsystems:* family alliances and their effects on family stability
- *Family rules:* rules that foster stability, maladaptive rules, appropriateness of rules to child's developmental level, consequences if rules are broken
- *Physical and emotional needs:* family's ability to meet the child's physical and emotional needs
- *Developmental stage:* changes in relationships between family members; ability of family to adapt to change; family conflicts and coping patterns; evidence of physical, emotional, and sexual abuse

- *Socioeconomic factors:* economic status of family, family members, sense of adequacy and self-worth, employment status, attitudes toward work
- *Family health history:* anxiety disorders, antisocial behavior, incarcerations, personality disorders
- *Diagnostic test:* Family Genogram

Parental status
- *History:* knowledge of normal growth and development, agreement on appropriate disciplinary measures, stability of parental relationship, available support systems

Psychological status
- *History:* ability to play with others, current level of development, recent separation or divorce of parents or other losses
- *Psychiatric history:* age at onset of illness, type and severity of symptoms, impact on functioning, response to treatment
- *Developmental history:* birth order; number of siblings; developmental milestones; past separations, losses, moves, changes in school; personality traits; school performance; social interactions; involvement in church, synagogue, or clubs
- *Medications:* anxiolytics, stimulants, mood stabilizers, beta-adrenergic blockers, alpha-adrenergic antagonists
- *Signs and symptoms:* anxiety, aggression, or withdrawal; frequent teasing of others; impulsive gestures and talk; changes in self-image, self-esteem, or mood; hyperactivity
- *Diagnostic tests:* Revised Children Manifest Anxiety Scale, Children De-

pression Inventory, Behavioral Checklists (Achenbach, Conners Rating Scale, Gordon Diagnostic System, Matching Familiar Figures)

Social status
- *History:* social skills, ability to cope with group activities
- *Signs and symptoms:* withdrawal, lack of eye contact, intrusiveness, inappropriate responses, aggressiveness, inappropriate sexual behavior, frequent time-outs or need to separate from group

DEFINING CHARACTERISTICS
- Behavior that is unacceptable to dominant cultural group
- Expressed feelings of loneliness, exclusion, or rejection
- Family environment that fails to foster child's social development as indicated by maladaptive or rigid family rules, inability of family members to adapt to change, poor understanding of child's developmental needs, inconsistent discipline, inability to nurture child, lack of social contact, poor communication between family members, recent traumatic event such as separation or divorce, evidence of physical, sexual, or emotional abuse
- Frequent aggressive outbursts or inability to play with others
- Frequent life changes throughout life span, such as frequent moving or losses through separation or death
- Frequent mood changes
- High level of anxiety
- Inability to concentrate or function in school
- Lack of peer group contact
- Poor sense of self

- Preoccupation with personal thoughts or repetitive, meaningless activities or actions
- Uncommunicative or withdrawn behavior; lack of eye-contact

ASSOCIATED DISORDERS

Anxiety disorders, Asperger's disorder, attention deficit-disorder, child or adolescent antisocial behavior, communication disorder, conduct disorder, eating disorders, learning disorder, mental retardation, mood disorders, obsessive-compulsive disorder, oppositional defiant disorder, parent-child relational problem, pervasive developmental disorder, separation anxiety disorder

EXPECTED OUTCOMES

Initial outcome
- Child makes adequate adjustment to hospital environment.

Interim outcomes
- Child uses play to express feelings that are difficult to articulate directly.
- Child participates in structured group activities.
- Child identifies behaviors that alienate peers.
- Child describes socially appropriate behaviors.
- Child expresses positive perceptions of himself.
- Child and family discuss relationships at home.

Discharge outcomes
- Child demonstrates improvement in social skills.

- Child and family plan to continue treatment.

INTERVENTIONS AND RATIONALES

Initial interventions
- Orient the child to unit routine and surroundings *to help him acclimate to the unit.*
- Introduce the child to the staff and other children slowly, taking into account his developmental level and ability to tolerate a new environment *to minimize anxiety.*
- Inform the child of safety rules and explain the consequences if rules are not followed *to provide structure and enhance his feelings of security.*
- Use time-outs or separate the child from others as needed *to decrease stimulation and place limits on aggressive behavior.*

Interim interventions
- Prepare the child for anticipated changes in his daily routine by offering simple, honest explanations *to help the child incorporate changes and foster trust.*
- Avoid getting involved in trivial arguments or power struggles with the child *to provide a more solid foundation for the development of interpersonal skills.*
- Reassure the child and set aside specific periods for one-to-one talks. *This demonstrates that the child is worthwhile to you and encourages him to express thoughts and feelings.*
- Use toys, such as puppets or games, *to encourage the child to act out thoughts and feelings he may be unable to talk about.*

- Encourage the child to attend group outings and activities *to help him practice and master social skills.*
- Help the child identify positive personal characteristics and then plan to use these characteristics in relationships with peers. *Recognizing positive personality characteristics enhances self-esteem.*
- Structure activities to provide opportunities for interacting with other children. Encourage taking turns and playing cooperatively *to provide a structure to help ensure success with mastering social skills.*
- Encourage family members to discuss their perceptions of the child's strengths and weaknesses *to help them develop a more balanced view of the child's behavior.*
- Encourage the family members to attend family therapy sessions *to explore family dynamics and investigate their relationship to the child's behaviors.*
- Help the child identify situations in which peers are alienated because of his behavior *to help him identify areas where improvement is needed.*
- Help the child pinpoint socially appropriate behaviors and provide positive reinforcement for all attempts to modify behavior *to encourage the use of adaptive behaviors.*
- Ask the child to identify one peer who accepts him unconditionally and encourage daily interaction with this individual *to foster social skills and reduce isolation.*

Discharge interventions
- Engage the child in role playing of social situations *to help him incorporate social skills to use at home and school.*

- Describe successful interventions to teachers and parents *to provide continuity of care.*
- Tell therapists or others who will provide follow-up care about the child's and family members' achievements while in the hospital *to encourage them to continue successful interventions and foster compliance with follow-up care.*

EVALUATION STATEMENTS

Child:
- follows directions to maintain safety.
- follows the unit routine.
- participates in one-to-one interactions and group activities.

   Child and family members:
- participate in family treatment.
- state their commitment to continuing treatment following discharge.

DOCUMENTATION

- Frequency of participation in group activities
- Specific actions and expressions that cause social isolation
- Nursing interventions to enhance social interaction and self-esteem
- Child's response to nursing interventions
- Education provided to parents and teachers
- Communication with treatment team members and representatives from community agencies regarding follow-up care
- Evaluation statements.

Verbal communication impairment

related to psychological or developmental factors

DEFINITION

Impaired ability to use or understand verbal communication in the absence of diagnosed pathophysiological impairment

ASSESSMENT

Family status

- *Demographics:* age, sex, developmental and grade level of child and siblings; level of education, occupation, and socioeconomic status of parents; developmental stage of the family
- *Cultural influences:* nationality and ethnic and religious affiliation; values, beliefs, and practices regarding health, illness, and child rearing
- *Family communication:* family communication patterns, usual methods of coping, methods of conflict resolution
- *Parents' child rearing skills:* level of knowledge regarding normal childhood growth and development (especially speech development); usual coping mechanisms and disciplinary measures; level of understanding and frustration concerning their child's speech problem; expectations for their child; ability to meet the child's basic physical, social, and emotional needs; available support systems
- *Diagnostic tests:* Family Genogram, Cultural Assessment Guide

Respiratory status

- *Physical examination:* use of accessory muscles, respiratory pattern, dyspnea

Neurologic status

- *Mental status:* level of consciousness, orientation, cognition, memory, insight and judgment, speech or verbal communication patterns (including use of signing, pen and pencil, picture or alphabet board)
- *Auditory examination:* auditory acuity, auditory canal, tympanic membrane, excess cerumen
- *Physical examination:* eye contact, tone of voice, response to verbal directions
- *Signs and symptoms:* lack of eye contact, agitation, speaking in a loud voice, poor response to verbal directions, expressive and receptive deficits
- *Laboratory tests:* drug toxicology screen, electrolyte levels
- *Diagnostic test:* magnetic resonance imaging

Musculoskeletal status

- *Physical examination:* range of motion, manual dexterity

Psychological status

- *History of verbal impairment:* age at onset, type and severity of symptoms, level of verbal communication, impact on functioning, patient's response to treatment, reliance on adaptive communication techniques or equipment
- *Childhood development:* maladaptive behaviors, academic performance, relationship with peers, social skills, usual recreational activities

- *Diagnostic tests:* Achenbach and Conners Behavioral Checklists, Weschler Intelligence Scales for Children (WISC-III)

Social status

- *Social skills:* interpersonal skills (communication, behavior), quality of relationships, ability to trust others, level of self-esteem, level of social functioning (school and play)
- *Signs and symptoms:* withdrawal, lack of eye contact, intrusiveness, inappropriate responses, aggressiveness

DEFINING CHARACTERISTICS

- Behavior indicating trouble speaking or hearing
- Congenital anomaly or mechanical impairment to forming sounds
- Developmental delays
- Dyspnea, tachypnea, stridor
- Inadequate interpersonal skills
- Inappropriate responses to questions
- Lack of peer relationships
- Low self-esteem, poor self-concept
- Poor academic performance
- Poor communication patterns in the home
- Poor parental coping and problem-solving skills
- Poor parental understanding of normal childhood growth and development and of their child's problem
- Social withdrawal or isolation

ASSOCIATED DISORDERS AND TREATMENTS

This diagnosis may be associated with any disorder or treatment that alters the child's ability to speak or hear. Examples include acute respiratory dis-

tress, autistic disorder, brain tumor, cleft palate or lip, head injury, hearing loss or impairment, mental retardation, mixed receptive-expressive language disorder, pervasive developmental disorders, premature birth, psychotic disorders, seizure disorders, speech disorders, substance-related disorder, Tourette's disorder, treatment with neuroleptics, antimanic agents, or anticonvulsants.

EXPECTED OUTCOMES

Initial outcomes

- Child remains safe during hospital stay.
- Staff member accurately describes alternative communication techniques favored by child.

Interim outcomes

- Parents demonstrate an improved understanding of normal childhood growth and development.
- Parents describe techniques for assessing their child's needs.
- Parents demonstrate skills necessary to enhance their child's communication skills.
- Child receives positive reinforcement for his efforts to communicate.

Discharge outcomes

- Child demonstrates improved ability to use and understand language.
- Parents receive appropriate referrals for obtaining ongoing care for their child.
- Parents explain their child's needs to family members, teachers, and social contacts as appropriate.

INTERVENTIONS AND RATIONALES

Initial interventions

- Observe the child's ability to communicate personal needs *to assess techniques used to compensate for verbal communication impairment.*
- Provide the child with clear directions using familiar techniques (verbal, written, pictures, hand signs) *to promote understanding and encourage a trusting therapeutic relationship.*

Interim interventions

- Assess the parents' understanding of the speech development process and correct any misconceptions. For example, explain that children develop language skills at different rates. Also explain that toddlers have limited language skills and must be given one direction at a time and that preschoolers have a limited vocabulary and often communicate with gestures and symbols. If a language or cognitive impairment is diagnosed, describe methods of nonverbal communication. *This information improves the parents' understanding of normal developmental processes and their child's status.*
- Teach the parents common methods of assessing the needs of speech-delayed children. For example, explain that toddlers and preschoolers can communicate by using dolls and stuffed animals in role playing. School-age children may communicate by drawing. Explain how to use the pictorial (faces) pain scale when assessing their child's level of discomfort. *These techniques help the parents communicate more effectively with their child.*

- Describe techniques the parents can use to stimulate language development, for example, talking and reading with their child, playing music, repeating sounds the child makes, pointing to objects and naming them, *to help the parents understand their child's problem and possible solutions, reduce their anxiety, and promote a sense of control.*
- Demonstrate to parents how to ask open-ended questions, such as "What would you like to wear today?" rather than closed-ended questions, such as "Do you want to wear the red shirt?" *Open-ended questions require the child to express complete thoughts; closed-ended questions simply require him to shake his head or say yes or no.*
- Praise the child each time he attempts to use verbal communication to describe his needs. *Positive reinforcement encourages improvement by promoting confidence and self-esteem.*

Discharge interventions

- Provide appropriate referrals to medical professionals and community resources, as necessary, *to improve the parents' knowledge and foster the child's development of age-appropriate language skills.*
- Suggest that the parents discuss the child's problem with teachers, family members, and other key people in the child's life *to promote a consistent approach to helping the child develop language skills.*

EVALUATION STATEMENTS

Child:
- participates in group or other pre-scribed activities to enhance his communication skills.
- demonstrates appropriate verbal and nonverbal methods of expressing his feelings and needs.

Parents:
- demonstrate acceptance of their child's verbal communication impairment.
- demonstrate alternative methods of assessing the needs of their speech-delayed child.
- accurately describe the stages of speech development.
- identify and use techniques to enhance their child's speech development.
- acknowledge the need for ongoing treatment if appropriate.

DOCUMENTATION

- Diagnostic test results
- Methods the child uses to communicate needs
- Coping skills of parents
- Parents' understanding of the speech development process
- Parents' ability to assess the needs of their speech-delayed child
- Parents' understanding of alternative methods of communicating with their child
- Nursing interventions to enhance the child's verbal communication skills and the parents' ability to adapt
- Parents' and child's response to interventions
- Referrals for continued treatment
- Evaluation statements.

PART THREE

GERIATRIC MENTAL HEALTH

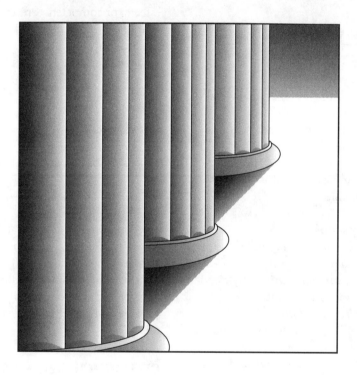

Adjustment impairment

related to chronic illness

DEFINITION

Patient's and family's inability to modify behavior to meet the demands of changing health status

ASSESSMENT

Cultural status

- *Demographics:* age, sex, level of education, occupation, nationality, race, ethnic group
- *History:* beliefs, values, and attitudes about health and illness; health customs, practices, and rituals
- *Diagnostic test:* Cultural Assessment Guide

Family status

- *Family roles:* formal and informal roles and role performance
- *Family communication:* style and quality of communication
- *Developmental stage of family:* adaptability, changes in problem-solving methods over time
- *Physical and emotional needs:* ability of family to meet patient's essential physical, social, and emotional needs; disparities between patient's needs and family's ability to meet them
- *Coping patterns:* usual coping patterns, family's perception of effectiveness of coping patterns
- *Diagnostic tests:* Family Adjustment Device, Family Genogram

Neurologic status

- *Mental status:* appearance and attitude, thought and speech, mood and affect, perceptions, orientation, attention span, abstraction, judgment and insight
- *Diagnostic test:* Folstein Mini-Mental Status Examination

Psychological status

- *History:* changes in self-image, self-esteem, or competence; recent life changes; past psychiatric illness or hospitalization
- *Diagnostic tests:* Problem Solving Inventory, Self-Efficacy Scale, Rosenberg Self-Esteem Scale

Self-care status

- *Prior medical conditions:* neurologic, sensory, or psychological impairment
- *History:* use of adaptive equipment, devices, or supplies
- *Observation:* functional ability (muscle tone, size, and strength; range of motion; coordination), daily activities (dressing, grooming, bathing, toileting, and hygiene)
- *Diagnostic test:* Self-Care Assessment Tool

DEFINING CHARACTERISTICS

- Altered cognitive function
- Diminishing self-care abilities
- Extended period of shock, disbelief, or anger at progression of chronic illness
- Inability of family to adapt to demands of ill member
- Inability of family to meet patient's physical, social, or emotional needs

- Inability to anticipate and plan for changes in health status
- Lack of movement toward independence
- Lack of successful problem-solving strategies
- Poor family communication
- Refusal to accept chronic illness

ASSOCIATED DISORDERS

This diagnosis may be associated with a chronic medical illness, such as arthritis, chronic obstructive pulmonary disease, diabetes, heart disease, neurologic disorders, or spinal cord injury. It may also be associated with psychiatric diagnoses, such as an adjustment disorder with anxiety, with depressed mood, or with mixed disturbance of emotions and conduct.

EXPECTED OUTCOMES

Initial outcomes

- Patient becomes aware of the need for improved coping skills.
- Patient modifies his lifestyle to minimize disability.

Interim outcomes

- Patient develops adaptive coping and problem-solving skills.
- Patient makes decisions about treatment.
- Patient learns about illness and anticipates health status changes.
- Patient becomes as independent as possible.

Discharge outcome

- Patient assumes responsibility for using social service and community health resources.

INTERVENTIONS AND RATIONALES

Initial interventions

- Provide an open and accepting environment and encourage the patient and family to express feelings about the illness *to help them work through such emotions as anxiety, denial, fear, and depression.*
- Help family members identify their strengths and successes in fulfilling roles *to promote a sense of control over their current situation.*
- Teach patient and family members about the illness and provide strategies for enhancing the patient's control over his self-care needs *to reduce fear and foster hope.*

Interim interventions

- Help the patient and family identify coping skills and problem-solving strategies used successfully in the past *to promote a sense of mastery and hope.*
- Assist the patient and family in using problem-focused coping strategies. Provide information about the patient's illness. Encourage discussion with other patients with the same illness and their families. Refer them to appropriate support groups *to improve their emotional adjustment to the illness and provide opportunities for effective role modeling.*
- Actively involve the family in the patient's rehabilitation *to enhance their sense of commitment.*
- Encourage the patient to help make health care decisions *to promote autonomy.*
- Monitor the family's willingness and ability to support the patient as his health care changes and to provide on-

going care *to ensure that his health care needs are met and to determine if outside intervention is necessary.*

Discharge intervention
- Identify appropriate social service and community resources *to help the patient locate needed resources as his illness progresses.*

EVALUATION STATEMENTS

Patient and family members:
- start learning to live with demands of chronic illness.
- accept grief as normal reaction to changes in health status.
- use adaptive coping mechanisms and problem-solving strategies.
- share their concerns with patients with similar conditions and their families.
- discuss strategies to manage care that foster independence and maintain family functioning.
    Patient:
- participates in his own health care.

DOCUMENTATION

- Diagnostic test results
- Patient's and family members' statements indicating difficulty adjusting to the patient's diagnosis
- Patient's and family members' expressions and behaviors that indicate their understanding of course of chronic illness
- Nursing interventions used to improve coping mechanisms and problem-solving strategies
- Patient's and family's responses to nursing interventions

- Referrals to social service and community health resources
- Family's ongoing ability to manage demands of chronic illness
- Evaluation statements.

Body image disturbance
related to negative attitudes about aging

DEFINITION

Disruption in self-perception as a result of normal physical changes associated with aging

ASSESSMENT

Cultural status
- *Demographics:* age, sex, level of education, occupation, nationality, race, ethnic group
- *History:* beliefs, values, and attitudes about health and illness; health customs, practices, and rituals; attitudes about aging and elderly people

Family status
- *Family composition:* presence of spouse; length of marriage, divorce, or widowhood; location of children and grandchildren
- *Family roles:* formal and informal roles, role performance, degree of family agreement on roles
- *Family communication:* style and quality of communication, methods of conflict resolution

• *Family values and aspirations:* extent to which family permits pursuit of individual goals and values

Integumentary status
• *Personal habits:* daily hygienic practices for skin, hair, and nails; use of creams, lotions, and other skin products; environmental or occupational exposure to skin toxins
• *Physical examination:* skin color, elasticity, sensation, temperature, texture, turgor, and hygiene; hair distribution; description of incisions, scars, and lesions; presence or absence of edema; characteristics of nails and nailbeds; presence of rashes, nevi, angiomas, keloids, and moles

Musculoskeletal status
• *History:* ability to carry out activities of daily living, exercise and activity patterns, participation in sports, occupational hazards, mobility aids
• *Physical examination:* range of motion of all joints; joint and muscle symmetry; evidence of swelling, masses, or deformity; pain or tenderness on movement; coordination and gait; muscle size, strength, and tone; functional mobility
• *Signs and symptoms:* pain, joint swelling, stiffness, limitation of movement, weakness, tenderness, inflammation, falls, contractures, subluxation, masses, joint deformity, dislocation, muscle atrophy

Neurologic status
• *Mental status:* appearance and attitude, level of consciousness, motor activity, thought and speech, mood and affect, perceptions, orientation, memory, general information, visual-

spatial ability, attention span, abstraction, judgment and insight, capacity to read, write, and perform calculations

Sensory status
• *Visual examination:* visual acuity, visual fields, pupillary action
• *Auditory examination:* ear position, size, and symmetry; skin color and texture; auditory canal, tympanic membrane, and cerumen

DEFINING CHARACTERISTICS
• Extreme sensitivity to remarks about advancing age
• Frequent, disparaging remarks about aging and its physical effects
• Reluctance or refusal to wear hearing aids or corrective lenses
• Unwillingness to accept physical changes associated with aging, or to view aging in a positive light

ASSOCIATED DISORDERS
Cataracts, depressive disorder, hearing and visual deficits, impotence, osteoarthritis, osteoporosis, psoriasis, rheumatoid arthritis, sexual dysfunctions

EXPECTED OUTCOMES
Initial outcomes
• Patient discusses physical changes caused by aging.
• Patient alters skin care routine to reflect age-related changes.

Interim outcomes
• Patient uses visual and auditory aids appropriately.

- Patient demonstrates increased interest in personal appearance.
- Patient identifies at least one positive aspect of aging.

Discharge outcomes

- Patient demonstrates increased interest in participating in social activities.
- Patient exercises and engages in safe, appropriate physical activities.

INTERVENTIONS AND RATIONALES

Initial interventions

- Encourage the patient to express feelings about physical changes associated with aging. *Active listening conveys a caring and accepting attitude.*
- Suggest an age-appropriate skin care routine, including use of skin lotions to combat dryness and less frequent bathing *to promote good health.*

Interim interventions

- Provide information on appropriate self-care activities, such as maintenance of a proper diet and age-appropriate exercise. *These will promote overall good health and will help maintain muscle mass, bone strength, and cardiopulmonary health.*
- Encourage the patient to consider new grooming styles, perhaps seeking advice from a cosmetologist on updating hair and makeup styles. *Attractive, tasteful grooming may help the older patient achieve a sense of control over the aging process.*
- Provide the patient with referrals for corrective lenses and auditory aids *to address sensory deficits.*

- Provide the patient with positive role models. For example, share literature that emphasizes the capabilities of older adults *to form a more positive view of the elderly population.*
- While conversing with the patient, focus on his strengths; emphasize the positive aspects of aging *to increase his self-esteem.*

Discharge interventions

- Encourage the patient to engage in social activities with people from all age-groups *to foster opportunities for increased human interaction, positive feedback, and development of new interests.*
- Refer the patient to a physical therapist or qualified physical education instructor *to learn about safe, age-appropriate exercises.*

EVALUATION STATEMENTS

Patient:
- keeps skin clean and well cared for.
- identifies an age-related physical change and comments on it positively.
- identifies at least one personal advantage to growing older.
- identifies one aspect of his life or personality that is better than it was 10 years ago.
- uses visual and auditory aids comfortably and consistently.
- participates in at least one social activity or group regularly.
- makes a positive statement about a new interest, idea, or activity.
- makes a positive statement about another older adult.
- identifies at least one activity that he does well.

- engages in regular, appropriate exercise.

DOCUMENTATION

- Patient's statements about appearance, ability, and age
- Mental status assessment (baseline and ongoing)
- Physical assessment
- Nursing interventions directed toward improving the patient's body image
- Patient's response to nursing interventions
- Evaluation statements.

Caregiver role strain

related to caring for an aging family member

DEFINITION

Feeling of difficulty in caring for an aging family member resulting from actual or perceived complexities

ASSESSMENT

Cultural status
- *Demographics:* caregiver's age, sex, level of education, occupation, general health status, nationality, area of residence (rural, suburban, urban), relationship to elderly family member
- *History:* affiliation with racial, ethnic, or religious group; beliefs, values, and attitudes about health and illness; health customs, practices, and rituals; beliefs and attitudes about aging and elderly people

- *Diagnostic test:* Cultural Assessment Guide

Family status
- *Family roles:* formal and informal roles and role performance, degree of family agreement on roles, interrelationships of various roles
- *Family rules:* rules that foster stability, maladaptive rules, methods of rule modification
- *Family communication:* style and quality of communication, methods of conflict resolution
- *Family subsystems:* family alliances, effect of alliances on family stability
- *Physical and emotional needs:* ability of family to meet caregiver's and elderly relative's physical and emotional needs
- *Social and economic factors:* economic status of family, sense of adequacy and self-worth of members, employment and attitudes toward work, influence of religious beliefs on values and practices
- *Coping patterns:* major life events and their meaning to each family member, usual coping patterns, family's perception of effectiveness of coping patterns
- *Evidence of abuse:* physical and behavioral indicators
- *Family health history:* depressive disorder, suicide, substance use disorder, stress-related illness, medical illness
- *Diagnostic tests:* Family Environment Scale, Family Adjustment Device, Family Genogram

Caregiver's psychological status
- *History:* family life, quality of relationship with elderly family member,

ability to accept health changes in aging family member, sense of self-worth, hobbies, recreational activities, psychiatric history
- *Recent life changes:* divorce, illness, job loss, or loss of loved one; changes in elderly family member's health status
- *Signs and symptoms:* changes in appetite, energy level, motivation, hygiene, self-image, self-esteem, sleep pattern, or sexual drive; alcohol or drug abuse
- *Diagnostic test:* Hamilton Rating Scale for Depression

Elderly family member's self-care status
- *Medical conditions:* neurologic, physical, sensory, or psychological impairment
- *History:* use of adaptive equipment, devices, or supplies
- *Observation:* functional ability (muscle tone, size, and strength; range of motion; coordination), daily activities (dressing, grooming, bathing, toileting, and hygiene)
- *Diagnostic tests:* Functional Ability Scale, Self-Care Assessment Tool

Caregiver's spiritual status
- *History:* religious or church affiliation; current perception of faith and religious practices; perceptions about life, death, and suffering; support network (family, clergy, friends)
- *Diagnostic test:* Spiritual Well-Being Scale

DEFINING CHARACTERISTICS
- Excessive involvement with elderly family member

- Feeling of loss because elderly family member has changed drastically
- Feeling that providing care for elderly family member interferes with other aspects of life, including career and social activities
- High level of dependency between elderly family member and caregiver
- Ineffective coping skills
- Perceived or actual inadequate physical, psychological, and social support from family and community
- Poor family communication; inadequate conflict resolution; inability of family to meet physical, psychological, and social needs

ASSOCIATED DISORDERS

Chronic fatigue syndrome, constipation, depressive disorder, diarrhea, eating disorders, headache, insomnia, obsessive-compulsive disorder, peptic ulcer disease

EXPECTED OUTCOMES

Initial outcomes
- Caregiver describes her current obligations.
- Caregiver distinguishes obligations she must fulfill from those that can be controlled or limited.

Interim outcomes
- Caregiver identifies coping skills used to deal with past crises.
- Caregiver describes informal and formal support systems that can help meet current obligations.
- Caregiver acknowledges codependency and takes appropriate steps to receive help and support.

- Caregiver demonstrates improved time management skills.

Discharge outcome
- Caregiver uses informal and formal support systems to get relief.

INTERVENTIONS AND RATIONALES

Initial interventions
- Help the caregiver identify her obligations, including caring for an aging family member and other family, work, and social responsibilities *to evaluate her perception of her situation.*
- Help the caregiver distinguish obligations she has no control over from those that she has the ability to limit *to enhance her feeling of control.*

Interim interventions
- Help the caregiver identify past experiences with similar stressful situations and how she coped *to promote recognition of coping skills.*
- If the caregiver seems overly anxious or distraught, gently point out the facts about the aging family member's mental and physical condition. *Many times, the caregiver's perspective is clouded by a long history of emotional involvement. Your input may help the caregiver view the situation more objectively.* If you believe that excessive emotional involvement is hindering the caregiver's ability to function, consider recommending Co-dependent's Anonymous, a support group for people whose preoccupation with a relationship leads to chronic suffering and diminished effectiveness *to provide ongoing support.*
- Encourage the caregiver to participate in a support group. Provide information on an organization such as the Alzheimer's Disease and Related Disorders Association or Children of Aging Parents *to foster mutual support and provide an opportunity for the caregiver to discuss personal feelings with empathetic listeners.*
- Suggest ways for the caregiver to use time more efficiently. For example, the caregiver may be able to save time by filling out insurance forms while visiting and chatting with the care recipient. *Better time management may help the caregiver reduce stress.*
- Find out which obligations the caregiver considers difficult to fulfill *to identify areas where additional support may be required.*

Discharge interventions
- Help the caregiver contact informal sources of support, such as church groups, extended family, and community volunteers *for support and relief.*
- Encourage the caregiver to use formal support agencies, such as social service and home health care agencies, clinics, and adult day care centers, *to get additional relief.*
- Refer the caregiver to appropriate agencies *to help provide continuity of care.*

EVALUATION STATEMENTS

Caregiver:
- develops a realistic assessment of her obligations.
- exhibits a positive sense of self-worth.
- describes her emotional response to caring for an aging family member.
- identifies coping skills that can help her deal with stress.

- uses available informal and formal support systems and resources.
- expresses less role strain.

DOCUMENTATION

- Diagnostic test results
- Caregiver's description of her current obligations
- Caregiver statements indicating her difficulty coping with an aging family member
- Participation in Co-dependent's Anonymous or other support group
- Informal and formal support systems and resources identified by the caregiver
- Referrals to formal agencies
- Evaluation statements.

Coping, ineffective family

related to unresolved emotional conflict between patient and family members

DEFINITION

Inability of family members to make the adjustments necessary to care for an elderly relative because of unresolved conflicts

ASSESSMENT

Cultural status
- *Family demographics:* age, sex, level of education, and occupation of members; nationality, race, and ethnic group; relationship to patient
- *Health care habits:* beliefs, values, and attitudes about health and illness;

health customs, practices, and rituals; attitudes about responsibility for caring for aging parents and other relatives
- *Diagnostic test:* Cultural Assessment Guide

Family status
- *Family roles:* formal and informal roles and role performance, degree of family agreement on roles, interrelationships of various roles
- *Family rules:* rules that foster stability, maladaptive rules, methods of rule modification
- *Family communication:* style and quality of communication, methods of conflict resolution
- *Family subsystems:* family alliances, long-standing family conflicts, effect of alliances on family stability
- *Physical and emotional needs:* ability of family to meet patient's physical and emotional needs; ability of family members to meet each others' physical and emotional needs
- *Social and economic factors:* economic status of family, sense of adequacy and self-worth, employment and attitudes toward work, financial pressures brought on by patient's illness and increased health care needs
- *Coping patterns:* major life events and their meaning to each family member, usual coping patterns, perceptions regarding effectiveness of coping patterns
- *Evidence of abuse:* physical and behavioral indicators
- *Family health history:* depressive disorder, suicide, substance use disorder, stress-related illness, medical illness
- *Family developmental and emotional history:* patient's and family mem-

bers' relationship before illness, frequency of contact between patient and family members, family members' perceptions about patient's role in family history (supportive, interfering, uninvolved, highly critical, tyrannical), patient's awareness of family resentments, effect of patient's illness on family members, willingness and ability of other relatives to share burden of caring for aging family member
▪ *Diagnostic tests:* Family Environment Scale, Family Adjustment Device, Family Genogram

Spiritual status
▪ *History:* patient's and family members' perceptions about life, death, and suffering; membership and participation in church or synagogue; additional sources of spiritual support
▪ *Diagnostic tests:* Spiritual and Religious Concerns Questionnaire, Spiritual Well-Being Scale

Elderly family member's self-care status
▪ *Prior medical conditions:* neurologic, sensory, or psychological impairment
▪ *History:* use of adaptive equipment, devices, or supplies
▪ *Observation:* functional ability (muscle tone, size, and strength; range of motion; coordination), daily activities (dressing, grooming, toileting, bathing, and hygiene)
▪ *Diagnostic test:* Self-Care Assessment Tool

Elderly family member's neurologic status
▪ *Mental status:* appearance and attitude, level of consciousness, motor

activity, thought and speech, mood and affect, perceptions, orientation, memory, general information, visual-spatial ability, attention span, abstraction, judgment and insight, capacity to read, write, and perform calculations

DEFINING CHARACTERISTICS

▪ Expressions of anger, resentment, disrespect, or ambivalence toward patient by family members
▪ Expressions of powerlessness, helplessness, hopelessness, guilt, or anxiety by patient
▪ Fluctuation of family members' attitudes regarding patient; for example, family members may be supportive one day and then angry the next day
▪ Frequent statements by family members about events that happened in the past
▪ Inadequate family communication patterns, problem-solving skills, or coping techniques
▪ Lack of mutual emotional support among family members
▪ Neglect of patient's emotional and physical needs by family members
▪ Prevalence of stress-related illness among family members

ASSOCIATED DISORDERS

This diagnosis may accompany any condition that results in temporary or permanent dependence on family members, such as Alzheimer's disease, anxiety disorders, arthritis, cancer, cerebrovascular accident, cirrhosis, hip fracture, mood disorders, Parkinson's disease, rheumatoid arthritis, schizophrenia, somatoform disorders.

EXPECTED OUTCOMES

Initial outcomes
- Patient receives appropriate physical and emotional care.
- Family members honestly express feelings about caring for the patient.

Interim outcomes
- Patient expresses grief related to unresolved conflicts with family members.
- Patient identifies sources of social support outside of family.
- Family members listen to suggestions for dealing with unresolved issues from their past without expressing anger or denial.
- If appropriate, patient and family members attend a conference to discuss better ways to communicate and explore health-related concerns.

Discharge outcome
- Family members identify and contact social service agencies to assist with caring for aging family member.

INTERVENTIONS AND RATIONALES

Initial interventions
- Assess the effects of the patient's disease on family functioning *to plan interventions.*
- Maintain objectivity when dealing with family conflicts. Do not become embroiled in the dynamics of a dysfunctional family *to uphold your ability to intervene effectively.* Dysfunctional family coping patterns evolve over many years and are unlikely to change just because the patient is elderly or his health is deteriorating. Accepting your limitations will enable you to provide better care.
- Act as a patient advocate, when necessary. Take steps to guard the patient's rights, including the right to be free of abuse and, if legally competent, to make autonomous decisions regarding health care. Take any reports of abuse seriously *to ensure safety.*
- Provide necessary information about health care options to the patient *to facilitate decision making and ensure autonomy.*
- Encourage family members to express their feelings about caring for the patient and the reasons for their anger toward the patient. Be especially careful to communicate a nonjudgmental attitude *to promote honest, effective communication. Family members may not express their true feelings if they sense they are under pressure to act as a model family.*

Interim interventions
- Provide the patient with opportunities to express grief over unresolved conflicts with family members. The patient may have to grieve over the loss of the "ideal" family, which he was never able to achieve. *Therapeutic listening helps the patient to understand himself and his family better and to come to terms with his past.*
- Encourage the patient to contact a support group, senior services agency, or adult day care center to help him obtain the emotional support his family is unable to provide.
- If your observations of family members suggest they are psychologically hampered by unresolved emotional conflict from the past, share your insights with them gently. If appropri-

ate, suggest they consider counseling *to work through their feelings.*

- Assess whether the patient and family members could benefit from a family conference. If there is sufficient understanding and patience on the part of all parties, conduct family discussions *to explore ways to communicate more effectively and resolve immediate health-related concerns.* However, if anger and resentment appear to be overwhelming, don't attempt to act as a moderator. Instead, provide referral for family counseling.

Discharge interventions

- Refer the family members to a home health care agency, homemaker service, Meals On Wheels, adult day care center, or other appropriate outside agencies for assistance and follow-up. *Use of community services may help to reduce the burden on family members and thereby help ease resentment.*
- Depending on the patient's level of self-care and the attitudes of family members, explore the possibility of placing the patient in a long-term care facility *to facilitate appropriate treatment of chronic illness.*

EVALUATION STATEMENTS

Family members:
- honestly express feelings about caring for the patient.
- listen to suggestions for dealing with unresolved issues from their past without expressing anger or denial.
  Patient:
- receives appropriate physical and emotional care.
- expresses grief related to unresolved conflicts with family members.

- identifies sources of social support outside of family.
  Patient and family members:
- attend a conference to discuss better ways to communicate and explore immediate health-related concerns, if they are emotionally ready.
- identify and contact social service agencies to assist with caring for aging family member.

DOCUMENTATION

- Diagnostic test results
- Family members' responses to patient's illness
- Observations of patient's interactions with family members
- Patient's expressions of grief, anger, or disappointment over unresolved conflicts with family members
- Family members' statements of anger, hostility, resentment, rage, or other feelings toward the patient
- Referrals made to support groups and community services (patient and family members)
- Patient's and family members' reaction to possible placement in long-term care facility.
- Evaluation statements.

Coping, ineffective individual

related to difficulty meeting demands of daily living

DEFINITION

Inability to use adaptive behaviors in response to difficult life situations

ASSESSMENT

Cultural status
- *Demographics:* age, sex, marital status, level of education, occupation, nationality, race, ethnic group
- *History:* beliefs, values, and attitudes about health and illness; health customs, practices, and rituals

Family status
- *Family composition:* presence of spouse; length of marriage, divorce, or widowhood; location of children and grandchildren
- *Family roles:* formal and informal roles, role performance, degree of family agreement on roles, interrelationships of various roles
- *Family rules:* rules that foster stability, maladaptive rules, methods of rule modification
- *Family communication:* style and quality of communication, methods of conflict resolution
- *Developmental stage of family:* changes in relationships between family members, shifts in role responsibility over time, problems adjusting to change
- *Family subsystems:* family alliances, effect of family alliances on family stability
- *Family needs:* ability of family to meet patient's physical, social and emotional needs; disparities between patient's needs and family's willingness or ability to meet them
- *Values and aspirations:* extent to which family permits pursuit of individual goals and values
- *Social and economic factors:* economic status of family, sense of adequacy and self-worth, employment, attitudes toward work; influence of religious beliefs on values and practices
- *Coping patterns:* major life events and their meaning to each family member, usual coping patterns, family members' perception of effectiveness of coping patterns, evidence of abuse
- *Family health history:* bipolar disorder, depressive disorder, suicide, schizophrenia, mental retardation, substance use disorder, stress-related illness, medical illness
- *Diagnostic tests:* Family Environment Scale, Family Adjustment Device, Family Genogram, Dyadic Adjustment Scale, Family Awareness Scale, Primary Communication Inventory, Index of Family Relations

Psychological status
- *Life changes:* recent divorce, illness, job loss, or loss of loved one; deterioration in health status
- *Psychiatric history:* age at onset of illness, impact on functioning, type of treatment, patient's response to treatment
- *Signs and symptoms:* changes in appetite, energy level, motivation, personal hygiene, self-image, self-esteem, sleep patterns, sexual drive, competence; alcohol or drug abuse
- *Laboratory tests:* urinalysis, hemoglobin and hematocrit, electrolyte and blood glucose levels, thyroid and liver function tests, blood and urine drug toxicology screen, dexamethasone suppression test, thyrotropin-releasing hormone test
- *Diagnostic tests:* Brief Psychiatric Rating Scale, Hamilton Rating Scale for Depression, Thematic Apperception Test, Self-Rating Anxiety Scale, Automatic Thoughts Questionnaire,

Fear Questionnaire, Impact of Event Scale, The Problem Solving Inventory, Reasons for Living Inventory, Revised UCLA Loneliness Scale, Self-Efficacy Scale, and State-Trait Anger Scale

DEFINING CHARACTERISTICS

- Disheveled appearance
- Disorganized behavior that may be mistaken for senility
- Frequent accidents or illness
- Heightened sense of fear and anxiety
- Hypersensitivity to normal aging changes
- Inability to meet basic needs or solve problems
- Inability to meet role expectations
- Isolation
- Poor personal hygiene
- Verbal expressions indicating inability to cope with present demands

ASSOCIATED DISORDERS

Alcohol use disorder; Alzheimer's disease; amyotrophic lateral sclerosis; cancer; cataracts; cor pulmonale; depressive disorder; diabetes mellitus; end-stage renal, pulmonary, or cardiac disease; paralysis; Parkinson's disease; rheumatoid arthritis

EXPECTED OUTCOMES

Initial outcome
- Patient identifies and contacts resources to enhance coping ability.

Interim outcomes
- Patient expands support network to meet social and emotional needs.
- Patient locates and uses appropriate resources for help in problem solving.

- Patient reports increased success in meeting demands of daily living.

Discharge outcome
- Patient changes environment to ensure enhanced coping or moves into a long-term care facility.

INTERVENTIONS AND RATIONALES

Initial intervention
- Refer the patient to social service agencies, such as geriatric assessment centers, adult day care programs, and home health care agencies, *to expand his support network and help him cope with physical, psychological, and economic stressors.*

Interim interventions
- Help the patient become involved with informal community programs, such as volunteer, foster grandparent, or religious groups. *Increased community involvement provides peer and social contact, thereby decreasing loneliness and isolation.*
- Encourage the patient to reminisce *to help him recall past challenges and successful coping strategies.*
- Provide the patient with information about the aging process, how to cope with stress, and techniques used by other older adults to meet the demands of daily living, *to enhance his coping strategies.*
- If the patient must enter a long-term care facility or undergo a lengthy home-based convalescence, help him put the situation in perspective. Explain to the patient that extreme stress can overwhelm anyone, even well-adapted individuals with strong sup-

port systems. Mention that when stress becomes overwhelming, rehabilitation in a secure environment may be the best option. Entering a long-term care facility is not "the beginning of the end," as many people think, but rather an additional mechanism for ensuring optimal recovery. *Taking the time to provide a carefully worded explanation may help the patient come to terms with his situation.*

Discharge interventions
- If treatment in a long-term care facility is required, provide the least restrictive environment possible *to reduce the patient's fear and anxiety, help him retain a sense of control, and encourage him to use his abilities to the maximum.*
- Discuss with the patient the possibility of making lifestyle changes. For example, suggest moving closer to relatives, moving to a retirement community, or hiring someone to help with housework. *These adjustments can improve his ability to cope.*

EVALUATION STATEMENTS

Patient:
- identifies resources to help him cope with the demands of daily living.
- describes strategies to improve coping ability.
- reports success in developing support network to meet social and emotional needs.
- reports increased ability to meet demands of daily living.
- identifies lifestyle changes that will improve his ability to cope.

- states that he understands and accepts need to move to a long-term care facility if necessary.

DOCUMENTATION

- Diagnostic test results
- Patient's statements about present life situation and difficulty coping
- Sources of support identified to help patient cope with demands of daily living
- Observations of patient's behavior in response to stressful situations
- Teaching provided and patient's response
- Evaluation statements.

Decisional conflict

related to advance directives

DEFINITION

State of uncertainty regarding health-related course of action; in this instance, whether or not to limit the use of heroic life-sustaining measures in terminal illness or incapacitation

ASSESSMENT

Cultural status
- *Demographics:* age, sex, marital status, level of education, occupation, nationality, race, ethnic group, religion
- *History:* beliefs, values, and attitudes about health and illness; health customs, practices, and rituals
- *Diagnostic test:* Cultural Assessment Guide

Family status
- *Family composition:* presence of spouse; length of marriage, divorce, or widowhood; location of children and grandchildren; extended family, companion, or others who function as family for the patient; decision maker in family
- *Family communication:* style and quality of communication, methods of resolving conflicts
- *Values and aspirations:* extent to which family permits its members to pursue individual goals and values
- *Coping patterns:* major life events, usual coping patterns
- *Diagnostic test:* Family Genogram

Neurologic status
- *Mental status:* appearance and attitude, level of consciousness, motor activity, thought and speech, mood and affect, perceptions, orientation, memory, visual-spatial ability, attention span, abstraction, judgment and insight, general information, capacity to read, write, and perform calculations
- *Motor function:* muscle tone, strength, and symmetry; gait; cerebellar function
- *Sensory function:* cortical function

Psychological status
- *Psychiatric history:* age at onset of illness, type and severity of symptoms, impact on functioning, treatment and patient's response
- *Recent events:* divorce, illness, loss of job or loved one
- *Current illness:* prognosis, understanding of medical history and options regarding advance directives

- *Adult development:* academic, military, and occupational history; marital history; hobbies and recreation; reactions to illness and disability
- *Signs and symptoms:* changes in appetite, energy level, motivation, personal hygiene, self-image, self-esteem, sleep pattern, sexual drive, or level of competence
- *Diagnostic tests:* Brief Psychiatric Rating Scale, Hamilton Rating Scale for Depression

Social status
- *History:* interpersonal skills, quality of relationships, ability to trust others, comfort level in social settings

Spiritual status
- *History:* religious affiliation and education; beliefs about significance of life, suffering, illness, and death; influence of religious beliefs on choice of treatment options

DEFINING CHARACTERISTICS

- Feelings of anxiety or indecision regarding treatment options
- Indecision caused by difficulty reconciling conflicting recommendations regarding health care choices (health care team, family members, clergy)
- Lack of knowledge regarding the content or purpose of advance directives
- Limited history of autonomous decision making
- Procrastination in making health-related decisions

ASSOCIATED DISORDERS

This diagnosis may accompany any terminal illness or potentially incapacitating condition. Examples include end-stage renal or cardiopulmonary disease, cancer, Parkinson's disease, and multiple sclerosis.

EXPECTED OUTCOMES

Initial outcomes
- Patient discusses potential outcomes of his disorder and associated treatment options.
- Patient asks for help in understanding the content and purpose of advance directives.

Interim outcomes
- Patient receives information describing his options regarding advance directives.
- Patient receives appropriate referral for help in executing advance directive, if he wishes to do so.
- Patient provides a copy of his advance directive to people likely to be involved in his care (family members, surrogate decision maker, doctors).

Discharge outcome
- Patient reviews and updates his advance directive annually.

INTERVENTIONS AND RATIONALES

Initial interventions
- Encourage the patient to express his feelings about his illness, his prognosis, and the possibility that he may undergo extraordinary or painful life-sustaining treatments. Listen to his fears and concerns without conveying judgment *to help him express his wishes concerning health care.*
- Assess the patient's understanding of his right to participate in treatment decisions and his options regarding advance directives *to determine his learning needs.*

Interim interventions
- Explain to the patient that an advance directive (for example, a living will or durable power of attorney for health care) is a legal document. It states his preferences for medical interventions if he is irreversibly comatose or vegetative or suffering with end-stage terminal illness *to help him make informed decisions.*
- Using simple terms, describe options for limiting treatment in a realistic but positive context. Reassure the patient that he'll continue to receive supportive care and pain medication *to provide guidance and reduce anxiety.*
- If the patient expresses interest in drafting an advance directive, recommend that he talk to his attorney, or refer him to your health care facility's legal department or local legal aid society. *Legal requirements regarding the content and execution of advance directives vary from state to state. The patient may need legal counsel to ensure the document is properly written and executed.*
- If the patient decides to draft a living will or other advance directive while under your care, document his decision in your notes. Describe the circumstances under which the document was drawn up and signed. Review your nursing or hospital manual for any additional steps to take; for ex-

ample, you may need to inform the doctor or your health care facility's administrative and legal departments *to help ensure that the patient's rights are respected.*
- Encourage the patient to inform key people, such as doctors or family members who would care for him if he were terminally ill, that he has executed an advance directive *to help ensure their cooperation if the advance directive must be carried out.*
- If the patient is unable to decide about future treatment options or chooses not to draft an advance directive, demonstrate that you respect his choice. *The patient has the right to refuse to participate in health care decisions.*

Discharge intervention
- Encourage the patient to review his advance directive annually and update it as needed *to ensure that it continues to accurately reflect his preferences.*

EVALUATION STATEMENTS

Patient:
- discusses potential outcomes of his illness and the types of extraordinary measures that may be required to sustain life.
- asks for information about the purpose and content of advance directives.
- obtains appropriate guidance for executing an advance directive, if he chooses to do so.
- provides a copy of his advance directives to people likely to be involved in his care if he becomes terminally ill.
- periodically reviews the advance directive to be sure it continues to reflect his preferences and best interests.

DOCUMENTATION

- Diagnostic test results
- Evidence of decisional conflict regarding whether to execute an advance directive
- Patient's expressed preferences for care (verbatim, whenever possible)
- Teaching provided to improve the patient's understanding of advance directives
- Discussions with the doctor or nursing supervisor regarding the patient's desire to draft advance directives
- If appropriate, the patient's decision to draft an advance directive and the circumstances under which the document was drawn up and signed
- Referrals to appropriate legal counsel
- Evaluation statements.

Fear
related to aging and potential disability

DEFINITION

Physiologic or emotional disruption related to anxiety over the possibility of losing one's capacities

ASSESSMENT

Cultural status
- *Demographics:* age, sex, marital status, level of education, occupation, nationality, race, ethnic group
- *History:* beliefs, values, and attitudes about health, aging, and illness; health customs, practices, and rituals

Cardiovascular status
- *Physical examination:* vital signs, blood pressure, respirations, facial expressions, skin temperature
- *Signs and symptoms:* tachycardia, rapid respirations or hyperventilation, chest pain, fatigue, palpitations, dyspnea, cough, shortness of breath

Gastrointestinal status
- *Physical examination:* abdominal inspection, palpation, and auscultation; stool characteristics; bowel sounds
- *Signs and symptoms:* constipation or diarrhea, decreased appetite, dry mouth
- *Laboratory test:* Hemoccult
- *Diagnostic tests:* upper and lower GI series

Genitourinary status
- *History:* history of urinary tract infections, urine characteristics, urinary frequency and urgency
- *Physical examinations:* pelvic, abdominal, genital, and rectal examinations
- *Laboratory tests:* urinalysis, culture and sensitivity testing, urine specific gravity
- *Diagnostic tests:* urodynamic tests

Integumentary status
- *Physical examination:* inspection of skin, skin and body temperature
- *Signs and symptoms:* diaphoresis, pruritus

Musculoskeletal status
- *History:* accidents or trauma, degenerative joint disease, daily activities
- *Signs and symptoms:* limited movement, muscle tension

Neurologic status
- *Mental status:* appearance and attitude, thought and speech, mood and affect, perceptions, orientation, attention span, abstraction, judgment and insight
- *Physical examination:* motor system, reflexes, pupillary response
- *Signs and symptoms:* restlessness, incoordination
- *Laboratory tests:* drug toxicity screening, thyroid function test, electrolyte levels
- *Diagnostic tests:* Folstein Mini-Mental Status Examination, Abnormal Involuntary Movement Scale

Peripheral vascular status
- *Physical examination:* superficial vasoconstriction, peripheral skin temperature and sensation, capillary refill time

Psychological status
- *History:* self-esteem; response to changes in health status; changes in appetite, motivation, or energy level; recent illness, hospitalization, or surgery; recent divorce, loss of job, death of loved one, or other major life changes; spiritual resources; ability to accept change
- *Diagnostic tests:* Brief Psychiatric Rating Scale, Hamilton Rating Scale for Depression, Behavior Checklist

Self-care status
- *Prior medical conditions:* neurologic, sensory, or psychological impairment
- *History:* use of adaptive equipment, devices, or supplies
- *Observation:* functional ability (muscle tone, size, and strength; range

of motion; coordination), daily activities (dressing, grooming, bathing, toileting, and hygiene)
- *Diagnostic test:* Self-Care Assessment Tool

Family status
- *History:* family composition, proximity to family members, involvement with children or other family members, family alliances and conflicts, family coping patterns, ability of family members to cope with change
- *Social and economic factors:* financial resources, proximity to health care services
- *Diagnostic test:* Family Adjustment Device

DEFINING CHARACTERISTICS

- Chronic illness that may eventually cause disability or incapacitation
- Expressions of fear
- Inadequate financial resources
- Increased speaking or questioning
- Lack of friends or family
- Perceived loss of control
- Physical manifestations of fear, such as diaphoresis, high blood pressure, increased pulse rate, or increased respirations
- Recent death of loved one
- Sad, dull affect
- Voice tremors or pitch changes

ASSOCIATED DISORDERS

Alzheimer's disease, chronic obstructive pulmonary disease, congestive heart failure, dementia, head injury, multiple sclerosis, Parkinson's disease, rheumatoid arthritis, transient ischemia

EXPECTED OUTCOMES

Initial outcome
- Patient identifies fear and other feelings related to the possibility of future disability or incapacitation.

Interim outcomes
- Patient states plans to adjust to changes in health status.
- Patient contacts community resources for help with activities of daily living.
- Patient uses available support systems to aid coping.
- Patient employs coping mechanism to reduce fear each day.
- Patient reports improved ability to cope with changes associated with aging or illness.

Discharge outcomes
- Physical signs or symptoms of fear are decreased.
- Patient receives information about composing a living will or other advance directives.

INTERVENTIONS AND RATIONALES

Initial interventions
- Encourage the patient to express fear related to the possibility of becoming disabled or incapacitated, such as fear of being kept alive in a comatose state, *to help him cope with his feelings and detect misconceptions.*
- Spend time with the patient each shift *to encourage expression of feelings and emotions and to increase trust.*

Interim interventions

- Regularly provide the patient with information about his health status *to increase his feeling of control, decrease his anxiety, and promote cooperation.*
- Involve the patient in care decisions when possible *to reduce feelings of powerlessness and victimization.*
- Teach relaxation techniques, such as guided imagery and progressive muscle relaxation, *to reduce anxiety.*
- Allow a family member or friend to participate in care and planning *to increase the patient's support system.*
- Provide consultation with a minister, priest, or rabbi *to enhance spiritual support.*
- Encourage family members to tell the patient he is still important to them even if his health deteriorates *to encourage him to focus on positive aspects of life and ways he will still be able to contribute if his health declines.*
- Being careful to convey a nonjudgmental attitude, discuss with the patient the importance of accepting life's changes to spiritual and emotional well-being. *Sharing thoughts and feelings can provide comfort and help the patient gain insight.*

Discharge interventions

- Discuss available community resources, such as Meals On Wheels, home health services, and rehabilitative services, *to promote independence and a sense of control.*
- Explain the patient's fears to family or friends *to help them understand and respond appropriately.*
- Provide information about a living will, power of attorney, and advance directives *to help the patient maintain control over his future if he becomes incapacitated.*

EVALUATION STATEMENTS

Patient:
- states cause of fear.
- reports feeling less fearful of incapacitation.
- demonstrates at least one coping mechanism daily.
- discusses health concerns.
- reports increased feeling of control.
- exhibits blood pressure, pulse rate, and respiration rate within specified ranges.

DOCUMENTATION

- Diagnostic test results and laboratory findings
- Patient's expressions of fear
- Behavioral and physiologic evidence of fear
- Nursing interventions
- Patient's response to interventions
- Available support systems to help patient cope with fear
- Patient's response to help from family, friends, or other caregivers
- Evaluation statements.

Grieving, anticipatory
related to preparation for death

DEFINITION

Grief in anticipation of death

ASSESSMENT

Cultural status
- *Demographics:* age, sex, level of education, occupation, nationality, race, ethnic group
- *History:* beliefs, values, and attitudes about health, illness, life, and death; health customs, practices, and rituals

Family status
- *Family composition:* marital status, ages of members, proximity of patient to family members
- *Family roles:* formal and informal roles, role performance, degree of family agreement on roles, interrelationships of roles
- *Family communication:* style and quality of communication, methods of conflict resolution
- *Developmental stage of family:* length of patient's relationships with family members, family's adaptation to change and shifts in role responsibility, problem-solving methods
- *Family alliances:* effects on stability of family unit
- *Physical and emotional needs:* ability of family to meet patient's physical and emotional needs
- *Family goals and values:* degree to which family permits members to pursue individual goals and values
- *Socioeconomic factors:* economic status; sense of adequacy and self-worth of members; employment and attitudes toward work; sense of belonging to racial, cultural, or ethnic group; influence of religious beliefs on values and practices
- *Coping patterns:* major life events and their meanings to each member,

usual coping patterns, family member's perception of effectiveness of coping patterns
- *Family health history:* bipolar disorder, depressive disorder, suicide, schizophrenia, mental retardation, substance use disorder, stress-related illness, medical illness

Psychological status
- *Signs and symptoms:* changes in appetite, energy level, motivation, personal hygiene, self-image, self-esteem, sleep pattern, or sexual drive
- *Alcohol or drug abuse:* type of substance, effects on mood and behavior, evidence of abuse or withdrawal
- *Psychiatric history:* presence of illness, age at onset, type and severity of symptoms, type of treatment and patient's response
- *Developmental history:* major life events, reactions to losses throughout life
- *Diagnostic tests:* Hamilton Rating Scale for Depression, Beck Depression Inventory

Sleep status
- *History:* presence of sleep pattern disturbances
- *Medications:* sleep aids, caffeine, alcohol, amphetamines, benzodiazepines

Social status
- *History:* size of social network, quality of relationships, trust in others, level of self-esteem, ability to function in social roles
- *Signs and symptoms:* withdrawal from social relationships

Spiritual status

- *History:* current perception of faith and religious practices, religious affiliation, perceptions about life and death, support network

DEFINING CHARACTERISTICS

- Altered communication patterns
- Anger
- Difficulty in expressing loss
- Expressions of distress over possible death
- Guilt, sorrow, or anxiety
- Physical deterioration
- Weight loss

ASSOCIATED DISORDERS

This diagnosis may be associated with exacerbation of any chronic or terminal illness, such as bronchopneumonia; cancer; end-stage pulmonary, cardiac, or renal disease; or influenza A.

EXPECTED OUTCOMES

Initial outcome

- Patient expresses feelings about anticipated death.

Interim outcomes

- Patient progresses through the stages of grieving process in his own way.
- Patient practices religious rituals or uses other coping mechanisms.

Discharge outcome

- Family members or companion provide supportive care and comfort to patient.

INTERVENTIONS AND RATIONALES

Initial outcomes

- Provide time for the patient to express feelings about death or terminal illness. Do not appear to be rushed or harried while he speaks. *Active listening alleviates feelings of isolation.*
- Establish a relationship that encourages the patient to express concerns about death. *Basic nursing care combined with genuine interest in the patient fosters trust and understanding.*

Interim outcomes

- Guide the patient in reviewing his life. Encourage him to write or tape his life history as a lasting gift to family members. *This allows the patient to give events from his past a meaningful interpretation.*
- Involve the interdisciplinary team, including a psychologist, nurse, nutritionist, doctor, physical therapist, and chaplain, in providing care for the dying patient. *Each team member offers unique expertise for meeting the dying patient's needs.*
- Encourage family members to become involved in the care of the dying patient. Communicate with the patient and family members honestly and compassionately. *Giving family members a role in patient care helps to relieve anxiety and lessen feelings of regret and guilt. Honest communication is important because family members need an opportunity to acknowledge loss and to say farewell.*
- Demonstrate acceptance of the patient's response to his anticipated death, whatever it may be: crying, sadness, anger, fear, or denial. *Each pa-*

tient responds to dying in his own way. Helping him express his feelings freely will enhance his ability to cope.
- Help the patient progress through the psychological stages associated with anticipated death: shock and denial, anger, bargaining, depression, and acceptance. *Knowing these stages will help you anticipate the dying patient's psychological needs, but note that not all dying patients will go through each stage.*
- Support the patient's spiritual coping behaviors. For example, arrange for the patient to have at the bedside objects that provide spiritual comfort, such as a Bible, a prayer shawl, pictures, statues, or rosary beads. *Even nonobservant patients frequently turn to religion when confronted by death or serious illness.*

Discharge outcomes
- Discuss hospice services with the patient. *Hospice services emphasize symptomatic relief and caring, with the aim of improving patient and family comfort until death occurs, instead of prolonging life for its own sake.*
- Provide referrals for home health care assistance, if requested, *to support the patient's decision to remain at home.*

EVALUATION STATEMENTS

Patient:
- expresses feelings about anticipated death.
- accepts feelings brought about by the possibility of death.
- progresses through stages of grief in his own way.

- participates in religious rituals or uses other appropriate coping mechanisms.
- receives adequate support during end of life from family members, friends, and health care team.

DOCUMENTATION

- Diagnostic test results
- Patient's feelings about anticipated death
- Observations of emotional responses, such as crying, anger, and withdrawal
- Nursing interventions performed to help patient cope with anticipated death
- Patient's requests for assistance in achieving spiritual comfort, such as spiritual objects or visits from clergy
- Patient's response to interventions
- Evaluation statements.

Hopelessness

related to decline in physical capabilities

DEFINITION

Feelings of despair as a result of debilitating physical symptoms

ASSESSMENT

Cultural status
- *Demographics:* age, sex, level of education, occupation, nationality, race, ethnic group

- *History:* beliefs, values, and attitudes about health and illness; health customs, practices, and rituals

Neurologic status

- *Mental status:* speech patterns, intellectual functioning, thought processes, general orientation, perception, mood and affect, attention span, insight and judgment
- *Motor system:* muscle tone, strength, and symmetry; gait; cerebellar function; pupillary response
- *Signs and symptoms:* lethargy, restlessness, tremors, falls, syncope, irritability
- *Laboratory tests:* drug toxicology screening, thyroid function test, electrolyte levels
- *Diagnostic tests:* computed tomography, magnetic resonance imaging, memory loss scale

Nutritional status

- *History:* use of drugs or alcohol, use of laxatives, refusal to eat, history of malabsorption or nutritional deficiencies
- *Physical examination:* height and weight, abdominal examination
- *Medications:* multivitamins with iron, nutritional supplements
- *Signs and symptoms:* weight loss, nausea, vomiting, fainting, constipation, diarrhea
- *Laboratory tests:* hemoglobin and hematocrit, serum iron level, nitrogen balance, creatinine-height index
- *Diagnostic tests:* upper GI series, barium enema, barium swallow

Psychological status

- *History:* appetite, energy level, motivation, personal hygiene, self-image,

self-esteem, sleep pattern, sexual drive, level of competence, relationship with family, relationship with peers and social groups
- *Life changes:* recent divorce, job loss, loss of loved ones, move to long-term care facility
- *Psychiatric history:* age at onset, type and severity of symptoms, impact on functioning, type of treatment, patient's response to treatment
- *Signs and symptoms:* changes in appetite, low energy level, lack of motivation, poor personal hygiene, low self-concept, changes in sleep patterns, changes in libido, abuse of chemical substances, dangerous mixing of medications, changes in mood and behavior, depression, self-destructiveness
- *Laboratory tests:* blood profile, complete blood count, thyroid and liver function tests, urinalysis, blood and urine toxicology screening
- *Diagnostic tests:* Geriatric Hopelessness Scale, Miller Hope Scale, Philadelphia Geriatric Center Morale Scale, Lohmann Life Satisfaction Scale, Cornell Personal Adjustment Scale, Cavan Attitude Inventory

Self-care status

- *Prior medical conditions:* neurologic, sensory, or psychological impairment
- *History:* use of adaptive equipment, devices, or supplies
- *Observation:* functional ability (muscle tone, size, and strength; range of motion; coordination), daily activities (dressing, grooming, bathing, toileting, and hygiene)
- *Signs and symptoms:* inability to perform activities of daily living without assistance, inability to perform

self-care and follow prescribed treatment, deliberate disregard for safety
- *Diagnostic tests:* Index of Activities of Daily Living, Barthel Index, Instrumental Activities of Daily Living

Sleep pattern status
- *History:* sleep and wake patterns, rest and relaxation patterns, living arrangements, caffeine use, alcohol consumption
- *Medications:* sedative-hypnotics, antihistamines, barbiturates
- *Signs and symptoms:* irritability, change in sleep patterns, early morning awakening, insomnia, confusion, sunrise syndrome, excessive day napping, poor sleep habits, diminished ability to achieve rapid eye movement (REM) sleep, inability to maintain REM sleep, tired feeling after sleep
- *Diagnostic test:* sleep electroencephalography

Social status
- *History:* size of social network; employment status; length of marriage, divorce, or widowhood; length of time in current community; recent losses
- *Medications:* antidepressants
- *Signs and symptoms:* withdrawal, irritability, agitation

Spiritual status
- *History:* religious affiliation, attendance at religious services, religious practices, relationship with clergy and members of church or synagogue
- *Signs and symptoms:* despair, crying, withdrawal, resignation, feeling of unfulfillment in life, doubts about previously held beliefs, feeling that life has no meaning, negative attitude about God, expression of regret

- *Diagnostic tests:* Spiritual and Religious Concerns Questionnaire, Spiritual Well-Being Scale

DEFINING CHARACTERISTICS

- Expressions of hopelessness
- Lack of motivation
- Past suicidal history
- Poor compliance with medical regimen
- Presence of risk factors for hopelessness, including experience of multiple losses, isolation, physical deterioration, tenuous family connections
- Sleep disturbances

ASSOCIATED DISORDERS

Alcohol or substance use disorders, arthritis, cancer, chronic illness, depressive disorder, diabetes mellitus, dyssomnia, end-stage renal disease, hypertension, multiple sclerosis, Parkinson's disease, physical disabilities, recurrent and primary degenerative dementia of the Alzheimer's type, schizophrenia, terminal illness

EXPECTED OUTCOMES

Initial outcomes
- Patient remains safe in a therapeutic environment.
- Patient interacts at least three times a day with peers and staff.

Interim outcomes
- Patient participates in the therapeutic environment, attending group sessions and auxiliary therapies.
- Patient discusses feelings of hopelessness and his physically debilitating condition.

- Patient expresses improved feelings about self and begins to feel hopeful in spite of limited physical capabilities.

Discharge outcomes
- Patient identifies appropriate coping skills that he can use after discharge.
- Patient expresses awareness of available resources.

INTERVENTIONS AND RATIONALES

Initial interventions
- Maintain a safe environment; remove any of the patient's belongings with which he could hurt himself. *This will help the patient feel protected from himself and give him control over harmful feelings.*
- Encourage the patient to talk to staff members and other patients *to reduce his sense of isolation.*

Interim interventions
- Explain the purpose of the therapeutic environment and prescribed therapy, such as art therapy, to the patient and encourage his participation. *This shows him that this environment has been designed to offer support and foster feelings of hope.*
- Allow time for the patient to express his feelings, and approach him with short, frequent contacts *to build a trusting relationship and establish rapport. Because an older person may require frequent rest periods, short contacts are advisable.*
- As the patient shows signs of improvement, point out how he has developed *to reassure him that hope is valid in spite of limitations.*

- Encourage participation in a reminiscence group *to promote pride in past accomplishments.*
- Discuss ways for the patient to continue activities meaningful to himself, such as writing to a grandchild or putting together a scrapbook for family members, *to help reaffirm his contributions to others.*
- Encourage the patient to participate in group activities, such as a bridge club, *to reduce social isolation.*

Discharge interventions
- Make sure the patient is aware of resources available in the community. Stress the importance of follow-up treatment *to ease the transition from a controlled environment to the community.*
- Assess whether the patient is comfortable using new coping skills *to help ensure that he will be able to manage his feelings in the future.*

EVALUATION STATEMENTS

Patient:
- no longer uses phrases that convey hopelessness.
- expresses a willingness to participate in therapies and verbalizes feelings freely.
- no longer feels hopeless about his physical limitations.
- shows increased feelings of self-worth.
- discusses the desire to return home and use the coping skills attained in the hospital.

DOCUMENTATION

- Diagnostic test results
- Patient's statements of hopelessness
- Patient's behavior
- Patient's response to the therapeutic environment
- Instruction in coping techniques provided to the patient
- Nursing interventions and the patient's response
- Evaluation statements.

Injury, high risk for

related to elder abuse

DEFINITION

Risk of physical, emotional, or psychological harm due to abuse or poor care

ASSESSMENT

Patient status
- *History:* age, sex, care requirements, physical and emotional needs, mental health, substance use or abuse
- *Evidence of physical abuse:* imprint of hand or fingers; marks from restraints; unexplained bruises, burns, welts, cuts, dislocations, or abrasions
- *Evidence of emotional abuse:* observation or reports of insults, ridicule, or humiliation

Self-care status
- *Prior medical conditions:* neurologic, musculoskeletal, sensory, or psychological impairment
- *Observation:* functional ability (muscle tone, size, and strength; range

of motion; coordination), daily activities (dressing, grooming, bathing, toileting, and hygiene), meal preparation, clothing, sanitation, availability of medication and physical aids
- *Evidence of neglect:* inappropriate clothing; unsanitary living conditions; inadequate food supplies; lack of medication; absence of needed eyeglasses, hearing aids, cane, or walker
- *Diagnostic test:* Self-Care Assessment Tool

Nutritional status
- *Physical examination:* weight and weight changes, skin tone, daily diet, evidence of malnutrition

Family status
- *Caregiver:* relationship to patient; proximity to patient; time and resources available for caregiving; willingness and ability to meet patient's physical, social, and emotional needs; feelings of frustration; family health history
- *Family development:* family composition, family dynamics, changes in roles and responsibilities, ability to adapt to change, history of abuse of any family member
- *Socioeconomic factors:* economic status of family, changes in patient's financial status, responsibility for patient's finances
- *Evidence of financial abuse:* unexplained changes in bank accounts, transfer of funds to caregivers
- *Diagnostic tests:* Family Environment Scale, Family Adjustment Device

RISK FACTORS

- Caregiver expresses frustration over responsibilities of caring for older family member.
- Family has limited education or inadequate financial resources.
- Family is isolated from community, without relatives living nearby.
- Patient is forced to depend on family members for daily care.
- Patient reports lack of social contacts outside family.
- Patient suffers from deteriorating health, frailty, or impaired mobility.

ASSOCIATED MEDICAL DIAGNOSES

Alzheimer's disease, bipolar disorder, cardiovascular disease, cerebrovascular accident, dementia, fractures, malnutrition, osteoarthritis, rheumatoid arthritis, schizophrenia

EXPECTED OUTCOMES

Initial outcomes

- Patient remains free of injury.
- Patient states that incidents of abuse do not occur.
- Patient expresses understanding of right to be free from abuse.

Interim outcomes

- Patient maintains control over mail, telephone, and other personal effects.
- Patient reports increased social contact outside the family.
- Patient establishes a mutual "buddy system," whereby he and a friend visit or telephone each other at regularly scheduled intervals.

Discharge outcomes

- Caregiver states intention to contact respite care services, support groups, and other community resources.
- Patient and caregiver report improved communication patterns.

INTERVENTIONS AND RATIONALES

Initial interventions

- Monitor the patient closely at each visit for evidence of physical or mental abuse or neglect. Observe for bruises or abrasions, body odor, or dirty, unkempt appearance *to ensure his safety and well-being.* Question him privately about findings *to encourage trust and promote open communication.*
- Encourage the patient to discuss incidents of abuse or threats of abuse. Be willing to listen and be careful to convey a nonjudgmental attitude. *Older patients may be reluctant to discuss abuse or threats of abuse because of fear of retaliation, embarrassment, or reluctance to report family members to authorities. By communicating that you care and are willing to listen, you may help the patient overcome these barriers.*
- Educate the patient regarding his right to be free from abuse. Discuss the responsibility of law enforcement agencies to investigate incidents of abuse. Provide a list of social service agencies that are available to provide counseling. *Education may help empower patient to resist or prevent episodes of abuse.*
- Report actual or suspected elder abuse to local authorities and provide follow-up or emergency care if needed. *Nearly every state has laws mandat-*

ing that suspected elder abuse be reported to the authorities.

Interim interventions
- Encourage the patient to maintain use of a personal telephone and open his own mail *to promote his sense of control and self-worth and to maintain contact with people outside the home.*
- Encourage the patient to participate in community activities, such as church groups and retired senior volunteer organizations, *to establish social contacts necessary for a strong support network.*
- Suggest use of Meals On Wheels or community geriatric outreach for the homebound patient *to prevent isolation and provide respite for the family caregiver.*
- Encourage friends to visit the patient at home. Suggest that the patient and a friend develop a "buddy system," whereby each takes turns telephoning or visiting the other at regular intervals *to provide social contact, respite for the caregiver, and an additional safeguard against abuse.*

Discharge interventions
- If appropriate, encourage the patient and family members to periodically hold conferences. Help them identify productive topics for discussion, such as strategies for dealing with the patient's self-care deficits or scheduling respite care, *to foster open communication, diffuse tension, and develop solutions to the practical problems of caring for an older family member.*
- Inform the caregiver about state and county services for elderly people, respite services, adult day care, support groups for children of aging parents,

and other community resources *to enhance the caregiver's ability to cope and thereby diminish the likelihood of abuse.*

EVALUATION STATEMENTS

Patient:
- does not exhibit injuries and states that incidents of abuse have stopped.
- expresses understanding of right to be protected from abuse.
- reports satisfaction with ability to maintain or increase social contacts outside family.
- establishes "buddy system" with a friend outside the home.
- maintains control over mail, telephone, and other personal effects.
  Caregiver:
- regularly attends a community support group and contacts appropriate social service agencies and other sources of support.
- reports increased ability to cope with responsibilities of caring for an older family member.
  Patient and caregiver:
- report improved communication.

DOCUMENTATION

- Diagnostic test results
- Evidence of emotional, physical, or financial neglect or abuse
- Patient's statements that indicate risk for abuse
- Caregiver's statements indicating feelings about caring for an older family member
- Caregiver's statements indicating willingness to attend support groups or use community resources

- Patient's and caregiver's expressions indicating understanding of teaching provided by nurse
- Nursing interventions
- Patient's response to nursing interventions
- Evaluation statements.

Poisoning, high risk for

related to medication use

DEFINITION

Heightened risk of toxicity because of excessive drug doses or multiple drug use

ASSESSMENT

Cultural status
- *Demographics:* age, sex, level of education, nationality, race, ethnic group
- *History:* beliefs, values, and attitudes about health and illness; health practices, customs, and rituals

Cardiovascular status
- *Signs and symptoms:* elevated or decreased blood pressure, orthostatic hypotension, tachycardia or bradycardia, chest pain, palpitations
- *Medications:* digoxin, antihypertensives, beta blockers, calcium channel blockers, anticoagulants
- *Laboratory tests:* electrolyte levels, especially sodium and potassium; complete blood count; hemoglobin and hematocrit; lipid profile; prothrombin time; partial thromboplastin time
- *Diagnostic test:* electrocardiography

Gastrointestinal status
- *Signs and symptoms:* nausea, vomiting, diarrhea, constipation, abdominal pain; blood in stool; dry mouth or gums; tongue irritation or lesions; changes in appetite
- *Laboratory tests:* glucose, serum creatinine, and blood urea nitrogen levels; liver function tests

Genitourinary status
- *Symptoms:* urine retention
- *Laboratory findings:* high or low urine pH, elevated creatinine clearance

Integumentary status
- *Signs and symptoms:* rash, lesions, discoloration, bruises, induration, inflammation, pruritus

Musculoskeletal status
- *Signs and symptoms:* altered gait; tremor, shakiness, or rigidity; weakness
- *Medications:* systemic corticosteroids, nonsteroidal anti-inflammatory drugs

Neurologic status
- *Mental status:* appearance and attitude, thought and speech, mood and affect, perceptions, orientation, attention span, abstraction, judgment and insight
- *Signs and symptoms:* sluggishness or slow movement, peripheral neuropathy, headache, ataxia, dizziness, slurred speech, garbled speech, pinpoint pupils, hyperactive or impaired reflexes

Psychological status
- *Signs and symptoms:* confusion, delirium, agitation, altered level of consciousness, lethargy, fatigue, behavior

changes, depression, sleep disorder, drowsiness

Family status
- *Family composition:* presence of spouse; length of marriage, divorce, or widowhood; location of children and grandchildren

RISK FACTORS

- Age-related physiologic changes, such as decreased body fluid, hepatic blood flow, glomerular filtration rate; increased body fat; muscle weakness
- Cognitive or emotional difficulty, including forgetfulness or confusion
- Decreased visual acuity, difficulty reading medication labels
- Large supplies of drugs in house
- Multiple disorders
- Multiple health care providers, multiple prescriptions, and use of multiple pharmacies
- Poor understanding of drug interactions, usage, and precautions
- Unsafe medication storage

ASSOCIATED DISORDERS

Alzheimer's disease, arteriosclerotic heart disease, cataracts, cerebrovascular accident, chronic obstructive pulmonary disease, congestive heart failure, degenerative joint disease, depressive disorder, diabetes mellitus, diverticulitis, glaucoma, hepatic disease, hypertension, myocardial infarction, pneumonia, renal disease, rheumatoid arthritis, urinary tract infections

EXPECTED OUTCOMES

Initial outcomes
- Patient and family members demonstrate knowledge of purpose of all medications.
- Patient states correct dosages and times medications are to be taken.

Interim outcomes
- Patient and family members describe plan to reduce the risk of excessive medication use.
- Patient and caregivers express an understanding of the risk when multiple health care providers prescribe medications.
- Patient and family members retain a home care agency, nurse practitioner, or doctor to coordinate medication regimen.
- Patient uses weekly pill box, calendar, or other mechanism to regulate medication regimen.
- Patient and family members describe how aging process can affect prescribed medication dosages.

Discharge outcome
- Patient doesn't experience episodes of toxicity.

INTERVENTIONS AND RATIONALES

Initial interventions
- Instruct the patient or family members in the patient's drug regimen, including reasons for taking the drugs and safety precautions, *to increase compliance.*
- Review and document the patient's entire medication regimen regularly *to assess whether certain prescriptions*

should be reevaluated, and to monitor for drug interactions.
- Make sure all medication labels are inscribed in large print and include dosage instructions *to avoid medication errors.*

Interim interventions
- Provide written instructions for use of medications, including size, frequency, and number of doses, *to enhance understanding of the medication regimen and increase compliance.*
- Make sure instructions are clearly written in black or blue ink. *Older patients can read black or blue type more easily.*
- Instruct the patient or family members to store drugs in a secure area away from the bedside to prevent accidental ingestion. *Often, older patients will keep medications at their bedside to decrease the need to arise during the night and may inadvertently ingest incorrect doses or drugs.*
- When color-coding medications, use only bright contrasting colors. *Older patients can't distinguish pastel colors well.*
- Help the patient or family members identify behaviors that may contribute to the risk of toxicity, for example, obtaining prescriptions from various health care providers or using different pharmacies, *to raise awareness of potential hazards.*
- Encourage the patient or family members to retain a nurse, nurse practitioner, or doctor to coordinate care. *Older patients with multiple health problems may receive care from various providers who are unaware of each other's treatment plans and drug regimens.*

- Help the patient maintain an accurate and effective system for following his medication regimen, such as a check-off calendar system or separate pill boxes labeled for each day of the week, *to reduce errors.* Encourage the patient to work with his pharmacist and health care provider when developing this system.
- Educate the patient or family members about age-related changes, such as atrophy, loss of protein, decreased liver and kidney functions, and change in body mass, that can influence how medications affect the body *to increase their knowledge and to prevent drug interactions or toxicity.*

Discharge intervention
- Monitor the patient's urine and serum drug levels as necessary. *Age-related changes in bodily function may lead to decreased renal, liver, and GI clearance of drugs, thereby increasing the patient's risk of toxicity. In addition, the variety of drugs commonly used by the older patient increases the risk of drug interactions.*

EVALUATION STATEMENTS

Patient or family member:
- expresses understanding of danger from simultaneous use of prescribed medication, over-the-counter medication, and home remedies to treat chronic conditions.
- demonstrates knowledge of dose, schedule, and purpose of medications.
- describes mechanisms to aid adherence to medication regimen.
- retains a nurse, nurse practitioner, or doctor to coordinate medication regimen.

- expresses understanding of age-related changes that may affect medication administration.

DOCUMENTATION

- Results of laboratory and diagnostic tests
- Patient's statements that indicate risk for drug interaction or toxicity
- Observations and evidence of unsafe practices
- Physical findings
- Nursing interventions
- Patient's response to nursing interventions
- Evaluation statements.

Powerlessness

related to perceived loss of control over life situations

DEFINITION

Feelings of helplessness, hopelessness, and lack of control

ASSESSMENT

Cultural status
- *Demographics:* age, sex, level of education, occupation, marital status, nationality, race, ethnic group, place of residence, economic status (including retirement income), medical expenses, insurance coverage or Medicare
- *History:* beliefs, values, and attitudes about health and illness; health practices, customs, and rituals
- *Diagnostic test:* Cultural Assessment Guide

Family status
- *Family composition:* presence of spouse; length of marriage, divorce, or widowhood; location of children and grandchildren; relatives or others living with patient
- *Coping patterns:* major life events, meaning of these events to each family member, usual coping patterns, family's perception of the effectiveness of coping patterns
- *Family communication:* style and quality of communication, methods of conflict resolution
- *Family subsystems:* family alliances, effect of family alliances on family stability
- *Diagnostic tests:* Family Awareness Scale, Index of Family Relations

Psychological status
- *History:* recent illness; loss of a loved one; financial problems; change in residence; reactions to illness, disability, or other change
- *Psychiatric history:* age at onset, type and severity of symptoms, impact on functioning, type of treatment, patient's response to treatment
- *Signs and symptoms:* changes in appetite, energy level, motivation, personal hygiene, self-image, self-esteem, sleep patterns, sexual drive, or feelings of competence; alcohol abuse
- *Diagnostic tests:* Hamilton Rating Scale for Depression, Wechsler Adult Intelligence Inventory

Self-care status
- *Prior medical conditions:* neurologic, sensory, or psychological impairment
- *History:* use of adaptive equipment, devices, or supplies

- *Observation:* functional ability (muscle tone, size, and strength; range of motion; coordination), daily activities (dressing, grooming, toileting, bathing, and hygiene)
- *Diagnostic test:* Self-Care Assessment Tool

Social status
- *History:* conversational and interpersonal skills, degree of trust in others, level of self-esteem, ability to function in social roles
- *Signs and symptoms:* withdrawal, lack of eye contact, intrusiveness, inappropriate responses, aggressiveness
- *Diagnostic test:* Social Adjustment Scale

Spiritual status
- *History:* religious affiliation; religious practices; beliefs about life, death, and suffering; religious support network
- *Diagnostic tests:* Spiritual and Religious Concerns Questionnaire, Spiritual Well-Being Scale

DEFINING CHARACTERISTICS

- Angry outbursts
- Emotional withdrawal and passivity
- Expressions of loss of control over life situation
- Hopelessness
- Lack of interest in improving or modifying own care
- Lack of participation in activities of daily living, including personal hygiene and nutrition
- Perceived lack of control over life situation
- Unwarranted dependency on others

ASSOCIATED DISORDERS

Adjustment disorder, anxiety disorders, blindness, cancer, cerebrovascular accident, chronic obstructive pulmonary disease, cirrhosis, congestive heart failure, degenerative joint disease, dementia, diabetes mellitus, macular degeneration, mood disorders, osteoporosis, Parkinson's disease, rheumatoid arthritis, schizophrenia, substance-related disorders

EXPECTED OUTCOMES

Initial outcomes
- Patient identifies aspects of life still under his control.
- Patient accepts that some areas are out of his control.

Interim outcome
- Patient helps develop schedule for self-care activities.

Discharge outcome
- Patient participates in decisions about own care and lifestyle.

INTERVENTIONS AND RATIONALES

Initial interventions
- Ask the patient open-ended questions rather than questions that can be answered yes or no. *Open-ended questions encourage him to assert his opinions and thus regain a feeling of control.*
- Identify factors that make the patient feel powerless *to help him realign his expectations.*
- Help the patient identify aspects of his life that are still under his control. For example, offer him the opportuni-

ty to request changes to the arrangement of furniture in the room. *This can show the patient that he still retains some control over his life.*
- Recognize the patient's right to express feelings. *Venting may prevent feelings of powerlessness from becoming overwhelming.*
- Guide the patient through life review. Encourage him to reflect on past achievements *to foster a sense of satisfaction and promote acceptance of his current status.*

Interim interventions
- Assist the patient in establishing realistic goals. *Realistic expectations help avoid failures, which might exacerbate feelings of powerlessness.*
- Encourage the patient to make his own choices in scheduling his daily routine and self-care activities. Emphasize that the patient, not the staff, has the authority to make scheduling decisions. *This helps the patient reassert control.*
- Encourage staff members to express interest in the patient's progress. *Set aside time to listen attentively to the patient to acknowledge and reinforce his efforts to regain control.*

Discharge interventions
- Encourage the patient to choose social and recreational activities *to enhance his lifestyle and further diminish his feelings of powerlessness.*
- Support the patient in expressing realistic feelings of regained control. *Expression of feelings can promote healthy adjustment and hope for the future.*

EVALUATION STATEMENTS

Patient:
- describes actions that improve or modify his routine.
- displays an appropriate sense of responsibility in scheduling self-care activities.
- expresses more realistic expectations and increased satisfaction with current situation.
- selects appropriate social and recreational activities.

DOCUMENTATION

- Diagnostic test results
- Patient's verbal and behavioral expressions of powerlessness
- Patient's level of involvement in self-care activities
- Patient's level of participation in the therapeutic and social milieu
- Nursing interventions
- Patient's response to nursing interventions
- Patient's statements indicating increased feelings of control
- Evaluation statements.

Relocation stress syndrome

related to temporary or permanent reduction in functional level

DEFINITION

Physiologic or psychosocial disturbances caused by relocation to an environment where the patient is dependent on others

ASSESSMENT

Cultural status
- *Demographics:* age, sex, marital status, educational and occupational history, economic status (including retirement income), medical expenses, insurance coverage, Medicare or Medicaid
- *History:* beliefs, values, and attitudes about health and illness; health practices, customs, and rituals

Psychological status
- *History:* recent changes in medical or psychiatric status, affect, attitude toward move, reasons for relocation, conditions in original and new environments, social attachments in original environment
- *Diagnostic tests:* Hamilton Rating Scale for Depression or Zung Self-Rating Depression Scale, Folstein Mini-Mental Status Examination

Family status
- *Family composition:* presence of spouse; length of marriage, divorce, or widowhood; location of children and grandchildren; relatives who live with patient
- *History:* relationships with family members, family members' involvement in the relocation decision, efforts to convince patient of necessity for move, family traditions and expectations regarding independence in older adults
- *Diagnostic test:* Family Genogram

Self-care status
- *Prior medical conditions:* neurologic, sensory, or psychological impairment

- *History:* use of adaptive equipment, devices, or supplies
- *Observation:* functional ability (muscle tone, size, and strength; range of motion; coordination), daily activities (dressing, grooming, bathing, toileting, and hygiene)
- *Diagnostic test:* Self-Care Assessment Tool

Sensory status
- *Physical examinations:* visual, auditory, and tactile examinations
- *Signs and symptoms:* visual, auditory, and tactile deficits

DEFINING CHARACTERISTICS

In patient:
- Anger or lack of trust toward family members promoting move
- Anxiety or depression
- Change in eating habits
- Expressions of unwillingness to relocate
- Loss of cognitive or self-care capabilities in elderly adult
- Recent and enduring decompensation in adult with mental illness
- Sleep disturbance
- Withdrawal
  In family:
- Anxiety
- Conflict among family members regarding move
- Inability of family to settle on adequate discharge plan
- Repeated attempts to convince patient of need for relocation

ASSOCIATED DISORDERS

Any disorders that may prevent patient from living on his own, such as cerebrovascular accident, dementia of the Alzheimer's type, head trauma, or Parkinson's disease

EXPECTED OUTCOMES

Initial outcomes
- Family members seek assistance of treatment team in planning for patient's relocation.
- Patient tolerates discussions of possibility of relocation.

Interim outcomes
- Family member takes steps to prepare for relocation.
- Patient participates in discussions of his options regarding living arrangements.
- Patient discusses situation with family members and staff without becoming enraged or withdrawn.

Discharge outcomes
- Patient expresses understanding of need for relocation.
- Patient expresses satisfaction with relocation plans.

INTERVENTIONS AND RATIONALES

Initial interventions
- Assign a primary nurse to the patient *to help him and family members develop trust.*
- Assist family members in finding appropriate placement for the patient *to help reduce their sense of isolation and frustration.*
- Encourage the patient to express his feelings about members of the treatment team and family members who recommend relocation *to lessen his*

anxiety and help prepare him for discussion with the family.

Interim interventions
- Offer the family and patient an appropriate place to meet, with team participants if desired, to discuss relocation *in order to reinforce the importance of this issue and to show support for all participants.*
- Offer information about the patient's status and abilities and about placement options *to help ensure adequate placement and continuity of care.*
- If appropriate, encourage the patient to look forward to regaining a greater level of independence in the future *to promote confidence.* Otherwise, allow the patient to express his feelings about his loss of independence *to help him work through the grieving process.*
- If possible, allow the patient and family members to visit the new location and meet the new staff *to help ease the amount of stress they will experience during relocation.*

Discharge interventions
- Encourage the patient to express feelings associated with relocation *to provide an opportunity to correct misconceptions and reduce anxiety.*
- Educate the family and patient about relocation stress syndrome *to encourage family members to offer emotional support and to help them understand the patient's feelings and forgive his angry outbursts.*
- Communicate all aspects of the patient's discharge plan to appropriate staff at the patient's new residence *to ensure continuity of care.*
- Assist family members in communicating with personnel at the patient's

new residence *to ensure continuity of care.*

EVALUATION STATEMENTS

Patient:
- has fewer symptoms of anxiety, anger, or withdrawal.
- collaborates with his family to make adequate plans for relocation.
- expresses understanding of reasons for relocation.
- interacts with family members without becoming enraged or withdrawn.
- expresses increased acceptance of the plan for relocation.

DOCUMENTATION

- Diagnostic test results
- Changes in patient's health status that indicate need for relocation
- Patient's and family members' comments regarding need for relocation
- Plans for relocation as they are developed
- Results of meetings with patient, staff, and family members
- Information conveyed to staff at new place of residence
- Evaluation statements.

Role performance alteration

related to declining health

DEFINITION

Disruption in ability to perform social, vocational, and family roles because of deteriorating health

ASSESSMENT

Cultural status
- *Demographics:* age, sex, marital status, level of education, occupation, nationality, race, ethnic group
- *History:* beliefs, values, and attitudes about health and illness; health practices, customs, and rituals
- *Diagnostic test:* Cultural Assessment Guide

Family status
- *Family composition:* presence of spouse; length of marriage, divorce, or widowhood; location of children and grandchildren
- *Family roles:* formal and informal roles and role performance, degree of family agreement on roles, interrelationships of various roles
- *Family communication:* style and quality of communication, methods of conflict resolution
- *Developmental stage of family:* shifts in role responsibility over time, ability to adapt to change
- *Values and aspirations:* extent to which family permits pursuit of individual goals and values
- *Social and economic factors:* economic status of family, sense of adequacy and self-worth, employment and attitudes toward work, religious affiliation, influence of religious beliefs on daily practices
- *Coping patterns:* major life events and their meaning to family members, usual coping patterns, family's perception of effectiveness of coping patterns
- *Evidence of abuse*
- *Family health history:* bipolar disorder, depressive disorder, suicide, schizophrenia, mental retardation,

substance use disorder, stress-related illness, medical illness
- *Diagnostic tests:* Family Environment Scale, Family Adjustment Device, Family Genogram

Social status
- *History:* employment status, size of social network, quality of relationships, trust in others, level of self-esteem, ability to function in social roles
- *Living conditions:* residence (rural, suburban, or urban), dwelling (single family, multifamily), site of activities, available transportation

Musculoskeletal status
- *History:* ability to carry out activities of daily living, exercise and activity patterns, occupational hazards, sports, use of mobility aids
- *Prior medical conditions:* neuromuscular or skeletal accidents or trauma, degenerative joint diseases
- *Medications:* aspirin, anti-inflammatory agents, muscle relaxants
- *Physical examination:* range of motion of all joints; joint and muscle symmetry; evidence of swelling, masses, or deformity; pain or tenderness on movement; coordination and gait; muscle size, strength, and tone; functional mobility
- *Signs and symptoms:* pain, joint swelling, stiffness, limitation of movement, muscle weakness, tenderness, inflammation, falls, contractures, subluxation, masses, joint deformity, dislocation, muscle atrophy
- *Laboratory tests:* serum uric acid levels, rheumatoid factor level, erythrocyte sedimentation rate
- *Diagnostic tests:* Functional Mobility Scale, Muscle Strength Scale

DEFINING CHARACTERISTICS
- Change in ability to perform social, vocational, and family roles
- Change in mental or physical capacity that affects ability to perform usual roles

ASSOCIATED DISORDERS
Any chronic medical condition or age-related change, such as angina pectoris; arteriosclerosis; blindness; bursitis; chronic obstructive pulmonary disease; congestive heart failure; deafness; dementia of the Alzheimer's type or other dementias; diabetes mellitus; end-stage renal, cardiac, or pulmonary disease; hip fracture; Parkinson's disease; or rheumatoid arthritis

EXPECTED OUTCOMES

Initial outcome
- Patient identifies factors that make it difficult to fulfill usual social, family, and vocational roles.

Interim outcomes
- Patient discusses ways of revising his goals to adapt to changes in his physical or mental status.
- Family members agree to assume responsibilities previously performed by patient.
- Family members express willingness to provide emotional support as patient adjusts to altered role performance.

Discharge outcomes
- Patient identifies resources for forming new social relationships.

- Patient continues to engage in usual social activities to the extent possible.

INTERVENTIONS AND RATIONALES

Initial interventions

- Discuss with the patient factors that make it difficult to fulfill his usual family and vocational roles. For example, if the patient has recently been retired, how does he cope with his free time? How does he feel about no longer being the family breadwinner? *Discussion helps the patient gain insight and rationally define problems and potential solutions.*
- Discuss factors that interfere with the patient's ability to fulfill usual social roles, such as the death of close friends or lack of transportation, *to help him identify the causes of his diminished social interaction.*

Interim interventions

- Explore ways in which the patient can continue to contribute to society, such as volunteer work, *to help restore his own sense of purpose.*
- Give the patient and family members information about the developmental tasks of aging. These include accepting changes in mental and physical capacities, giving up past roles, creating new social relationships, substituting new activities and interests for overly difficult ones, and revising goals, values, and self-concept to accommodate the patient's lifestyle changes. *Helping the patient and family members understand that these tasks are a normal part of the aging process may enhance their coping abilities.*

- Discuss with family members ways they can help the patient cope with altered role performance, including frequent visits, providing emotional support, and requesting the patient's input into family decisions *to help maintain his self-esteem.*
- Encourage family members to express feelings about the patient's altered role performance. Discuss how family members may partially or fully assume roles once performed by the patient *to enhance family coping.*

Discharge interventions

- Investigate support groups, senior citizen centers, and other community resources *to help the patient find new outlets for forming social relationships.*
- Encourage the patient to continue his social activities within the constraints imposed by aging *to maintain his sense of purpose and preserve his connection with others.*

EVALUATION STATEMENTS

Patient:
- makes plans to adapt to changes related to aging and chronic illness.
- expresses desire to fulfill family, social, and vocational responsibilities to extent possible.
- describes new activities designed to maintain a sense of purpose in life.
  Family members:
- agree to take on responsibilities formerly held by the patient.
- are willing to provide emotional support to the patient.

DOCUMENTATION

- Diagnostic test results and laboratory findings
- Patient's expressions of feelings and concern associated with altered role performance
- Nursing interventions
- Patient's response to nursing interventions
- Statements by family members indicating their attitude toward patient's altered role performance
- Referrals to support services for patient and family members
- Evaluation statements.

Self-esteem, situational low

related to increased dependence on caregivers during hospitalization

DEFINITION

Negative feelings about oneself during hospitalization brought on by increased dependence on caregivers

ASSESSMENT

Cultural status

- *Demographics:* age, sex, level of education, occupation, nationality, race, ethnic group
- *History:* beliefs, values, and attitudes about health and illness; health practices, customs, and rituals; influence of religious beliefs on values and practices

Family status

- *Family composition:* presence of spouse; length of marriage, divorce, or widowhood; location of children and grandchildren; relatives who live with patient
- *Family roles:* formal and informal roles and role performance, degree of family agreement on roles, interrelationships of family roles
- *Family rules:* rules that foster stability, maladaptive rules, methods of rule modification
- *Family communication:* style and quality of communication, methods of conflict resolution
- *Developmental stage:* changes in relationships between family members, shifts in role responsibility over time, problems adapting to change
- *Family subsystems:* conflict between family members, supportive relationships, effect of alliances on family stability
- *Needs fulfillment:* ability of family to meet patient's physical, social, and emotional needs; disparities between patient's needs and family's willingness or ability to meet them
- *Values and aspirations:* extent to which family permits pursuit of individual goals and values
- *Social and economic factors:* economic status of family, sense of adequacy and self-worth, employment status, attitudes toward work
- *Coping patterns:* major life events, meaning of life events to each family member, usual coping patterns, family's perception of effectiveness of coping patterns
- *Evidence of abuse:* physical and behavioral indicators

• *Diagnostic tests:* Family Environment Scale, Family Adjustment Device, Family Genogram, Dyadic Adjustment Scale, Family Awareness Scale, Index of Spouse Abuse, Primary Communication Inventory, Index of Family Relations

Neurologic status

• *Mental status:* appearance and attitude, level of consciousness, motor activity, thought and speech, mood and affect, perceptions, orientation, memory, visual-spatial ability, attention span, abstraction, judgment and insight, general information, capacity to read, write and perform calculations

Self-care status

• *Prior medical conditions:* neurologic, sensory, or psychological impairment
• *History:* use of adaptive equipment, devices, or supplies
• *Observation:* functional ability (muscle tone, size, and strength; range of motion; coordination), daily activities (dressing, grooming, bathing, toileting, and hygiene)
• *Diagnostic test:* Self-Care Assessment Tool

Sleep pattern status

• *Personal habits:* usual hours of sleep, circadian pattern, energy level after sleep, rest and relaxation patterns, caffeine and alcohol intake
• *Medications:* sleeping aids, amphetamines
• *Signs and symptoms:* difficulty falling asleep, nocturnal awakening, early morning awakening, hypersomnia, insomnia, sleep pattern reversal

Social status

• *Personal habits:* conversational and interpersonal skills, size of social network, quality of relationships, degree of trust in others, level of self-esteem, ability to function in social roles
• *Signs and symptoms:* withdrawal, lack of eye contact, intrusiveness, inappropriate responses, aggressiveness

DEFINING CHARACTERISTICS

• Difficulty making decisions
• Feelings of helplessness or uselessness
• Frustration, sadness, or regret over inability to handle life events
• Negative view of self in response to life events

ASSOCIATED DISORDERS

Acute exacerbation of any chronic illness, such as arthritis, cardiovascular disease, cataracts, hypertension, obesity, or varicose veins

EXPECTED OUTCOMES

Initial outcomes

• Patient maintains eye contact and initiates conversations.
• Patient participates in self-care to the extent possible.

Interim outcomes

• Patient's environment is enhanced to promote feelings of self-esteem, for example, by providing mobility aids or placing personal items in view.
• Patient discusses past accomplishments.
• Patient discusses chronic illness and aging and their impacts on his lifestyle.

- Patient reports that he feels more independent.

Discharge outcomes
- Patient expresses increased acceptance of changes caused by chronic illness or aging and increased self-esteem.
- Patient obtains referrals for ongoing care.

INTERVENTIONS AND RATIONALES

Initial interventions
- Ask permission to enter the patient's personal space, including areas around the bed, bedside tables, and closet. *As the patient's self-esteem decreases, significance of personal space increases. Asking permission to enter personal space provides the patient with a sense of control.*
- Spend non-care-related time with the patient *to encourage ongoing conversations.*
- Encourage the patient to care for himself to the greatest extent possible. Assess whether he needs help initiating self-care and provide only when the patient has difficulty *to foster feelings of independence.*

Interim interventions
- Encourage the patient to wear his own pajamas or gowns and robes *to foster a positive self-identity.*
- Arrange the patient's personal items on the bedside stand within easy reach *to maintain the patient's independence.*
- Incorporate appropriate exercise activities into the patient's daily care *to enhance strength, endurance, and coordination, all of which affect self-esteem.*

- Encourage the patient to reminisce *to help focus his attention on past accomplishments.*
- If the patient's mobility is limited, install an over-the-bed trapeze *to promote feelings of independence.*
- Incorporate therapeutic touch into daily activities with back rubs, foot massages, or touching of the patient's hand or arm. *Frequent touch enhances the patient's sense of worth.*
- Encourage the patient to express feelings about chronic illness or the aging process. Also encourage him to discuss fears about loss of independence and diminished ability to participate in work and leisure activities. *This allows him to gain insight and to rationally define problems and potential solutions.*

Discharge intervention
- Provide information about appropriate support groups or senior services. *Interacting with people who have successfully adapted to aging or chronic illness may enhance the patient's coping skills.*

EVALUATION STATEMENTS

Patient:
- carries out activities of daily living while in the hospital.
- initiates conversations and maintains eye contact.
- is open and receptive to others.
- states at least two ways hospitalization will change his lifestyle.
- discusses feelings associated with aging, chronic illness, loss of independence, and diminished ability to participate in work and leisure activities.

- makes statements reflecting greater self-esteem at least once each day.

DOCUMENTATION

- Diagnostic test results
- Patient's expressions of lowered self-esteem
- Mental status assessment (baseline and ongoing)
- Nursing interventions directed toward improving the patient's self-esteem
- Patient's response to nursing interventions
- Evaluation statements.

Self-esteem disturbance

related to social misconceptions about aging

DEFINITION

Negative self-evaluation as a result of living in a society that fails to acknowledge the contributions and capabilities of older adults

ASSESSMENT

Cultural status
- *Demographics:* age, sex, level of education, occupation, nationality, race, ethnic group
- *History:* beliefs, values, and attitudes about health and illness; health practices, customs, and rituals; attitudes about aging and elderly people

Psychological status
- *History:* presence of psychiatric illness, coping skills, ability to carry out voluntary activities, sense of adequacy and self-worth, body image, recent losses or stressors, ability to adapt to change, feelings about aging
- *Signs and symptoms:* depression, anxiety, negative statements about self, inability to make decisions, psychological impairment, drug and alcohol abuse

Social status
- *History:* hobbies and recreational activities, social network, ability to perform social roles

Neurologic status
- *Mental status:* appearance and attitude, level of consciousness, motor activity, thought and speech, mood and affect, perceptions, orientation, memory, visual-spatial ability, attention span, abstraction, judgment and insight, general information, capacity to read, write, and perform calculations

Family status
- *Family composition:* presence of spouse; length of marriage, divorce, or widowhood; location of children and grandchildren
- *Family roles:* formal and informal roles, role performance, degree of family agreement on roles, interrelationships of various roles
- *Family rules:* rules that foster stability, maladaptive rules, methods of rule modification
- *Family communication:* style and quality of communication, methods of conflict resolution

- *Developmental stage of family:* shifts in role responsibility over time, problems adjusting to change
- *Family subsystems:* family alliances, effect of alliances on family stability
- *Family needs:* ability of family to meet patient's physical, social, and emotional needs; disparities between patient's needs and family's willingness or ability to meet them
- *Values and aspirations:* extent to which family permits pursuit of individual goals and values

DEFINING CHARACTERISTICS

- Frequent negative comments about aging and elderly people
- Lying about age
- Refusal to acknowledge significance of signs and symptoms of aging or chronic illness
- Refusal to frequent places or participate in activities enjoyed by peers
- Refusal to talk about growing older

ASSOCIATED DISORDERS

This diagnosis may be associated with any disorder that causes physical disability or limitations. Examples include angina pectoris, arteriosclerosis, atherosclerosis, chronic obstructive pulmonary disease, chronic renal failure, fractured hip, hypertension, osteoporosis, presbycusis, presbyopia, renal calculi, and rheumatoid arthritis.

EXPECTED OUTCOMES

Initial outcome

- Patient discusses aging process and impact of aging on ability to participate in hobbies and other activities.

Interim outcomes

- Patient expresses a more positive view of growing older.
- Patient states intention to set aside time for reminiscing as part of daily routine.

Discharge outcome

- Patient obtains information about volunteer activities or other opportunities for increased involvement in community.

INTERVENTIONS AND RATIONALES

Initial interventions

- Discuss the challenge of being an older adult in today's youth-oriented society *to encourage the patient to express his feelings and to help him recognize that he does not have to accept society's prejudices with regard to aging.*
- Discuss with the patient and family members changes that normally occur as part of the aging process *to correct misconceptions.* Discuss how to adapt activities and hobbies to accommodate physiologic changes that occur with aging *to avoid excess physical stress.*

Interim interventions

- Discuss advantages of growing older, for example, having increased time to pursue hobbies and other interests, *to help the patient develop a positive view of aging.*
- Invite an active member of a senior citizens club, social group, senior sports league, or advocacy group to visit the patient *to provide a positive role model.*

- Emphasize the variety of activities that the patient can continue to do well *to enhance his self-esteem.*
- Encourage the patient to set aside time for reminiscing as part of his daily routine. *Reminiscing helps him affirm his past and promotes self-esteem.*

Discharge intervention
- Provide information about senior volunteer groups and part-time work or volunteer opportunities *to help the patient maintain physical and mental functioning and promote social interaction.*

EVALUATION STATEMENTS

Patient:
- states intention to attend an age-appropriate community activity.
- expresses positive and negative feelings about aging.
- expresses willingness to set aside time for reminiscing.
- adapts activities to avoid unnecessary physical stress on body.

DOCUMENTATION

- Evidence of patient's difficulty adjusting to the aging process
- Nursing interventions
- Referrals provided
- Patient's response to nursing interventions
- Patient's statements that indicate a more positive attitude toward growing older
- Evaluation statements.

Social isolation

related to physiologic, environmental, or emotional barriers

DEFINITION

Insufficient contact with others due to physical, psychological, or environmental factors

ASSESSMENT

Cultural status
- *Demographics:* age, sex, marital status, level of education, nationality, race, ethnic group, religion
- *History:* beliefs, values, and attitudes about health and illness; health customs, practices, and rituals
- *Diagnostic test:* Cultural Assessment Guide

Family status
- *Family composition:* presence of spouse; length of marriage, divorce, or widowhood; location of children and grandchildren
- *Family roles:* formal and informal roles and role performance
- *Family communication:* style, quality, and frequency of communication
- *Social and economic factors:* economic status of family, influence of religious beliefs on daily life
- *Evidence of abuse:* physical and behavioral indicators
- *Family health history:* bipolar disorder, depressive disorder, suicide, schizophrenia, mental retardation, substance use disorder, stress-related

illness, communication disorders, medical illness
- *Diagnostic tests:* Family Environment Scale, Family Adjustment Device, Family Genogram

Psychological status
- *Recent events:* illness, loss of loved one, retirement, move to new community, argument with family members
- *History:* self-esteem, hobbies and recreational activities, spirituality, reactions to illness and disability
- *Psychiatric history:* age at onset of illness, type and severity of symptoms, impact on functioning, type of treatment and patient's response
- *Signs and symptoms:* poor personal hygiene, lowered self-image and self-esteem, alcohol or drug abuse, low level of functioning
- *Laboratory tests:* urinalysis, hemoglobin and hematocrit, electrolyte and blood glucose levels, thyroid function tests, blood and urine drug toxicology screening
- *Diagnostic tests:* Brief Psychiatric Rating Scale, Hamilton Rating Scale for Depression

Self-care status
- *Observation:* functional ability (muscle tone, size, and strength; range of motion; coordination), daily activities (dressing, grooming, bathing, toileting, and hygiene)
- *Prior medical conditions:* neurologic, sensory, physical, or psychological impairment
- *Diagnostic tests:* Functional Ability Scale, Self-Care Assessment Tool

Sensory status
- *History:* use of tobacco, alcohol, or drugs; polypharmacy; use of glasses, hearing aids, walker, or wheelchair
- *Signs and symptoms:* visual hallucinations, blurred vision, ptosis, auditory hallucinations, tinnitus, vertigo, pain
- *Diagnostic tests:* Snellen eye chart, hearing acuity test

Social status
- *History:* conversational and interpersonal skills, size of social network, quality of relationships, degree of trust in others, ability to function in social roles
- *Living conditions:* residence area (rural, suburban, or urban) and type (single family, multifamily), site of activities, available transportation, available family and community support, safety of neighborhood, availability of telephone
- *Signs and symptoms:* withdrawal, lack of eye contact, inability to enjoy social activity because of environmental barriers
- *Diagnostic test:* Social Adjustment Scale

DEFINING CHARACTERISTICS

- Absence of support from family, friends, or other groups
- Barriers to social activity, such as unsafe neighborhood, lack of transportation, limited mobility
- Expressed lack of significant purpose in life
- Feelings that aloneness is not by choice
- History of institutionalization

- Inability or unwillingness to communicate
- Physical or mental handicap or ill health, limited sight or hearing
- Sad, dull affect; withdrawal

ASSOCIATED DISORDERS

Alzheimer's disease, arthritis, cancer, cerebrovascular accident, chronic disease, decreased muscle strength and endurance, depressive disorder, head or neck disorders requiring surgery, hepatitis, hip fracture, organic brain syndrome, osteoporosis, pain, Parkinson's disease, schizophrenia, spinal cord injuries, tuberculosis, urinary or fecal incontinence

EXPECTED OUTCOMES

Initial outcomes
- Patient discusses his inadequate social relationships and expresses desire to increase social activity.
- Patient communicates knowledge of his disorder and other circumstances that may limit social activity.

Interim outcomes
- Patient interacts with members of health care team.
- Patient and members of the health care team explore ways of reducing barriers to increased social activity.

Discharge outcomes
- Patient contacts appropriate resources for developing social relationships.
- Patient notes an improvement in social relationships.
- Patent reports feeling less socially isolated.

INTERVENTIONS AND RATIONALES

Initial interventions
- Assign a primary nurse to the patient *to provide consistency and promote trust.*
- Discuss with the patient the causes and contributing factors of his social isolation. Find out what factors he believes interfere most with his ability to develop relationships with others *to determine his wants and needs.*
- Find out if the patient is willing to make changes in his lifestyle or daily routine that would increase contact with others *to learn whether he is motivated enough for nursing interventions to be successful.*

Interim interventions
- Address any physical conditions that may limit the patient's social activity. For example, if he has a hearing deficit, refer him to an audiologist for a hearing aid. If a mobility impairment holds him back, refer the patient to a physical therapist for an exercise program or an assistive device. *Physical limitations may contribute to social isolation.*
- Investigate the availability and cost of public transportation and teach the patient the route to planned activities *to overcome transportation barriers that may isolate him.*
- Assess the influence of his home environment on the patient's social life. For example, if he feels threatened by neighborhood crime, consider options such as moving to a retirement community or residential care facility *to provide options for living and social contact he may not have considered.*

Discharge interventions

- Involve the patient and, if appropriate, his family in planning his social life *to individualize care and reduce his feelings of dependency.*
- Identify community resources for the patient, such as support groups, senior centers, and health education programs, and make referrals *to provide continuity of care.*
- Encourage the patient to make use of such resources as the American Association of Retired Persons or religious organizations *to increase his social involvement.*

EVALUATION STATEMENTS

Patient:
- seeks assistance in increasing social contacts.
- describes causes of social isolation.
- accepts assistance in increasing social contacts.
- reports an increase in social contacts.
- verbalizes decreased feelings of social isolation.

DOCUMENTATION

- Diagnostic test results
- Observations of patient's social interaction skills
- Identified causes of patient's social isolation
- Nursing interventions that encourage social interaction
- Patient's response to nursing interventions
- Appropriate resources identified for patient
- Referrals to social service agencies and support groups
- Evaluation statements.

Thought process alteration

related to memory deficits

DEFINITION

Decreased cognitive ability because of memory loss

ASSESSMENT

Cultural status
- *Demographics:* age, sex, level of education, occupation, nationality, race, ethnic group
- *History:* beliefs, values, and attitudes about health and illness; customs, rituals, and family practices

Neurologic status
- *Mental status:* appearance and attitude, level of consciousness, motor activity, thought and speech, mood and affect, perceptions, orientation, memory, comprehension, visual-spatial ability, attention span, abstraction, judgment and insight, general information, capacity to read, write, and perform calculations
- *Auditory status:* use of hearing aid, history of hearing deficits, presence of cerumen
- *Visual status:* use of eyeglasses, history of visual deficits, visual acuity (near and distant), visual fields
- *Medications:* prescribed, over-the-counter, and illicit drugs; recent changes in medication or dosage; use of outdated drugs
- *Speech pattern:* rate of speech, phrase length, effort, fluency, prosody,

repetition, information content, vocabulary, level of comprehension
- *Physical examination:* muscle tone, strength, and symmetry; gait; cerebellar function; cranial nerve function; sensation; reflexes
- *Signs and symptoms:* recent memory loss, forgetting names of familiar objects or people, communication problems, getting lost in familiar surroundings, decline in capabilities, inappropriate social behavior, attempts to hide or rationalize decline in mentation, disorientation to person, place, or time
- *Laboratory tests:* complete blood count; electrolyte, blood glucose, blood urea nitrogen, serum creatinine, serum phosphorus, and serum B_{12} levels; thyroid and liver function tests
- *Diagnostic tests:* computed tomography, magnetic resonance imaging, positron emission tomography, cerebral arteriography, digital subtraction angiography, electroencephalography, Glasgow Coma Scale, Folstein Mini-Mental Status Examination

Psychological status
- *Life changes:* recent divorce, illness, job loss, or loss of loved one; recent exposure to toxic substances; deterioration in health status
- *Current illness:* signs and symptoms including impact on functioning
- *Psychiatric history:* age at onset of illness, impact on functioning, type of treatment, patient's response to treatment
- *Signs and symptoms:* changes in appetite, energy level, motivation, personal hygiene, self-image, self-esteem, sleep patterns, sexual drive, or level of competence; lability of affect; incontinence; disinterest in hobbies; restlessness; pacing; outbursts of temper; suspicious delusions

Self-care status
- *History:* use of adaptive equipment, devices, or supplies
- *Observation:* functional ability (muscle tone, size, and strength; range of motion; coordination), daily activities (dressing, grooming, bathing, toileting, and hygiene)
- *Diagnostic test:* Self-Care Assessment Tool

Family status
- *Family composition:* presence of spouse; length of marriage, divorce, or widowhood; location of children and grandchildren; relatives who live with patient
- *Family roles:* formal and informal roles and role performance, degree of family agreement on roles, interrelationships of family roles
- *Family rules:* rules that foster stability, maladaptive rules, methods of rule modification
- *Family communication:* style and quality of communication, methods of conflict resolution
- *Developmental stage:* changes in relationships between family members, shifts in role responsibility over time, problems adapting to change
- *Family subsystems:* conflict between family members, supportive relationships, effect of alliances on family stability
- *Needs fulfillment:* ability of family to meet patient's physical, social, and emotional needs; disparities between patient's needs and family's willingness or ability to meet them

DEFINING CHARACTERISTICS

- Clinical evidence of impaired neurologic or psychological functioning
- Decreased ability to grasp ideas
- Disorientation to time, place, person, circumstances, and events
- Impaired ability to abstract or conceptualize, calculate, reason, make decisions, solve problems, follow instructions
- Inappropriate social behavior
- Memory deficit or problems

ASSOCIATED DISORDERS

Alzheimer's disease (dementia of the Alzheimer's type), chronic confusional states, delirium, dementias (all types), extrapyramidal disorders, head trauma, multi-infarct dementia (vascular dementia), pseudodementia

EXPECTED OUTCOMES

Initial outcomes

- Patient maintains orientation to time, place, and person.
- Patient's environment is enhanced to help him cope with memory deficits.
- Patient sustains no harm or injury.

Interim outcomes

- Patient voices feelings related to memory loss.
- Patient participates in activities that provide mental stimulation.
- Patient participates in self-care to the extent possible.
- Patient demonstrates appropriate skills for coping with memory loss.
- Patient communicates needs without excessive frustration.

Discharge outcomes

- Family members communicate an understanding of care required by patient.
- Family members demonstrate techniques for caring for patient, such as maintaining a safe environment and reorienting him as needed.
- Family members identify and contact appropriate support services.

INTERVENTIONS AND RATIONALES

Initial interventions

- Perform appropriate interventions *to foster communication:*
- Assess the patient's sight and hearing, and assist him with glasses or a hearing aid as necessary.
- Minimize distractions by turning off radios or television sets. When speaking to him, face him, maintain eye contact, and smile.
- Speak slowly in clear, low tones, using simple, direct language. Repeat your remarks as needed.
- Be aware that the patient may be sensitive to your unspoken feelings about him.
- Observe the patient's thought processes every shift. Document and report any changes. *Changes may indicate progressive improvement or decline in underlying condition.*
- Orient the patient to reality as needed.
- Call him by name.
- Tell him your name.
- Provide background information (place, time, date) frequently throughout the day, verbally and visually, using a reality orientation board.
- Orient him to his environment.

Reality orientation techniques foster his awareness of himself and his environment.

- Place the patient's photograph or name on the room door *to aid memory and help him find his room.*
- Keep items in the same places. *A consistent, stable environment reduces confusion, decreases frustration, and aids successful completion of activities of daily living.*
- Ask family members to provide the patient with photographs (labeled with the name and relationship on the back) and favorite belongings. *Belongings may his spark memory and promote a sense of security.*

Interim interventions

- Protect the patient from sensory overload; allow rest periods. *Sensory overload may increase his disability; frequent rest periods help avoid fatigue.*
- Provide a structured routine for the patient. List daily activities and post them in his room. Communicate his skill level to all personnel *to provide continuity and preserve his level of independent functioning.*
- Encourage the patient to care for himself to the greatest extent possible. Assess whether he needs help initiating self-care. For example, he may not brush his teeth unless you place the toothbrush in his hand. *Encouraging self-care helps preserve daily living skills.* Keep in mind that the patient may become increasingly dependent on others to maintain hygiene.
- Spend time daily with the patient and encourage discussion about his past. Encourage his participation in reminiscence groups. *Remote memory may be intact. Discussion of past events*

promotes a sense of continuity, aids memory, and promotes feelings of security. Joining in reminiscence groups provides diversional activity and may increase social skills.

- Correct the patient privately for inappropriate behavior; walk him to his room or initiate different behavior. *This avoids feelings of embarrassment and frustration. Redirection to appropriate activities reinforces desirable behavior.*
- Don't discourage the patient from wandering. *Wandering stimulates circulation, decreases contracture formation, reduces stress, and provides a feeling of freedom.* Place the patient in a room close to the nursing station, clear the area of as many hazards as possible, make sure he wears an identification bracelet, and provide hospital security with a recent photograph of him *to prevent the patient from getting lost or being injured.*
- Encourage the patient to voice his feelings and concerns about his loss of memory. *This helps reduce his anxiety, vents his frustrations, and promotes acceptance of the need for supervision and a treatment regimen.*
- Provide the patient with stimulation; for example, consider making puzzles or paint-by-number sets available *to help him occupy his time and use his remaining skills.*
- Encourage family members to take walks with the patient *to provide stimulation.*
- If the patient is diagnosed with pseudodementia, provide appropriate interventions for depression, including the following measures:
– administering prescribed antidepressant drug therapy.

– encouraging him to express his feelings, listening attentively, and allowing for slow responses.
– providing a structured routine with limited choices. For example, ask if he would like to shower before or after breakfast.
– encouraging involvement in group activities.
Pseudodementia closely resembles Alzheimer's disease. However, with proper treatment, symptoms may be reversible.

Discharge interventions
- Demonstrate reorientation techniques to family members and provide time for supervised return demonstrations *to prepare them to cope with the patient with altered thought processes.*
- Instruct family members on how to maintain a safe home environment for the patient. *The patient may be unable to consider his own safety needs.*
- Help family members identify appropriate community support groups or senior services *to assist in coping with the effects of the patient's illness.*

EVALUATION STATEMENTS

Patient:
- maintains orientation to time, place, and person.
- sustains no harm or injury.
- expresses feelings related to memory loss.
- demonstrates appropriate skills for coping with memory loss.
- communicates needs without excessive frustration.
  Family members:
- communicate an understanding of care required by patient.

- identify and contact appropriate support services.

DOCUMENTATION

- Diagnostic test results and laboratory findings
- Observations of patient's altered thought processes and response to treatment of underlying condition
- Nursing interventions
- Patient's response to nursing interventions
- Instructions to family members; their understanding of instructions and demonstrated ability to care for patient
- Referrals made for the patient or family members
- Evaluation statements.

Verbal communication impairment
related to physiologic or psychosocial changes

DEFINITION

Decreased ability to speak or understand language, caused by organic and environmental factors

ASSESSMENT

Cultural status
- *Demographics:* age, sex, level of education, occupation, nationality, race, ethnic group
- *History:* beliefs, values, and attitudes about health and illness; health customs, practices, and rituals

- *Diagnostic test:* Cultural Assessment Guide

Neurologic status
- *Mental status:* appearance and attitude, level of consciousness, motor activity, thought and speech, mood and affect, perceptions, orientation, memory, comprehension, visual-spatial ability, attention span, abstraction, judgment and insight, general information, capacity to read, write, and perform calculations
- *Auditory status:* use of hearing aid, history of hearing deficits, presence of cerumen
- *Visual status:* use of eyeglasses, history of visual deficits, visual acuity (near and distant), visual fields
- *Medications:* use of neuroleptics, anxiolytic agents, antidepressants, barbiturates, pain medications, alcohol, illicit drugs
- *Speech pattern:* rate of speech, phrase length, effort, fluency, prosody, repetition, information content, vocabulary, level of comprehension
- *Alternative forms of communication:* eye blinks, gestures, pictures, nods, written notes
- *Physical examination:* muscle tone, strength, and symmetry; gait; cerebellar function; cranial nerve function, reflexes
- *Laboratory tests:* hemoglobin and hematocrit, electrolyte and blood glucose levels, thyroid and liver function tests
- *Signs and symptoms:* aphasia (Broca's, global, receptive, transcortical, Wernicke's), dysarthria, garbled speech, echolalia, dysphasia
- *Diagnostic tests:* computed tomography, magnetic resonance imaging, positron emission tomography, cerebral arteriography, digital subtraction angiography, electroencephalography, Glasgow Coma Scale, Folstein Mini-Mental Status Examination

Psychological status
- *Life changes:* recent divorce, illness, job loss, or loss of loved one; deterioration in health status
- *Current illness:* signs and symptoms, including impact on functioning
- *Psychiatric history:* age at onset of illness, impact on functioning, type of treatment, patient's response to treatment
- *Signs and symptoms:* changes in appetite, energy level, motivation, personal hygiene, self-image, self-esteem, sleep patterns, sexual drive, level of competence; alcohol or drug abuse

DEFINING CHARACTERISTICS

- Decreased ability to comprehend language or to use meaningful language
- Difficulty producing speech sounds (phonation)
- Disorientation
- Dyspnea
- Garbled or incomprehensible speech
- Inability to identify objects, modulate speech, or speak in sentences
- Incessant, incoherent speech
- Stuttering or slurring

ASSOCIATED DISORDERS

Alcoholic cerebellar degeneration, Alzheimer's disease (dementia of the Alzheimer's type), amyotrophic lateral sclerosis, cerebrovascular accident, dementia, Huntington's disease, intracranial tumors, myasthenia gravis, normal pressure hydrocephalus, Parkinson's disease, septic meningitis, subacute spongiform encephalopathy (Creutzfeldt-Jakob disease)

EXPECTED OUTCOMES

Initial outcome
- Visitors and staff demonstrate appropriate respect when speaking with patient.

Interim outcomes
- Patient's environment is enhanced to foster communication.
- Staff members use appropriate methods to promote communication.
- Patient communicates needs, using gestures, writing, or speaking, without excessive frustration.
- Patient pursues opportunities to enhance social interaction.
- Patient reminisces about past as a means to stimulate communication.

Discharge outcome
- Patient or family member identifies and contacts appropriate support services, including speech therapist.

INTERVENTIONS AND RATIONALES

Initial interventions
- When first addressing the patient, face him, maintain eye contact, speak slowly, and enunciate clearly *to make it easier for him to receive and process your message.* Instruct visitors and other staff in appropriate techniques for communicating with the patient.
- Encourage family members and other staff to use speech appropriate for

adults with the patient and not to talk about him within his hearing *to convey respect.*

Interim interventions
- While providing care, use the following communication techniques:
– present one idea at a time
– use yes or no questions
– avoid abstract statements or controversial topics
– use a simple vocabulary
– allow longer response times
– guess at the meaning of incorrect words
– reduce distractions and noise
– encourage the patient to use gestures or other alternative communication techniques.
Your efforts to ease communication decrease the patient's frustration.
- If the patient's communication problems are worsened by hearing deficits, minimize glare in the room *to make it easier for the patient to read your lips* and speak at a normal level. *Shouting makes your voice frequency higher and does not assist hearing.*
- Check for proper use of hearing aids, including working batteries and proper placement, *to enhance his hearing.*
- If hearing is severely impaired, use paper and pencil *to provide an alternative means of communication.*
- If the patient does not follow your conversation, rephrase ideas using simpler wording *to overcome differences in language or culture that may block communication.*
- Do not rush the patient when he is struggling to express his thoughts. Even if you can't understand him, let him know you accept his efforts to

communicate and you empathize with his frustration. *The patient with impaired verbal communication experiences isolation, despair, and frustration. Demonstrating compassion and fostering a therapeutic relationship is the single most important step in improving communication.*

- Avoid talking with the patient when he is tired. *Fatigue may reduce his attention span and make his efforts to communicate even more frustrating.*
- Encourage the patient to engage in social activities, such as therapy sessions and meals with other patients *to reduce feelings of isolation.*
- If appropriate, help the patient rejoin family life by arranging for him to attend family gatherings *to help diminish his feelings of loneliness and anxiety.* The patient with impaired verbal communication usually can no longer perform his usual role within the family.
- Encourage the patient to reminisce. Use photographs, gestures, and visits from family members and friends to stimulate his desire to express himself. *Recalling meaningful experiences from the past may motivate him to try to communicate and enhance feelings of self-worth.*

Discharge interventions

- Refer the patient to a speech therapist and teach family members and companions about methods to enhance communication *to ensure continuity of care.*
- Refer the patient and family members to appropriate community resources, such as a club for stroke survivors or a support group for relatives of Alzheimer's patients, *to help them cope*

with his communication impairment after discharge.

EVALUATION STATEMENTS

Patient:
- improves communication skills to extent possible.
- attends sessions with speech therapist ____ times per week.
- is shown appropriate respect by visitors and staff.
- communicates needs without excessive frustration.
- takes steps to decrease isolation from friends and family members.
- identifies and contacts appropriate support services (with family member).
- indicates that he is coming to terms with his impaired ability to communicate.

DOCUMENTATION

- Diagnostic test results and laboratory findings
- Observations of impaired speaking ability, use of communication aids, and expressions of frustration
- Nursing interventions to reduce barriers to effective communication
- Patient's efforts to communicate using gestures, behavior, writing, or speech
- Patient teaching and patient's response to teaching efforts
- Referrals to speech therapist and other support services
- Evaluation statements.

APPENDICES
AND INDEX

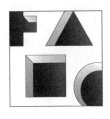
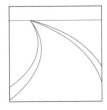
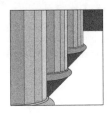
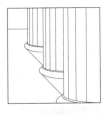
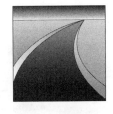
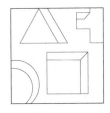
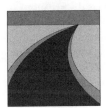
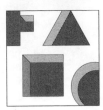
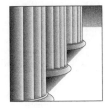

Nursing Diagnoses for Psychiatric Illnesses

ABUSE AND NEGLECT

Elder abuse (physical abuse of adult)
- Coping, ineffective family
- Family process alteration
- Injury, high risk for
- Posttrauma response
- Social interaction impairment

Neglect of child
- Coping, ineffective family
- Family process alteration
- Injury, high risk for
- Parenting alteration
- Sensory or perceptual alteration
- Social interaction impairment

Physical abuse of child
- Coping, ineffective family
- Family process alteration
- Injury, high risk for
- Parenting alteration
- Posttrauma response
- Social interaction impairment

Spouse abuse
- Coping, ineffective family
- Family process alteration
- Hopelessness
- Injury, high risk for
- Posttrauma response
- Powerlessness
- Rape-trauma syndrome: Compound reaction
- Rape-trauma syndrome: Silent reaction
- Social interaction impairment

ADJUSTMENT DISORDERS

All types
- Adjustment impairment
- Body image disturbance
- Coping, ineffective family
- Diversional activity deficit
- Hopelessness
- Personal identity disturbance
- Posttrauma response
- Powerlessness
- Role performance alteration
- Self-esteem disturbance

ANXIETY DISORDERS

All types
- Anxiety
- Adjustment impairment
- Body image disturbance
- Caregiver role strain
- Coping, ineffective family
- Coping, ineffective individual
- Coping, ineffective staff
- Denial, ineffective
- Family process alteration
- Fatigue
- Fear
- Grieving, dysfunctional
- Hopelessness
- Nutrition alteration: Less than body requirements
- Nutrition alteration: More than body requirements
- Posttrauma response
- Powerlessness
- Self-esteem, chronically low
- Self-esteem, situational low
- Sexual pattern alteration

- Sleep pattern disturbance
- Social interaction impairment
- Verbal communication impairment

Obsessive-compulsive disorder
- Anxiety
- Body image disturbance
- Caregiver role strain
- Caregiver role strain, high risk for
- Coping, ineffective individual
- Family process alteration
- Nutrition alteration: Less than body requirements
- Parenting alteration
- Posttrauma response
- Powerlessness
- Role performance alteration
- Social interaction impairment
- Social isolation

Panic disorder
- Anxiety
- Coping, ineffective individual
- Family process alteration
- Parenting alteration, high risk for
- Posttrauma response
- Role performance alteration
- Self-esteem disturbance
- Social isolation

Phobias
- Anxiety
- Coping, ineffective individual
- Family process alteration
- Health-seeking behaviors
- Parenting alteration, high risk for
- Posttrauma response
- Role performance alteration
- Self-esteem disturbance
- Social isolation

Posttraumatic stress disorder
- Coping, ineffective individual
- Fear
- Grieving, anticipatory
- Health-seeking behaviors
- Hopelessness
- Nutrition alteration: Less than body requirements
- Parenting alteration, high risk for

- Personal identity disturbance
- Posttrauma response
- Powerlessness
- Rape trauma syndrome
- Self-esteem disturbance
- Self-mutilation, high risk for
- Sensory or perceptual alteration
- Social interaction impairment
- Thought process alteration

COGNITIVE DISORDERS

Delirium
- Anxiety
- Injury, high risk for
- Sensory or perceptual alteration
- Thought process alteration
- Verbal communication impairment
- Violence, high risk for: Self-directed or directed at others

Dementia
- Anxiety
- Fear
- Grieving, dysfunctional
- Health maintenance alteration
- Injury, high risk for
- Powerlessness
- Role performance alteration
- Self-care deficit: Bathing, hygiene, dressing, grooming, toileting
- Sleep pattern disturbance
- Social isolation
- Thought process alteration
- Verbal communication impairment
- Violence, high risk for: Self-directed or directed at others

DISORDERS OF INFANCY, CHILDHOOD, AND ADOLESCENCE

Attention-deficit hyperactivity disorder
- Coping, family: Potential for growth
- Diversional activity deficit
- Family process alteration
- Injury, high risk for
- Posttrauma response
- Powerlessness

- Role performance alteration
- Social interaction impairment

Autistic disorder
- Health maintenance alteration
- Incontinence, functional
- Self-care deficit: Bathing, hygiene, dressing, grooming, toileting
- Self-mutilation, high risk for
- Thought process alteration
- Verbal communication impairment

Conduct disorder
- Coping, family: Potential for growth
- Diversional activity deficit
- Family process alteration
- Hopelessness
- Injury, high risk for
- Posttrauma response
- Powerlessness
- Self-esteem disturbance
- Social interaction impairment

Disruptive behavior disorder
- Anxiety
- Posttrauma response
- Social interaction impairment

Expressive language disorder
- Fear
- Powerlessness
- Role performance alteration
- Self-esteem disturbance
- Thought process alteration
- Verbal communication impairment

Learning disorders
- Knowledge deficit
- Self-esteem disturbance
- Thought process alteration

Mental retardation
- Health maintenance alteration
- Self-care deficit: Bathing, hygiene, dressing, grooming, toileting
- Social isolation
- Verbal communication impairment

Motor skills disorders
- Role performance alteration

- Self-esteem disturbance
- Social interaction impairment

Oppositional defiant disorder
- Coping, ineffective individual
- Injury, high risk for
- Parental role conflict
- Posttrauma response
- Powerlessness
- Role performance alteration
- Social interaction impairment

Pervasive developmental disorders
- Diversional activity deficit
- Fear
- Incontinence, functional
- Parental role conflict
- Role performance alteration
- Self-mutilation, high risk for
- Verbal communication impairment

Receptive language disorder
- Fear
- Powerlessness
- Role performance alteration
- Self-esteem disturbance
- Thought process alteration
- Verbal communication impairment

Separation anxiety disorder
- Anxiety
- Coping, family: Potential for growth
- Family process alteration
- Fear
- Self-esteem disturbance

Tourette's disorder
- Anxiety
- Injury, high risk for
- Powerlessness
- Social interaction impairment
- Verbal communication impairment

DISSOCIATIVE DISORDERS

All types
- Coping, ineffective individual
- Family process alteration
- Personal identity disturbance
- Posttrauma response

- Rape-trauma syndrome
- Self-mutilation, high risk for

Dissociative identity disorder
- Personal identity disturbance

EATING DISORDERS

All types
- Caregiver role strain
- Coping, ineffective individual
- Family process alteration
- Nutrition alteration: Less than body requirements
- Personal identity disturbance
- Posttrauma response
- Social isolation

Anorexia nervosa
- Body image disturbance
- Denial, ineffective
- Fluid volume deficit, high risk for
- Hyperthermia
- Nutrition alteration: Less than body requirements

Bulimia nervosa
- Body image disturbance
- Denial, ineffective
- Fluid volume deficit, high risk for
- Nutrition alteration: Less than body requirements

IMPULSE-CONTROL DISORDERS

Intermittent explosive disorder
- Anxiety
- Coping, ineffective family
- Fear
- Grieving, anticipatory
- Grieving, dysfunctional
- Parenting alteration, high risk for
- Posttrauma response
- Self-esteem, chronically low
- Social interaction impairment
- Violence, high risk for: Directed at others

MOOD DISORDERS

All types
- Anxiety
- Caregiver role strain
- Coping, ineffective individual
- Coping, ineffective staff
- Diversional activity deficit
- Fatigue
- Grieving, anticipatory
- Health-seeking behaviors
- Injury, high risk for
- Noncompliance
- Nutrition alteration: Less than body requirements
- Personal identity disturbance
- Posttrauma response
- Powerlessness
- Self-esteem disturbance
- Sexual pattern alteration
- Social interaction impairment
- Social isolation
- Thought process alteration

Bipolar disorder
- Coping, ineffective individual
- Denial, ineffective
- Fatigue
- Fluid volume excess
- Grieving, dysfunctional
- Health maintenance alteration
- Hopelessness
- Injury, high risk for
- Management of therapeutic regimen, ineffective
- Noncompliance
- Nutrition alteration: Less than body requirements
- Parenting alteration
- Parenting alteration, high risk for
- Personal identity disturbance
- Self-care deficit: Bathing, hygiene, dressing, grooming, toileting
- Self-esteem, chronically low
- Sexual pattern alteration
- Sleep pattern disturbance
- Social interaction impairment
- Thought process alteration
- Verbal communication impairment

Depressive disorder
- Adjustment impairment
- Anxiety
- Body image disturbance
- Caregiver role strain
- Caregiver role strain, high risk for
- Coping, ineffective family
- Coping, ineffective individual
- Denial, ineffective
- Diversional activity deficit
- Fatigue
- Grieving, dysfunctional
- Health maintenance alteration
- Health-seeking behaviors
- Hopelessness
- Hyperthermia
- Noncompliance
- Nutrition alteration: Less than body requirements
- Nutrition alteration: More than body requirements
- Pain
- Parenting alteration
- Parenting alteration, high risk for
- Personal identity disturbance
- Posttrauma response
- Powerlessness
- Self-esteem, chronically low
- Self-esteem, situational low
- Sensory or perceptual alteration
- Sexual dysfunction
- Sleep pattern disturbance
- Social interaction impairment
- Social isolation
- Thought process alteration
- Violence, high risk for: Self-directed

PERSONALITY DISORDERS

All types
- Adjustment impairment
- Coping, ineffective individual
- Coping, ineffective staff
- Family process alteration
- Grieving, anticipatory
- Grieving, dysfunctional
- Noncompliance
- Parenting alteration, high risk for
- Personal identity disturbance
- Posttrauma response

- Powerlessness
- Role performance alteration
- Self-esteem, chronically low
- Sexual pattern alteration
- Social interaction impairment
- Social isolation
- Violence, high risk for: Self-directed

Antisocial
- Coping, ineffective family
- Parenting alteration
- Posttrauma response
- Social interaction impairment
- Social isolation
- Violence, high risk for: Directed at others

Borderline
- Anxiety
- Body image disturbance
- Coping, defensive
- Coping, ineffective family
- Coping, ineffective individual
- Denial, ineffective
- Hopelessness
- Parenting alteration
- Personal identity disturbance
- Posttrauma response
- Powerlessness
- Self-mutilation, high risk for
- Sexual pattern alteration
- Thought process alteration
- Violence, high risk for: Self-directed or directed at others

Paranoid
- Anxiety
- Family process alteration
- Coping, ineffective family
- Management of therapeutic regimen, ineffective
- Parenting alteration, high risk for
- Powerlessness
- Self-esteem, chronically low
- Social interaction impairment
- Social isolation
- Thought process alteration
- Violence, high risk for: Self-directed or directed at others

Schizoid
- Anxiety
- Coping, ineffective family
- Personal identity disturbance
- Powerlessness
- Self-esteem, chronically low
- Self-mutilation, high risk for
- Sensory or perceptual alteration
- Social interaction impairment
- Thought process alteration
- Violence, high risk for: Self-directed or directed at others

RELATIONAL PROBLEMS

Parent-child relational problem
- Coping, ineffective family
- Diversional activity deficit
- Fear
- Hopelessness
- Incontinence, functional
- Injury, high risk for
- Parenting alteration
- Posttrauma response
- Powerlessness
- Self-esteem disturbance

SCHIZOPHRENIA AND OTHER PSYCHOTIC DISORDERS

All types
- Anxiety
- Coping, ineffective staff
- Diversional activity deficit
- Fluid volume excess
- Noncompliance
- Self-care deficit: Bathing, hygiene, dressing, grooming, toileting
- Social isolation
- Thought process alteration
- Verbal communication impairment

Brief psychotic disorder
- Coping, ineffective individual
- Parenting alteration, high risk for
- Self-esteem disturbance
- Sensory perceptual alteration
- Social interaction impairment
- Social isolation

Schizophrenia
- Body image disturbance
- Coping, ineffective individual
- Coping, ineffective staff
- Family process alteration
- Fluid volume excess
- Health maintenance alteration
- Hopelessness
- Injury, high risk for
- Knowledge deficit
- Management of therapeutic regimen, ineffective
- Noncompliance
- Parenting alteration, high risk for
- Personal identity disturbance
- Poisoning, high risk for
- Posttrauma response
- Role performance alteration
- Sexual dysfunction
- Social isolation
- Verbal communication impairment
- Violence, high risk for: Self-directed

SEXUAL AND GENDER IDENTITY DISORDERS

All types
- Family process alteration
- Grieving, anticipatory
- Sexual pattern alteration

Gender identity disorders
- Personal identity disturbance
- Sexual pattern alteration

Male erectile disorder
- Body image disturbance
- Self-esteem disturbance
- Sexual dysfunction

Sexual desire disorders
- Posttrauma response
- Sexual dysfunction

Sexual masochism
- Self-mutilation, high risk for
- Sexual dysfunction
- Sexual pattern alteration

SLEEP DISORDERS

Insomnia
- Activity intolerance, high risk for
- Caregiver role strain
- Caregiver role strain, high risk for
- Fatigue
- Health maintenance alteration
- Sleep pattern disturbance

Parasomnia
- Activity intolerance, high risk for
- Body image disturbance
- Fatigue
- Health maintenance alteration
- Sleep pattern disturbance

SOMATOFORM DISORDERS

All types
- Activity intolerance
- Caregiver role strain
- Coping, ineffective individual
- Coping, ineffective staff
- Denial, ineffective
- Family process alteration
- Parenting alteration, high risk for
- Role performance alteration
- Sexual dysfunction
- Sleep pattern disturbance
- Social interaction impairment

Hypochondriasis
- Body image disturbance
- Coping, ineffective staff
- Pain
- Role performance alteration

Somatization disorder
- Coping, ineffective staff
- Fatigue
- Pain

SUBSTANCE-RELATED DISORDERS

All types
- Caregiver role strain
- Fatigue
- Powerlessness
- Role performance alteration

- Self-esteem, chronically low
- Sensory or perceptual alteration
- Social isolation
- Thought process alteration
- Violence, high risk for: Self-directed or directed at others

Alcoholism
- Anxiety
- Caregiver role strain
- Coping, defensive
- Coping, ineffective family
- Coping, ineffective individual
- Coping, ineffective staff
- Denial, ineffective
- Family process alteration
- Fatigue
- Grieving, dysfunctional
- Health maintenance alteration
- Injury, high risk for
- Parenting alteration
- Personal identity disturbance
- Posttrauma response
- Powerlessness
- Self-care deficit: Bathing, hygiene, dressing, grooming, toileting
- Sensory or perceptual alteration
- Sexual dysfunction
- Sleep pattern disturbance
- Social interaction impairment
- Social isolation
- Verbal communication impairment
- Violence, high risk for: Self-directed or directed at others

Drug or alcohol withdrawal
- Coping, ineffective individual
- Injury, high risk for
- Sensory or perceptual alteration
- Social interaction impairment
- Thought process alteration
- Verbal communication impairment

ADDITIONAL CONDITIONS

Malingering
- Coping, ineffective individual
- Posttrauma response
- Self-mutilation, high risk for

Psychiatric Nursing Diagnoses and Medical Illnesses

CARDIOVASCULAR DISORDERS

All types
- Adjustment impairment
- Anxiety
- Health-seeking behaviors
- Hopelessness
- Knowledge deficit
- Management of therapeutic regimen, ineffective
- Parental role conflict
- Powerlessness
- Self-esteem, situational low
- Sexual dysfunction

Angina pectoris
- Anxiety
- Pain
- Role performance alteration

Cardiac disease: End-stage
- Coping, ineffective individual
- Decisional conflict
- Denial, ineffective
- Family process alteration
- Fear
- Grieving, anticipatory
- Hopelessness
- Role performance alteration

Congestive heart failure
- Anxiety
- Fear
- Hopelessness
- Powerlessness
- Role performance alteration
- Social isolation

Hypertension
- Anxiety
- Noncompliance
- Self-esteem, situational low
- Sexual dysfunction

Myocardial infarction
- Anxiety
- Coping, defensive
- Coping, ineffective family
- Coping, ineffective individual
- Denial, ineffective
- Pain
- Sexual dysfunction

Peripheral vascular disorder
- Diversional activity deficit
- Management of therapeutic regimen, ineffective
- Sexual dysfunction

ENDOCRINE DISORDERS

All types
- Grieving, anticipatory
- Health-seeking behaviors
- Hopelessness
- Sexual dysfunction
- Social isolation

Diabetes mellitus
- Adjustment impairment
- Coping, ineffective individual
- Health-seeking behaviors
- Hopelessness
- Management of therapeutic regimen, ineffective
- Powerlessness
- Role performance alteration

- Self-esteem, chronically low
- Sexual dysfunction
- Sexual pattern alteration
- Social isolation

Hyperthyroidism
- Adjustment impairment
- Anxiety
- Sleep pattern disturbance

Hypothyroidism
- Body image disturbance
- Coping, ineffective family
- Coping, ineffective individual
- Health-seeking behaviors

EYE, EAR, NOSE, AND THROAT DISORDERS

Cataracts
- Body image disturbance
- Coping, ineffective individual
- Diversional activity deficit
- Self-esteem, situational low
- Sensory or perceptual alteration
- Social isolation

Hearing loss
- Body image disturbance
- Diversional activity deficit
- Fear
- Role performance alteration
- Sensory or perceptual alteration
- Social isolation
- Verbal communication impairment

Vision loss
- Body image disturbance
- Diversional activity deficit
- Fear
- Powerlessness
- Role performance alteration
- Sensory or perceptual alteration
- Social isolation

GASTROINTESTINAL DISORDERS

Constipation or diarrhea
- Anxiety

- Management of therapeutic regimen, ineffective
- Pain

Diverticulitis
- Pain
- Management of therapeutic regimen, ineffective

Hemorrhoids
- Pain

Malabsorption syndrome
- Anxiety
- Body image disturbance
- Coping, ineffective individual

Pancreatic carcinoma
- Grieving, anticipatory
- Hopelessness
- Pain

Peptic ulcer disease
- Anxiety
- Caregiver role strain
- Caregiver role strain, high risk for
- Pain
- Personal identity disturbance

GENITOURINARY DISORDERS

All types
- Body image disturbance
- Knowledge deficit
- Sexual dysfunction

HEPATOBILIARY DISORDERS

Cirrhosis
- Coping, ineffective family
- Coping, ineffective individual
- Denial, ineffective
- Health maintenance alteration
- Noncompliance
- Powerlessness
- Social isolation

Gallbladder disorders
- Denial, ineffective
- Pain

Hepatitis
- Hopelessness
- Social isolation

IMMUNE DISORDERS

Acquired immunodeficiency syndrome
- Adjustment impairment
- Anxiety
- Coping, defensive
- Coping, ineffective family
- Coping, ineffective individual
- Decisional conflict
- Denial, ineffective
- Fatigue
- Hopelessness
- Knowledge deficit
- Noncompliance
- Parental role conflict
- Personal identity disturbance
- Role performance alteration
- Self-esteem, chronically low
- Sexual dysfunction
- Social interaction impairment
- Social isolation
- Verbal communication impairment

Rheumatoid arthritis and systemic lupus erythematosus
- Body image disturbance
- Coping, defensive
- Coping, ineffective family
- Coping, ineffective individual
- Fatigue
- Fear
- Pain, chronic
- Powerlessness
- Role performance alteration
- Sexual dysfunction
- Social isolation

INFECTION

All types
- Coping, ineffective family
- Coping, ineffective individual
- Fatigue
- Health maintenance alteration
- Management of therapeutic regimen, ineffective

- Sexual pattern alteration
- Social isolation

Pneumocystis carinii pneumonia
- Coping, ineffective family
- Coping, ineffective individual
- Personal identity disturbance
- Role performance alteration
- Thought process alteration

Sexually transmitted diseases
- Knowledge deficit
- Self-esteem disturbance
- Sexual pattern alteration
- Social isolation

INTEGUMENTARY DISORDERS

All types
- Body image disturbance
- Diversional activity deficit
- Knowledge deficit
- Self-esteem disturbance

METABOLIC AND NUTRITIONAL DISORDERS

Electrolyte imbalance
- Body image disturbance
- Sleep pattern disturbance
- Thought process alteration

Malnutrition
- Body image disturbance
- Family process alteration
- Health maintenance alteration
- Knowledge deficit
- Nutrition alteration: Less than body requirements
- Social isolation
- Thought process alteration

Obesity
- Body image disturbance
- Nutrition alteration: More than body requirements
- Self-esteem, situational low
- Social isolation

MULTISYSTEM DISORDERS

Chronic fatigue and immune dysfunction syndrome
- Caregiver role strain
- Caregiver role strain, high risk for
- Denial, ineffective
- Fatigue
- Hopelessness
- Management of therapeutic regimen, ineffective
- Self-esteem disturbance
- Sleep pattern disturbance

Chronic pain
- Coping, ineffective staff
- Hopelessness
- Knowledge deficit
- Management of therapeutic regimen, ineffective
- Noncompliance
- Pain, chronic
- Posttrauma response
- Powerlessness
- Social isolation

Deformities or disfigurement
- Body image disturbance
- Grieving, dysfunctional
- Self-esteem, chronically low
- Social isolation

Failure to thrive
- Grieving, dysfunctional
- Growth and development alteration
- Parental role conflict
- Parenting alteration
- Parenting alteration, high risk for

Long-term disability
- Noncompliance
- Management of therapeutic regimen, ineffective
- Role performance alteration
- Self-esteem, chronically low

Stress-related illnesses
- Caregiver role strain
- Caregiver role strain, high risk for
- Coping, ineffective family

- Management of therapeutic regimen, ineffective
- Pain
- Personal identity disturbance

MUSCULOSKELETAL DISORDERS

All types
- Growth and development alteration
- Hopelessness
- Parental role conflict
- Role performance alteration
- Social isolation

Chronic low back pain
- Denial, ineffective
- Management of therapeutic regimen, ineffective
- Pain, chronic

Osteoarthritis
- Adjustment impairment
- Body image disturbance
- Coping, defensive
- Health-seeking behaviors
- Knowledge deficit
- Management of therapeutic regimen, ineffective
- Pain
- Self-esteem, situational low
- Sexual dysfunction
- Social isolation

Osteoporosis
- Body image disturbance
- Powerlessness
- Social isolation

Paralysis
- Body image disturbance
- Coping, ineffective individual
- Powerlessness
- Role performance alteration
- Self-esteem disturbance
- Sexual dysfunction

NEONATAL DISORDERS

Prematurity
- Decisional conflict

- Growth and development alteration
- Parenting alteration, high risk for

NEOPLASMS

All types
- Adjustment impairment
- Anxiety
- Body image disturbance
- Coping, defensive
- Coping, ineffective family
- Coping, ineffective individual
- Decisional conflict
- Denial, ineffective
- Fear
- Grieving, anticipatory
- Grieving, dysfunctional
- Health-seeking behaviors
- Hopelessness
- Management of therapeutic regimen, ineffective
- Pain
- Powerlessness
- Sexual dysfunction
- Social interaction impairment
- Social isolation
- Spiritual distress
- Violence, high risk for: Self-directed

Brain tumor
- Anxiety
- Decisional conflict
- Fear
- Health maintenance alteration
- Hopelessness
- Powerlessness
- Thought process alteration
- Verbal communication impairment

Kaposi's sarcoma
- Coping, ineffective family
- Coping, ineffective individual
- Hopelessness
- Role performance alteration
- Thought process alteration

NEUROLOGIC DISORDERS

All types
- Adjustment impairment

- Coping, ineffective individual
- Fatigue
- Growth and development alteration
- Health maintenance alteration
- Health-seeking behaviors
- Knowledge deficit
- Pain, chronic
- Parental role conflict
- Sexual dysfunction
- Social interaction impairment
- Social isolation
- Thought process alteration
- Verbal communication impairment

Alzheimer's disease
- Anxiety
- Caregiver role strain
- Caregiver role strain, high risk for
- Coping, ineffective family
- Coping, ineffective individual
- Fear
- Health maintenance alteration
- Role performance alteration
- Social isolation
- Thought process alteration
- Verbal communication impairment

Amyotrophic lateral sclerosis
- Body image disturbance
- Hopelessness
- Powerlessness
- Social isolation
- Verbal communication impairment

Brain death
- Caregiver role strain
- Caregiver role strain, high risk for
- Decisional conflict
- Grieving, anticipatory
- Grieving, dysfunctional

Cerebrovascular accident
- Adjustment impairment
- Body image disturbance
- Coping, ineffective family
- Health maintenance alteration
- Powerlessness
- Social interaction impairment
- Social isolation
- Verbal communication impairment

Coma
- Decisional conflict
- Grieving, anticipatory

Epilepsy (seizure disorder)
- Body image disturbance
- Caregiver role strain
- Caregiver role strain, high risk for
- Coping, ineffective individual
- Hopelessness
- Management of therapeutic regimen, ineffective
- Noncompliance
- Parental role conflict
- Role performance alteration
- Social isolation
- Verbal communication impairment

Headache
- Anxiety
- Caregiver role strain
- Caregiver role strain, high risk for
- Denial, ineffective
- Pain
- Pain, chronic
- Personal identity disturbance

HIV encephalopathy
- Anxiety
- Coping, ineffective family
- Coping, ineffective individual
- Hopelessness
- Powerlessness
- Role performance alteration
- Social isolation
- Thought process alteration

Huntington's disease
- Body image disturbance
- Health maintenance alteration
- Hopelessness
- Powerlessness
- Self-esteem, chronically low
- Thought process alteration
- Verbal communication impairment

Multiple sclerosis
- Body image disturbance
- Coping, ineffective individual
- Fear

- Hopelessness
- Social isolation
- Verbal communication impairment

Organic brain syndrome
- Caregiver role strain
- Caregiver role strain, high risk for
- Health maintenance alteration
- Social interaction impairment
- Social isolation
- Thought process alteration
- Verbal communication impairment

Parkinson's disease
- Coping, ineffective family
- Coping, ineffective individual
- Fear
- Hopelessness
- Powerlessness
- Role performance alteration
- Social isolation
- Verbal communication impairment

Transient ischemic attack
- Fear
- Grieving, anticipatory
- Verbal communication impairment

OBSTETRIC AND GYNECOLOGIC DISORDERS

Abortion
- Anxiety
- Decisional conflict
- Grieving, dysfunctional

Birth of child with health problems
- Coping, ineffective family
- Denial, ineffective
- Fear
- Grieving, dysfunctional
- Knowledge deficit
- Parental role conflict
- Parenting alteration
- Parenting alteration, high risk for

Gynecologic disorders
- Anxiety
- Body image disturbance
- Coping, ineffective individual

- Fear
- Pain
- Pain, chronic
- Sexual dysfunction
- Sexual pattern alteration

Menopause or climacteric
- Coping, ineffective individual
- Fatigue
- Grieving, anticipatory
- Health-seeking behaviors
- Sleep pattern disturbance

Multiple pregnancy
- Coping, ineffective family
- Parenting alteration, high risk for

RENAL DISORDERS

Renal disease: End-stage
- Coping, defensive
- Coping, ineffective individual
- Decisional conflict
- Denial, ineffective
- Grieving, anticipatory
- Hopelessness
- Role performance alteration
- Sexual dysfunction

Renal failure
- Body image disturbance
- Decisional conflict
- Fear
- Powerlessness
- Sexual dysfunction
- Social isolation

RESPIRATORY DISORDERS

All types
- Coping, ineffective individual
- Grieving, anticipatory
- Health maintenance alteration
- Hopelessness
- Parental role conflict
- Social isolation
- Verbal communication impairment

Chronic obstructive pulmonary disease
- Adjustment impairment
- Coping, ineffective family
- Fear
- Knowledge deficit
- Noncompliance
- Powerlessness
- Role performance alteration
- Sleep pattern disturbance

Pulmonary disease: End-stage
- Coping, ineffective individual
- Decisional conflict
- Denial, ineffective
- Grieving, anticipatory
- Hopelessness
- Role performance alteration

Respiratory failure
- Anxiety
- Fear
- Thought process alteration

TRAUMA

All types
- Anxiety
- Body image disturbance
- Coping, ineffective family
- Coping, ineffective individual
- Fear
- Growth and development alteration
- Parenting alteration
- Parenting alteration, high risk for
- Personal identity disturbance
- Posttrauma response
- Powerlessness
- Thought process alteration

Burns
- Body image disturbance
- Diversional activity deficit
- Hopelessness
- Pain
- Parenting alteration, high risk for
- Powerlessness
- Social isolation

Drug overdose
- Coping, ineffective individual
- Decisional conflict
- Denial, ineffective
- Sensory or perceptual alteration
- Thought process alteration
- Verbal communication impairment
- Violence, high risk for: Self-directed

Fractures
- Coping, ineffective family
- Diversional activity deficit
- Pain
- Parenting alteration
- Role performance alteration

Head trauma
- Anxiety
- Diversional activity deficit
- Fear
- Health maintenance alteration
- Parenting alteration
- Self-care deficit: Bathing, hygiene, dressing, grooming, toileting
- Thought process alteration
- Verbal communication impairment

Orthopedic injury
- Hopelessness
- Sexual dysfunction

Sexual assault
- Posttrauma response
- Powerlessness
- Rape-trauma syndrome: Compound reaction
- Rape-trauma syndrome: Silent reaction

Spinal cord injuries
- Adjustment impairment
- Diversional activity deficit
- Fear
- Powerlessness
- Sexual dysfunction
- Social interaction impairment
- Social isolation

Nursing Diagnoses and Psychosocial Problems

AIDS patient care
- Coping, ineffective family
related to inability to support and care for patient with AIDS
- Role performance alteration
related to guilt brought on by transmission of HIV infection
- Thought process alteration
related to neuropsychiatric manifestations of AIDS

Codependency
- Caregiver role strain
related to caring for an aging family member (geriatric)
- Coping, ineffective family
related to codependence
- Social interaction impairment
related to codependence

Cross-cultural issues
- Noncompliance
related to cultural differences

Death and dying
- Decisional conflict
related to staff members' disagreement regarding end-of-life treatment decisions
- Grieving, anticipatory
related to potential loss of family member
- Grieving, anticipatory
related to potential loss of patient
- Grieving, anticipatory
related to preparation for death (geriatric)
- Spiritual distress
related to diagnosis of terminal illness

Domestic violence and abuse
- Injury, high risk for
related to elder abuse (geriatric)
- Parenting alteration
related to physical or psychological abuse (child)
- Parenting alteration, high risk for
related to mental illness
- Personal identity disturbance
related to a history of sexual abuse
- Posttrauma response
related to history of childhood incest
- Posttrauma response
related to incest (child)
- Powerlessness
related to physical, sexual, or emotional abuse by partner

Drug and alcohol abuse and addiction
- Coping, ineffective individual
related to substance abuse
- Decisional conflict
related to substance use (adolescent)
- Injury, high risk for
related to overdose or withdrawal

Drug therapy
- Fatigue
related to adverse effects of medications
- Knowledge deficit
related to drug therapy in cognitively impaired patients
- Poisoning, high risk for
related to medication use (geriatric)
- Thermoregulation, ineffective
related to neuroleptic malignant syndrome

Family counseling

- Caregiver role strain

related to caring for a chronically ill relative

- Caregiver role strain

related to caring for an aging family member (geriatric)

- Coping, family: Potential for growth

related to blending two existing families

- Coping, family: Potential for growth

related to marital conflict

- Coping, ineffective family

related to codependence

- Coping, ineffective family

related to inability to support and care for patient with AIDS

- Coping, ineffective family

related to unresolved emotional conflict between patient and family members (geriatric)

- Family process alteration

related to dysfunctional behavior

- Grieving, anticipatory

related to anticipated divorce or separation

- Grieving, anticipatory

related to potential loss of family member

- Self-esteem disturbance

related to adverse relationship with parents (adolescent)

Homelessness

- Powerlessness

related to homelessness

- Social isolation

related to homelessness

Law and ethics

- Decisional conflict

related to advance directives (geriatric)

- Decisional conflict

related to staff members' disagreement regarding end-of-life treatment decisions

- Injury, high risk for

related to use of restraints

- Knowledge deficit

related to informed consent

Organ transplantation

- Decisional conflict

related to family's choices regarding organ donation

- Family process alteration

related to organ transplantation (awaiting procedure)

- Family process alteration

related to organ transplantation (following procedure)

Parenting

- Parental role conflict

related to child's hospitalization

- Parental role conflict

related to home care of a child with special needs

- Parenting alteration

related to physical or psychological abuse (child)

- Parenting alteration, high risk for

related to lack of resources (child)

- Parenting alteration, high risk for

related to mental illness

- Self-esteem disturbance

related to adverse relationship with parents (adolescent)

Professional growth and development

- Caregiver role strain

related to caring for chronically ill patients

- Coping, ineffective staff

related to the special patient

- Decisional conflict

related to staff members' disagreement regarding end-of-life treatment decisions

- Grieving, anticipatory

related to potential loss of patient

Recovery from childhood trauma (in an adult patient)

- Personal identity disturbance

related to a history of sexual abuse

- Posttrauma response

related to history of childhood incest

- Posttrauma response

related to parent's alcoholism

Sexuality
- Decisional conflict
related to sexual activity (adolescent)
- Knowledge deficit
related to lack of information about safer
sex practices (adolescent)
- Sexual dysfunction
related to altered body structure or function
- Sexual dysfunction
related to decreased libido caused by depression
- Sexual dysfunction
related to impotence
- Sexual pattern alteration
related to hypersexuality caused by mania
- Sexual pattern alteration
related to psychological distress

Women's health
- Body image disturbance
related to an eating disorder (adolescent)
- Coping, family: Potential for growth
related to marital conflict
- Coping, ineffective individual
related to postpartum mood changes
- Decisional conflict
related to sexual activity (adolescent)
- Fatigue
related to postpartum state
- Grieving, anticipatory
related to anticipated divorce or separation
- Parenting alteration, high risk for
related to lack of resources (child)
- Personal identity disturbance
related to a history of sexual abuse
- Posttrauma response
related to history of childhood incest
- Powerlessness
related to physical, sexual, or emotional
abuse by partner
- Rape-trauma syndrome: Compound
reaction
- Rape-trauma syndrome: Silent reaction

DSM-IV Classification of Psychiatric Disorders

The following is an adapted version of the classification of mental disorders published in the fourth edition of the American Psychiatric Association's *Diagnostic and Statistical Manual of Mental Disorders (DSM-IV)*. Beside most diagnostic labels appears the associated numerical code from the *International Classification of Diseases*, Ninth Revision, Clinical Modification (ICD-9-CM). These codes are used by insurance companies to determine reimbursement for psychiatric services.

Because of the diverse clinical signs of mental disorders, a diagnostic nomenclature can't cover every possible situation. So, many diagnostic categories include a *not otherwise specified* (NOS) label. An *x* appearing in a diagnostic code indicates that a specific code number is required. An ellipsis (. . .) indicates that the name of a specific mental disorder or medical condition should be inserted (for example, 293.0, Delirium due to hypothyroidism).

ADJUSTMENT DISORDERS

309.xx	Adjustment disorder
.0	With depressed mood
.24	With anxiety
.28	With mixed anxiety and depressed mood
.3	With disturbance of conduct
.4	With mixed disturbance of emotions and conduct
.9	Unspecified (specify if acute or chronic)

ANXIETY DISORDERS

293.89	Anxiety disorder due to . . . (indicate the medical condition; specify if with generalized anxiety, panic attacks, or obsessive-compulsive symptoms)
300.00	Anxiety disorder NOS
300.01	Panic disorder without agoraphobia
300.02	Generalized anxiety disorder
300.21	Panic disorder with agoraphobia
300.22	Agoraphobia without history of panic disorder
300.23	Social phobia (specify if generalized)
300.29	Specific phobia (specify if animal, natural environment, blood-injection-injury, situational, or other type)
300.3	Obsessive-compulsive disorder (specify if with poor insight)
308.3	Acute stress disorder
309.81	Posttraumatic stress disorder (specify if acute, chronic, or with delayed onset)
——	Substance-induced anxiety disorder (refer to substance-related disorders for substance-specific codes; specify if with generalized anxiety, panic attacks, obsessive-compulsive symptoms, or phobic symptoms; and specify if onset occurred during intoxication or during withdrawal)

DELIRIUM, DEMENTIA, AND AMNESTIC AND OTHER COGNITIVE DISORDERS

Amnestic disorders

294.0 Amnestic disorder due to ... (indicate the medical condition; specify if transient or chronic)
294.8 Amnestic disorder NOS
—— Substance-induced persisting amnestic disorder (refer to substance-related disorders for substance-specific codes)

Delirium

293.0 Delirium due to ... (indicate the medical condition)
780.09 Delirium NOS
—— Delirium due to multiple etiologies (code each of the specific etiologies)
—— Substance intoxication delirium (refer to substance-related disorders for substance-specific codes)
—— Substance withdrawal delirium (refer to substance-related disorders for substance-specific codes)

Dementia

290.xx Dementia of the Alzheimer's type with early onset
.10 Uncomplicated
.11 With delirium
.12 With delusions
.13 With depressed mood (specify if with behavioral disturbance)
290.xx Dementia of the Alzheimer's type with late onset
.0 Uncomplicated
.3 With delirium
.20 With delusions
.21 With depressed mood (specify if with behavioral disturbance)
290.xx Vascular dementia
.40 Uncomplicated
.41 With delirium
.42 With delusions
.43 With depressed mood (specify if with behavioral disturbance)
290.10 Dementia due to Creutzfeldt-Jacob disease

290.10 Dementia due to Pick's disease
294.1 Dementia due to head trauma (also head injury)
294.1 Dementia due to Huntington's disease
294.1 Dementia due to Parkinson's disease
294.1 Dementia due to ... (indicate the medical condition not listed above)
294.8 Dementia NOS
294.9 Dementia due to HIV disease (also HIV infection affecting central nervous system)
—— Dementia due to multiple etiologies (code each of the specific etiologies)
—— Substance-induced persisting dementia (refer to substance-related disorders for substance-specific codes)

Other cognitive disorders

294.9 Cognitive disorder NOS

DISORDERS USUALLY FIRST DIAGNOSED IN INFANCY, CHILDHOOD, OR ADOLESCENCE

Attention-deficit and disruptive behavior disorders

312.8 Conduct disorder (specify onset as childhood or adolescent)
312.9 Disruptive behavior disorder NOS
313.81 Oppositional defiant disorder
314.xx Attention-deficit and hyperactivity disorder
.00 Predominantly inattentive type
.01 Combined type
.01 Predominantly hyperactive-impulsive type
314.9 Attention-deficit and hyperactivity disorder NOS

Communication disorders

307.0 Stuttering
307.9 Communication disorder NOS
315.31 Expressive language disorder
315.31 Mixed receptive-expressive language disorder
315.39 Phonological disorder

Elimination disorders
307.6   Enuresis unrelated to a medical
        condition (specify as nocturnal,
        diurnal, or nocturnal and diurnal)
307.7   Encopresis without constipation
        and overflow incontinence
787.6   Encopresis with constipation and
        overflow incontinence

Feeding and eating disorders of infancy or early childhood
307.52 Pica
307.53 Rumination disorder
307.59 Feeding disorder of infancy or
        early childhood

Learning disorders
315.00 Reading disorder
315.1   Mathematics disorder
315.2   Disorder of written expression
315.9   Learning disorder NOS

Mental retardation
317   Mild retardation
318.0   Moderate retardation
318.1   Severe retardation
318.2   Profound retardation
319   Unspecified severity

Motor skills disorder
315.4   Developmental coordination
        disorder

Pervasive developmental disorders
299.00 Autistic disorder
299.10 Childhood disintegrative disorder
299.80 Asperger's disorder
299.80 Rett's disorder
299.80 Pervasive developmental disorder
        NOS

Tic disorders
307.20 Tic disorder NOS
307.21 Transient tic disorder (specify as
        single episode or recurrent)
307.22 Chronic motor or vocal tic disorder
307.23 Tourette's disorder

Other disorders of infancy, childhood, or adolescence
307.3   Stereotypic movement disorder
        (specify if with self-injurious
        behavior)
309.21 Separation anxiety disorder
        (specify if early onset)
313.23 Selective mutism
313.89 Reactive attachment disorder of
        infancy or early childhood (speci-
        fy as inhibited or disinhibited)
313.9   Disorder of infancy, childhood, or
        adolescence NOS

DISSOCIATIVE DISORDERS
300.12 Dissociative amnesia
300.13 Dissociative fugue
300.14 Dissociative identity disorder
300.15 Dissociative disorder NOS
300.6   Depersonalization disorder

EATING DISORDERS
307.1   Anorexia nervosa (specify if
        restricting type or binge-eating
        and purging type)
307.50 Eating disorder NOS
307.51 Bulimia nervosa (specify if
        purging or nonpurging type)

FACTITIOUS DISORDERS
300.xx Factitious disorder
    .16 With predominantly psychological
        signs and symptoms
    .19 With predominantly physical signs
        and symptoms
    .19 With combined psychological and
        physical signs and symptoms
300.19 Factitious disorder NOS

IMPULSE-CONTROL DISORDERS NOT ELSEWHERE CLASSIFIED
312.30 Impulse-control disorder NOS
312.31 Pathological gambling
312.32 Kleptomania
312.33 Pyromania

312.34   Intermittent explosive disorder
312.39   Trichotillomania

MENTAL DISORDERS DUE TO A MEDICAL CONDITION NOT ELSE-WHERE CLASSIFIED

293.89   Catatonic disorder due to ... (indicate the medical condition)
293.9   Mental disorder NOS due to ... (indicate the medical condition)
310.1   Personality change due to... (indicate the medical condition; specify type: labile, disinhibited, aggressive, apathetic, paranoid, other, combined, or unspecified)

MOOD DISORDERS

Bipolar disorders
293.83   Mood disorder due to ...(indicate the medical condition; specify if with depressive features, with major depressive-like episode, with manic features, or with mixed features)
296.xx   Bipolar I disorder
.0x   Single manic episode (specify if mixed)
.40   Most recent episode hypomanic
.4x   Most recent episode manic
.5x   Most recent episode depressed
.6x   Most recent episode mixed
.7   Most recent episode unspecified
296.89   Bipolar II disorder (specify current or most recent episode as hypomanic or depressed)
296.80   Bipolar disorder NOS
296.90   Mood disorder NOS
301.13   Cyclothymic disorder
——   Substance-induced mood disorder (refer to substance-related disorders for substance-specific codes; specify if with depressive features, with manic features, or with mixed features; also specify if onset occurred during intoxication or during withdrawal)

Depressive disorders
296.xx   Major depressive disorder
.2x   Single episode
.3x   Recurrent
300.4   Dysthymic disorder (specify if early or late onset and if with atypical features)
311   Depressive disorder NOS

PERSONALITY DISORDERS

301.0   Paranoid personality disorder
301.4   Obsessive-compulsive personality disorder
301.6   Dependent personality disorder
301.7   Antisocial personality disorder
301.20   Schizoid personality disorder
301.22   Schizotypal personality disorder
301.50   Histrionic personality disorder
301.81   Narcissistic personality disorder
301.82   Avoidant personality disorder
301.83   Borderline personality disorder
301.9   Personality disorder NOS

SCHIZOPHRENIA AND OTHER PSYCHOTIC DISORDERS

95.xx   Schizophrenia
The following classification applies to all subtypes of schizophrenia: episodic with interepisode residual symptoms (specify if with prominent negative symptoms), episodic with no interepisode residual symptoms, continuous (specify if with prominent negative symptoms), single episode in partial remission (specify if with prominent negative symptoms or single episode in full remission), or other or unspecified pattern.
.10   Disorganized type
.20   Catatonic type
.30   Paranoid type
.60   Residual type
.90   Undifferentiated type
293.xx   Psychotic disorder due to ...(indicate the medical condition)
.81   With delusions
.82   With hallucinations
——   Substance-induced psychotic disorder (refer to substance-relat-

ed disorders for substance-specific codes; specify with onset during intoxication or during withdrawal)
295.40 Schizophreniform disorder (specify with or without good prognostic features)
295.70 Schizoaffective disorder (specify bipolar or depressive type)
297.1   Delusional disorder (specify erotomanic, grandiose, jealous, persecutory, somatic, mixed, or unspecified type)
297.3   Shared psychotic disorder
298.8   Brief psychotic disorder (specify with or without marked stressors, or with postpartum onset)
298.9   Psychotic disorder NOS

SEXUAL AND GENDER IDENTITY DISORDERS

Gender identity disorders
302.xx Gender identity disorder
.6   In children
.8   In adolescents or adults (specify if sexually attracted to males, females, both, or neither)
302.6   Gender identity disorder NOS

Paraphilias
302.2   Pedophilia (specify if sexually attracted to males, females, or both; specify if limited to incest; and specify if exclusive or nonexclusive type)
302.3   Transvestic fetishism (specify if with gender dysphoria)
302.4   Exhibitionism
302.81 Fetishism
302.82 Voyeurism
302.83 Sexual masochism
302.84 Sexual sadism
302.89 Frotteurism
302.9   Paraphilia NOS

Sexual dysfunctions
For all primary sexual dysfunctions, specify if lifelong or acquired type, generalized or situational type, and whether due to psychological factors or combined factors.
Orgasmic disorders
302.73 Female orgasmic disorder
302.74 Male orgasmic disorder
302.75 Premature ejaculation
Sexual arousal disorders
302.72 Female sexual arousal disorder
302.72 Male erectile disorder
Sexual desire disorders
302.71 Hypoactive sexual desire disorder
302.79 Sexual aversion disorder
Sexual dysfunction due to a medical condition
302.70 Sexual dysfunction NOS
607.84 Male erectile disorder due to ... (indicate the medical condition)
608.89 Male dyspareunia due to ... (indicate the medical condition)
608.89 Male hypoactive sexual desire disorder due to... (indicate the medical condition)
608.89 Other male sexual dysfunction due to ... (indicate the medical condition)
——   Substance-induced sexual dysfunction (refer to substance-related disorders for substance-specific codes; specify if with impaired desire, with impaired arousal, with impaired orgasm, or with sexual pain; and specify if onset occurred during intoxication)
625.0   Female dyspareunia due to ... (indicate the medical condition)
625.8   Female hypoactive sexual desire disorder due to ... (indicate the medical condition)
625.8   Other female sexual dysfunction due to ... (indicate the medical condition)
Sexual pain disorders
302.76 Dyspareunia (not due to a medical condition)
306.51 Vaginismus (not due to a medical condition)
Other sexual disorders
302.9   Sexual disorder NOS

SLEEP DISORDERS

Primary sleep disorders
Dyssomnias
307.42   Primary insomnia
307.44   Primary hypersomnia (specify if recurrent)
307.45   Circadian rhythm sleep disorder (specify if delayed sleep phase, jet lag, shift work, or unspecified type)
307.47   Dyssomnia NOS
347   Narcolepsy
780.59   Breathing-related sleep disorder
Parasomnias
307.46   Sleep terror disorder
307.46   Sleeping walking disorder
307.47   Nightmare disorder
307.47   Parasomnia NOS

Sleep disorders related to another mental disorder
307.42   Insomnia related to . . . (indicate the disorder)
307.44   Hypersomnia related to . . . (indicate the disorder)

Other sleep disorders
780.xx   Sleep disorder due to. . . (indicate the medical condition)
 .52   Insomnia type
 .54   Hypersomnia type
 .59   Mixed type
 .59   Parasomnia type
——-   Substance-induced sleep disorder (refer to substance-related disorders for substance-specific codes; specify if insomnia, hypersomnia, parasomnia, or mixed type; and specify if onset occurred during intoxication or withdrawal.)

SOMATOFORM DISORDERS

300.7   Body dysmorphic disorder
300.7   Hypochondriasis (specify if with poor insight)
300.11   Conversion disorder (specify if with motor symptom or deficit, sensory symptom or deficit, sei-

zures or convulsions, or mixed presentation)
300.81   Somatization disorder
300.81   Undifferentiated somatoform disorder
300.81   Somatoform disorder NOS
307.xx   Pain disorder
 .80   Associated with psychological factors
 .89   Associated with both psychological factors and a medical condition (specify if acute or chronic)

SUBSTANCE-RELATED DISORDERS

Alcohol-related disorders
Alcohol-induced disorders
291.0   Alcohol intoxication delirium
291.0   Alcohol withdrawal delirium
291.1   Alcohol-induced persisting amnestic disorder
291.2   Alcohol-induced persisting dementia
291.x   Alcohol-induced psychotic disorder
 .3   With hallucinations (specify if onset occurred during intoxication or withdrawal)
 .5   With delusions (specify if onset occurred during intoxication or withdrawal)
291.8   Alcohol-induced anxiety disorder (specify if onset occurred during intoxication or withdrawal)
291.8   Alcohol-induced mood disorder (specify if onset occurred during intoxication or withdrawal)
291.8   Alcohol-induced sexual dysfunction (specify with onset during intoxication)
291.8   Alcohol withdrawal (specify if with perceptual disturbances)
291.9   Alcohol-induced sleep disorder (specify if onset occurred during intoxication or withdrawal)
291.9   Alcohol-related disorder NOS
303.00   Alcohol intoxication

Alcohol use disorders

303.90   Alcohol dependence (specify with or without physiological dependence)
305.00   Alcohol abuse

Amphetamine-related disorders
Amphetamine-induced disorders

292.0   Amphetamine withdrawal
292.xx   Amphetamine-induced psychotic disorder
  .11   With delusions (specify if onset occurred during intoxication)
  .12   With hallucinations (specify if onset occurred during intoxication)
292.81   Amphetamine intoxication delirium
292.84   Amphetamine-induced mood disorder (specify if onset occurred during intoxication or withdrawal)
292.89   Amphetamine-induced anxiety disorder (specify if onset occurred during intoxication)
292.89   Amphetamine-induced sexual dysfunction (specify if onset occurred during intoxication)
292.89   Amphetamine-induced sleep disorder (specify if onset occurred during intoxication or withdrawal)
292.89   Amphetamine intoxication (specify if with perceptual disturbances)
292.9   Amphetamine–related disorder NOS

Amphetamine use disorders

304.40   Amphetamine dependence (specify with or without physiological dependence)
305.70   Amphetamine abuse

Caffeine-related disorders
Caffeine-induced disorders

292.89   Caffeine-induced anxiety disorder (specify if onset occurred during intoxication)
292.89   Caffeine-induced sleep disorder (specify if onset occurred during intoxication)

292.9   Caffeine-related disorder NOS
305.90   Caffeine intoxication

Cannabis-related disorders
Cannabis-induced disorders

292.xx   Cannabis-induced psychotic disorder
  .11   With delusions (specify if onset occurred during intoxication)
  .12   With hallucinations (specify if onset occurred during intoxication)
292.81   Cannabis intoxication delirium
292.89   Cannabis-induced anxiety disorder (specify if onset occurred during intoxication)
292.89   Cannabis intoxication (specify if with perceptual disturbances)
292.9   Cannabis-related disorder NOS

Cannabis use disorders

304.30   Cannabis dependence (specify with or without physiological dependence)
305.20   Cannabis abuse

Cocaine-related disorders
Cocaine-induced disorders

292.0   Cocaine withdrawal
292.xx   Cocaine-induced psychotic disorders
  .11   With delusions (specify if onset occurred during intoxication)
  .12   With hallucinations (specify if onset occurred during intoxication)
292.81   Cocaine intoxication delirium
292.84   Cocaine-induced mood disorder (specify if onset occurred during intoxication or withdrawal)
292.89   Cocaine-induced anxiety disorder (specify if onset occurred during intoxication or withdrawal)
292.89   Cocaine-induced sexual dysfunction (specify if onset occurred during intoxication)
292.89   Cocaine-induced sleep disorder (specify if onset occurred during intoxication or withdrawal)
292.89   Cocaine intoxication (specify if with perceptual disturbances)

292.9   Cocaine-related disorder NOS
Cocaine use disorders
304.20   Cocaine dependence (specify with or without physiological dependence)
305.60   Cocaine abuse

Hallucinogen-related disorders
Hallucinogen-induced disorders
292.xx   Hallucinogen-induced psychotic disorder
   .11   With delusions (specify if onset occurred during intoxication)
   .12   With hallucinations (specify if onset occurred during intoxication)
292.81   Hallucinogen intoxication delirium
292.84   Hallucinogen-induced mood disorder (specify if onset occurred during intoxication)
292.89   Hallucinogen-induced anxiety disorder (specify if onset occurred during intoxication)
292.89   Hallucinogen intoxication
292.89   Hallucinogen persisting perception disorder (flashbacks)
292.9   Hallucinogen-related disorder NOS
Hallucinogen use disorders
304.50   Hallucinogen dependence (specify with or without physiological dependence)
305.30   Hallucinogen abuse

Inhalant-related disorders
Inhalant-induced disorders
292.xx   Inhalant-induced psychotic disorder
   .11   With delusions (specify if onset occurred during intoxication)
   .12   With hallucinations (specify if onset occurred during intoxication)
292.81   Inhalant intoxication delirium
292.82   Inhalant-induced persisting dementia
292.84   Inhalant-induced mood disorder (specify if onset occurred during intoxication)
292.89   Inhalant-induced anxiety disorder (specify if onset occurred during intoxication)

292.89   Inhalant intoxication
292.9   Inhalant-related disorder NOS
Inhalant use disorders
304.60   Inhalant dependence (specify with or without physiological dependence)
305.90   Inhalant abuse

Nicotine-related disorders
Nicotine-induced disorder
292.0   Nicotine withdrawal
292.9   Nicotine-related disorder NOS
Nicotine use disorder
305.10   Nicotine dependence (specify with or without physiological dependence)

Opioid-related disorders
Opioid-induced disorders
292.0   Opioid withdrawal
292.xx   Opioid-induced psychotic disorder
   .11   With delusions (specify if onset occurred during intoxication)
   .12   With hallucinations (specify if onset occurred during intoxication)
292.81   Opioid intoxication delirium
292.84   Opioid-induced mood disorder (specify if onset occurred during intoxication)
292.89   Opioid-induced sexual dysfunction (specify if onset occurred during intoxication)
292.89   Opioid-induced sleep disorder (specify if onset occurred during intoxication or withdrawal)
292.89   Opioid intoxication (specify if with perceptual disturbances)
292.9   Opioid-related disorder NOS
Opioid use disorders
304.00   Opioid dependence (specify with or without physiological dependence)
305.50   Opioid abuse

Phencyclidine-related disorders
Phencyclidine-induced disorders
292.xx   Phencyclidine-induced psychotic disorder
   .11   With delusions (specify if onset occurred during intoxication)

.12 With hallucinations (specify if on-set occurred during intoxication)

292.81 Phencyclidine intoxication delirium

292.84 Phencyclidine-induced mood disorders (specify if onset occurred during intoxication)

292.89 Phencyclidine-induced anxiety disorders (specify if onset occurred during intoxication)

292.89 Phencyclidine intoxication (specify if with perceptual disturbances)

292.9 Phencyclidine-related disorder NOS

Phencyclidine use disorders

304.90 Phencyclidine dependence (specify with or without physiological dependence)

305.90 Phencyclidine abuse

Polysubstance-related disorder

304.80 Polysubstance dependence (specify with or without physiological dependence)

Sedative-, hypnotic-, or anxiolytic-related disorders

Sedative, hypnotic, or anxiolytic use disorders

304.10 Sedative, hypnotic, or anxiolytic dependence (specify with or without physiological dependence)

305.40 Sedative, hypnotic, or anxiolytic abuse

Sedative-, hypnotic-, or anxiolytic-induced disorders

292.0 Sedative, hypnotic, or anxiolytic withdrawal (specify if with perceptual disturbances)

292.xx Sedative-, hypnotic-, or anxiolytic-induced psychotic disorder

.11 With delusions (specify if onset occurred during intoxication)

.12 With hallucinations (specify if on-set occurred during intoxication)

292.81 Sedative, hypnotic, or anxiolytic intoxication delirium

292.81 Sedative, hypnotic, or anxiolytic withdrawal delirium

292.82 Sedative-, hypnotic-, or anxiolytic-induced persisting dementia

292.83 Sedative-, hypnotic-, or anxiolytic-induced persisting amnestic disorder

292.84 Sedative-, hypnotic-, or anxiolytic-induced mood disorder (specify if onset occurred during intoxication or withdrawal)

292.89 Sedative-, hypnotic-, or anxiolytic-induced anxiety disorder (specify if onset occurred during intoxication or withdrawal)

292.89 Sedative-, hypnotic-, or anxiolytic-induced sexual dysfunction (specify if onset occurred during intoxication)

292.89 Sedative-, hypnotic-, or anxiolytic-induced sleep disorder (specify if onset occurred during intoxication or withdrawal)

292.89 Sedative, hypnotic, or anxiolytic intoxication

292.9 Sedative-, hypnotic-, or anxiolytic-related disorder NOS

Other (or unknown) substance-related disorders

Other (or unknown) substance-induced disorders

292.0 Other (or unknown) substance withdrawal (specify if with perceptual disturbances)

292.xx Other (or unknown) substance-induced psychotic disorder

.11 With delusions (specify if onset occurred during intoxication)

.12 With hallucinations (specify if on-set occurred during intoxication)

292.81 Other (or unknown) substance-induced delirium

292.82 Other (or unknown) substance-induced persisting dementia

292.83 Other (or unknown) substance-induced persisting amnestic disorder

292.84 Other (or unknown) substance-induced mood disorder (specify if onset occurred during intoxication)

292.89   Other (or unknown) substance-induced anxiety disorder (specify if onset occurred during intoxication)

292.89   Other (or unknown) substance-induced sexual dysfunction (specify if onset occurred during intoxication)

292.89   Other (or unknown) substance-induced sleep disorder (specify if onset occurred during intoxication)

292.89   Other (or unknown) substance intoxication (specify if with perceptual disturbances)

292.9   Other (or unknown) substance-related disorder NOS

Other (or unknown) substance use disorders

304.90   Other (or unknown) substance dependence (specify with or without physiological dependence)

305.90   Other (or unknown) substance abuse

OTHER CONDITIONS

Abuse or neglect

V61.1   Physical abuse of adult (code 995.81 if focus is on victim)

V61.1   Sexual abuse of adult (code 995.81 if focus is on victim)

V61.21   Neglect of child (code 995.5 if focus is on victim)

V61.21   Physical abuse of child (code 995.5 if focus is on victim)

V61.21   Sexual abuse of child (code 995.5 if focus is on victim)

Medication-induced movement disorders

332.1   Neuroleptic-induced parkinsonism

333.1   Medication-induced postural tremor

333.7   Neuroleptic-induced acute dystonia

333.82   Neuroleptic-induced tardive dyskinesia

333.90   Medication-induced movement disorder NOS

333.92   Neuroleptic malignant syndrome

333.99   Neuroleptic-induced acute akathisia

Other medication-induced disorder

995.2   Adverse effects of medication NOS

Psychological factors affecting medical condition

316   Specified psychological factor affecting . . . (indicate the medical condition.) Choose name based on nature of mental disorder, psychological symptoms, personality traits or coping style, maladaptive health behaviors, stress-related physiological response, and other factors that affect medical condition.

Relational problems

V61.1   Partner relational problem

V61.20   Parent-child relational problem

V61.8   Sibling relational problem

V62.81   Relational problem NOS

V61.9   Relational problem related to a mental disorder or medical condition

Additional conditions

313.82   Identity problem

780.9   Age-related cognitive decline

V15.81   Noncompliance with treatment

V62.2   Occupational problem

V62.3   Academic problem

V62.4   Acculturation problem

V62.82   Bereavement

V62.89   Borderline intellectual functioning

V62.89   Phase of life problem

V62.89   Religious or spiritual problem

V65.2   Malingering

V71.01   Adult antisocial behavior

V71.02   Child or adolescent antisocial behavior

NANDA Taxonomy I, Revised

NANDA's Taxonomy I, Revised, organized around nine human response patterns, is the currently accepted classification system for nursing diagnoses. The complete taxonomic structure is listed below.

Pattern 1: Exchanging

1.1.2.1	Altered nutrition: More than body requirements
1.1.2.2	Altered nutrition: Less than body requirements
1.1.2.3	Altered nutrition: High risk for more than body requirements
1.2.1.1	High risk for infection
1.2.2.1	High risk for altered body temperature
1.2.2.2	Hypothermia
1.2.2.3	Hyperthermia
1.2.2.4	Ineffective thermoregulation
1.2.3.1	Dysreflexia
1.3.1.1	Constipation
1.3.1.1.1	Perceived constipation
1.3.1.1.2	Colonic constipation
1.3.1.2	Diarrhea
1.3.1.3	Bowel incontinence
1.3.2	Altered urinary elimination
1.3.2.1.1	Stress incontinence
1.3.2.1.2	Reflex incontinence
1.3.2.1.3	Urge incontinence
1.3.2.1.4	Functional incontinence
1.3.2.1.5	Total incontinence
1.3.2.2	Urinary retention
1.4.1.1	Altered (specify type) tissue perfusion (renal, cerebral, cardiopulmonary, gastrointestinal, peripheral)
1.4.1.2.1	Fluid volume excess
1.4.1.2.2.1	Fluid volume deficit
1.4.1.2.2.2	High risk for fluid volume deficit
1.4.2.1	Decreased cardiac output
1.5.1.1	Impaired gas exchange
1.5.1.2	Ineffective airway clearance
1.5.1.3	Ineffective breathing pattern
1.5.1.3.1	Inability to sustain spontaneous ventilation
1.5.1.3.2	Dysfunctional ventilatory weaning response
1.6.1	High risk for injury
1.6.1.1	High risk for suffocation
1.6.1.2	High risk for poisoning
1.6.1.3	High risk for trauma
1.6.1.4	High risk for aspiration
1.6.1.5	High risk for disuse syndrome
1.6.2	Altered protection
1.6.2.1	Impaired tissue integrity
1.6.2.1.1	Altered oral mucous membrane
1.6.2.1.2.1	Impaired skin integrity
1.6.2.1.2.2	High risk for impaired skin integrity

Pattern 2: Communicating

2.1.1.1	Impaired verbal communication

Pattern 3: Relating

3.1.1	Impaired social interaction
3.1.2	Social isolation
3.2.1	Altered role performance
3.2.1.1.1	Altered parenting
3.2.1.1.2	High risk for altered parenting
3.2.1.2.1	Sexual dysfunction
3.2.2	Altered family processes
3.2.2.1	Caregiver role strain
3.2.2.2	High risk for caregiver role strain
3.2.3.1	Parental role conflict
3.3	Altered sexuality patterns

Pattern 4: Valuing

4.1.1	Spiritual distress (distress of the human spirit)

Pattern 5: Choosing

5.1.1.1	Ineffective individual coping
5.1.1.1.1	Impaired adjustment
5.1.1.1.2	Defensive coping
5.1.1.1.3	Ineffective denial
5.1.2.1.1	Ineffective family coping: Disabling
5.1.2.1.2	Ineffective family coping: Compromised
5.1.2.2	Family coping: Potential for growth
5.2.1	Ineffective management of therapeutic regimen (individual)
5.2.1.1	Noncompliance (specify)
5.3.1.1	Decisional conflict (specify)
5.4	Health-seeking behaviors (specify)

Pattern 6: Moving

6.1.1.1	Impaired physical mobility
6.1.1.1.1	High risk for peripheral neurovascular dysfunction
6.1.1.2	Activity intolerance
6.1.1.2.1	Fatigue
6.1.1.3	High risk for activity intolerance
6.2.1	Sleep pattern disturbance
6.3.1.1	Diversional activity deficit
6.4.1.1	Impaired home maintenance management
6.4.2	Altered health maintenance
6.5.1	Feeding self-care deficit
6.5.1.1	Impaired swallowing
6.5.1.2	Ineffective breast-feeding
6.5.1.2.1	Interrupted breast-feeding
6.5.1.3	Effective breast-feeding
6.5.1.4	Ineffective infant feeding pattern
6.5.2	Bathing or hygiene self-care deficit
6.5.3	Dressing or grooming self-care deficit
6.5.4	Toileting self-care deficit
6.6	Altered growth and development
6.7	Relocation stress syndrome

Pattern 7: Perceiving

7.1.1	Body image disturbance
7.1.2	Self-esteem disturbance
7.1.2.1	Chronic low self-esteem
7.1.2.2	Situational low self-esteem
7.1.3	Personal identity disturbance
7.2	Sensory or perceptual alterations (specify visual, auditory, kinesthetic, gustatory, tactile, or olfactory)
7.2.1.1	Unilateral neglect
7.3.1	Hopelessness
7.3.2	Powerlessness

Pattern 8: Knowing

8.1.1	Knowledge deficit (specify)
8.3	Altered thought processes

Pattern 9: Feeling

9.1.1	Pain
9.1.1.1	Chronic pain
9.2.1.1	Dysfunctional grieving
9.2.1.2	Anticipatory grieving
9.2.2	High risk for violence: Self-directed or directed at others
9.2.2.1	High risk for self-mutilation
9.2.3	Posttrauma response
9.2.3.1	Rape-trauma syndrome
9.2.3.1.1	Rape-trauma syndrome: Compound reaction
9.2.3.1.2	Rape-trauma syndrome: Silent reaction
9.3.1	Anxiety
9.3.2	Fear

Selected References

Ackerman, R. J., and Gondolf, E.W. "Adult Children of Alcoholics: The Effects of Background and Treatment on ACOA Symptoms," *The International Journal of Addictions* 26(11):1159-72, 1991.

Affonso, D. "Postpartum Depression: A Nursing Perspective on Women's Health and Behaviors," *Image* 24(3):215-21, Fall 1992.

American Hospital Association. *Put It in Writing: A Guide to Promoting Advance Directives.* Chicago: American Hospital Association, 1991.

American Nurses Association. *Statement on Psychiatric and Mental Health Clinical Nursing Practice and Standards of Psychiatric and Mental Health Nursing Practice.* Washington, D.C.: American Nurses Association, 1994.

American Psychiatric Association. *Diagnostic and Statistical Manual of Mental Disorders*, 4th ed. Washington, D.C.: American Psychiatric Association, 1994.

Andreasen, N.C., and Black, D.W. *Introductory Textbook of Psychiatry.* Washington, D.C.: American Psychiatric Association, 1991.

Bartlett, J.G., and Finkbeiner, A.K. *The Guide to Living with HIV Infection*, 2nd ed. Baltimore: The Johns Hopkins University Press, 1991.

Batshaw, M., and Perret, Y. *Children with Disabilities: A Medical Primer,* 3rd ed. Baltimore: Paul H. Brookes Publishing, 1992.

Bazemore, P.H., et al. "Dysphagia in Psychiatric Patients: Clinical and Videofluoroscopic Study," *Dysphagia* 6(1):2-5, 1991.

Beattie, M. *Beyond Codependency.* Center City, Minn.: Hazelden Foundation, 1989.

Biegel, D.E., et al. *Family Caregiving in Chronic Illness.* Thousand Oaks, Calif.: Sage Publications, Inc., 1991.

Blair, D.T., and Dauner, A. "Neuroleptic Malignant Syndrome: Liability in Nursing Practice," *Journal of Psychosocial Nursing and Mental Health Services* 31(2):5-12, 34-35, February 1993.

Bruss, C.R. "Nursing Diagnosis of Hopelessness," *Journal of Psychosocial Nursing and Mental Health Services* 26(3):28-31, 38-39, March 1988.

Carrey, N.J., and Adams, L., "How to Deal with Sexual Acting-Out on the Child Psychiatric Inpatient Ward," *Journal of Psychosocial Nursing* 30(5):19-23, May 1992.

Caroff, S.N., and Mann, S.C. "Neuroleptic Malignant Syndrome," *Medical Clinics of North America* 77(1):185-202, January 1993.

Cate, F.H., and Gill, B.A. *The Patient Self-Determination Act: Implementation Issues and Opportunities.* Washington, D.C.: Annenberg Washington Program, 1991.

Derogatis, L.R., and Wise, T.N. *Anxiety and Depressive Disorders in the Medical Patient.* Washington, D.C.: American Psychiatric Association, 1989.

Donley, R. "Spiritual Dimensions of Health Care: Nursing Mission," *Nursing and Health Care* 12(4):178-83, April 1991.

Dubin, W.R., and Weiss, K.J. *Handbook of Psychiatric Emergencies.* Springhouse, Pa.: Springhouse Corp., 1991.

Elder, J.H. "Beliefs Held by Parents of Autistic Children," *Journal of Child and Adolescent Psychiatric Nursing and Mental Health* 7(1):9-16, January 1994.

Feetham, S.L., et al., eds. *The Nursing in Families: Theory/Research/Education/Practice.* Thousand Oaks, Calif.: Sage Publications, Inc., 1992.

Fogel, C.I., and Lauver, D. *Sexual Health Promotion.* Philadelphia: W.B. Saunders Co., 1990.

Grant, A.B. *The Professional Nurse: Issues and Actions.* Springhouse, Pa.: Springhouse Corp., 1994.

Guillory, B.A., and Riggin, O.Z. "Developing a Nursing Staff Support Group Model," *Clinical Nurse Specialist* 5(3):170-73, Fall 1991.

Gunzburg, J.C. *Unresolved Grief: A Practical Multicultural Approach for Health Professionals.* New York: Chapman & Hall, 1993.

Haber, J., et al. *Comprehensive Psychiatric Nursing,* 4th ed. St. Louis: Mosby–Year Book, Inc., 1992.

Hastings Center. *Guidelines on the Termination of Life-Sustaining Treatment and the Care of the Dying.* Bloomington, Ind.: Indiana University Press, 1988.

Heliker, D. "Reevaluation of a Nursing Diagnosis: Spiritual Distress," *Nursing Forum* 27(4):15-20, October-December 1992.

Hibbard, S. "Adult Children of Alcoholics: Narcissism, Shame and the Differential Effects of Paternal and Maternal Alcoholism," *Psychiatry* 56(2):153-62, May 1993.

Hogstel, M.O. *Geropsychiatric Nursing.* St. Louis: Mosby–Year Book, Inc., 1990.

Horne, A., and Saygerm, T. *Treating Conduct and Oppositional Defiant Disorder in Children.* New York: Pergamon Press, 1990.

Hsu, L.G. *Eating Disorders.* New York: Guilford Press, 1990.

Kluft, R. P. "Hospital Treatment of Multiple Personality Disorder: An Overview," *Psychiatric Clinics of North America* 14(3):695-719, September 1991.

Koller, P.A. "Family Needs and Coping Strategies During Illness Crisis," *AACN Clinical Issues in Critical Care Nursing* 2(2):338-45, May 1991.

Krupnick, S.L., and Wade, A.J. *Psychiatric Care Planning.* Springhouse, Pa.: Springhouse Corp., 1993.

Lamb, J., and Pusker, K.R. "School-based Adolescent Mental Health Project Survey of Depression, Suicidal Ideation, and Anger," *Journal of Child and Adolescent Psychiatric and Mental Health Nursing* 4(3): 101-104, September 1991.

Lewis, M., ed. *Child and Adolescent Psychiatry: A Comprehensive Textbook.* Baltimore: Williams & Wilkins, 1991.

Lubkin, I.M. *Chronic Illness: Impact and Intervention,* 2nd ed. Boston: Jones & Bartlett, Inc. 1991.

Mace, N., and Rabins, P. *The 36-Hour Day.* Baltimore: The Johns Hopkins University Press, 1991.

Miller, J.F. *Coping with Chronic Illness: Overcoming Powerlessness,* 2nd ed. Philadelphia: F.A. Davis Co., 1992.

Murray, R., and Zentner, J. *Nursing Assessment and Health Promotion: Strategies Through the Life Span.* East Norwalk, Conn.: Appleton & Lange, 1993.

Newcomb, P. "Tricyclic Antidepressants and Children," *Nurse-Practitioner* 16(5): 26-28, 30+, May 1991.

Norbeck, J.S., et al."Social Support Needs of Family Caregivers of Psychiatric Patients From Three Age Groups," *Nursing Research* 40(4):208-13, 1991.

Norris, M., and House, M., eds. *Organ and Tissue Transplantation: Nursing Care from Procurement through Rehabilitation*. Philadelphia: F. A. Davis Co., 1991.

Nurse's Handbook of Law & Ethics. Springhouse, Pa.: Springhouse Corp., 1992.

Resnick, T.J., and Rapin, I. "Language Disorders in Childhood," *Psychiatric Annals* 21(12):709-16, December 1991.

Scipien, G.M., et al. *Pediatric Nursing Care.* St. Louis: Mosby–Year Book, Inc., 1990.

Shalev, A., et al. "Levels of Trauma: A Multidimensional Approach to the Treatment of PTSD," *Psychiatry* 56(2):166-67, May 1993.

Sigardson-Poor, K.M., and Haggerty, L.M., eds. *Nursing Care of the Transplant Recipient.* Philadelphia: W.B. Saunders Co., 1990.

Solomon, M.Z., et al. "Decisions near the End of Life: Professional Views on Life-Sustaining Treatments," *American Journal of Public Health* 83(1):14-23, January 1993.

Sparks, S.M., and Taylor, C.M. *Nursing Diagnosis Reference Manual*, 3rd edition. Springhouse, Pa.: Springhouse Corp., 1995.

Stepnick, A., and Perry, T. "Preventing Spiritual Distress in the Dying Client," *Journal of Psychosocial Nursing and Mental Health Services* 30(1):17-24, 30-31, January 1992.

Stuart, G.W., and Sundeen, S.J., eds. *Principles and Practice of Psychiatric Nursing,* 4th ed. St. Louis: Mosby–Year Book, Inc., 1991.

Tarell, J.D. "Self-Regulation of Symptoms in Schizophrenia: A Psychoeducational Program for Patients and Families," *Chronic Mental Illness: Coping Strategies.* Edited by Maurin, J. Thorofare, N.J.: Charles B. Slack, 1989.

Tarell, J.D., and Schultz, S.C. "Nursing Assessment Using the Brief Psychiatric Rating Scale: A Structured Interview," *Psychopharmacology Bulletin* 24(1):105-15, 1988.

Taylor, C., et al. *Fundamentals of Nursing: The Art and Science of Nursing Care,* 2nd ed. Philadelphia: J.B. Lippincott, 1993.

Taylor-Loughran, A.E., et al. "Defining Characteristics of the Nursing Diagnoses Fear and Anxiety: A Validation Study," *Applied Nursing Research* 2(4):178-86, November 1989.

Walsh, F., and McGoldrich, M. *Living Beyond Loss: Death in the Family.* New York: W. W. Norton & Co., 1991.

Whitney, F., and Pfohl, D. "Nurses and Families: Partners in Care of the Patient with Alzheimer's Disease," *Journal of Advanced Medical-Surgical Nursing* 1(2):55-66, March 1989.

Yeomans, J.D., and Conway, S.P. "Biopsychosocial Aspects of Chronic Fatigue Syndrome (myalgic encephalomyelitis)," *Journal of Infection* 23(3):263-69, November 1991.

Index

Nursing diagnoses and related etiologies appear in italicized type.

Nursing diagnoses and related etiologies appear in italicized type.

Nursing diagnoses and related etiologies appear in italicized type.

Nursing diagnoses and related etiologies appear in italicized type.

Psychotic disorders, 253, 297, 338. *See also specific type.*
Psychotropics, 94
Pulmonary disease, end-stage, 61, 72, 74, 101, 104, 142, 244, 355, 358, 364, 381
Pulmonary embolism, 27

Q
Quadriplegia, 192

R
Radiation therapy, 216
Rape, 187, 189
Rape-trauma syndrome: Compound reaction, 186-188
Rape-trauma syndrome: Silent reaction, 188-191
Reactive attachment disorder of infancy or early childhood, 292, 331
Reading disorder, 321
Recovery from childhood trauma, 163, 170, 174
Relational problems, 97, 313, 318, 325, 328, 335
Relocation stress syndrome, 377-380
Renal calculi, 387
Renal disease, 94, 120, 288, 373
Renal disease, end-stage, 61, 68, 72, 74, 101, 104, 142, 244, 355, 358, 364, 367, 381
Renal failure, 81, 83, 138, 216, 387
Respiratory disease, chronic, 120
Respiratory disorders, 306
Respiratory distress, acute, 338
Respiratory failure, acute, 27, 259
Rheumatoid arthritis, 32, 192, 216, 345, 351, 355, 361, 370, 373, 376, 381, 387
Role performance alteration changed health status and, 191-193
declining health and, 380-383

Role performance alteration (continued)
guilt brought on by transmission of HIV infection and, 194-196
learning disability and, 320-324

S
Schizoid personality disorder, 208, 235
Schizophrenia, 18, 22, 40, 58, 64, 66, 79, 94, 109, 113, 120, 134, 138, 145, 159, 164, 172, 182, 192, 198, 208, 211, 213, 235, 237, 241, 249, 253, 261, 267, 331, 351, 367, 370, 376, 390
Schizophreniform disorder, 164, 208
Schizotypal personality disorder, 235
Sedatives, adverse effects of, 86
Seizure disorder, 283, 288, 297, 303, 338
Seizures, 58, 94
Self-care deficit: Bathing and hygiene, 196-199
Self-esteem, chronically low, 199-201
Self-esteem, situational low increased dependence on caregivers and, 383-386
life events and, 202-204
Self-esteem disturbance adverse relationship with parents and, 324-327
social misconceptions about aging and, 386-388
Self-mutilation, high risk for, 204-207
Sensory deprivation, 210, 259
Sensory disorders, 331
Sensory or perceptual alteration hallucinations and, 207-209
sensory deprivation and, 210-212
sensory overload and, 212-214
Separation anxiety disorder, 44, 292, 332, 335

Septicemia, 259
Sexual abuse of adult, 187, 189
Sexual abuse of child, 225, 318
Sexual arousal disorders, 164, 172, 220, 225
Sexual assault, 187, 189
Sexual aversion disorder, 218
Sexual desire disorders, 164, 218
Sexual dysfunction altered body structure or function and, 215-217
decreased libido and, 217-219
impotence and, 219-221
Sexual dysfunctions, 97, 225, 345. *See also specific type.*
Sexuality, 215, 217, 219, 221, 224, 276, 299
Sexually transmitted diseases, 277, 318
Sexual masochism, 205, 225
Sexual pattern alteration hypersexuality and, 221-224
psychological distress and, 224-227
Sexual sadism, 225
Shaken baby syndrome, 309
Single-gene defects, 283
Situational crisis, 27
Skeletal trauma, 309
Skin cancer, 32
Skin disorders, 182, 237
Skin grafting, 76
Sleep apnea, 88, 229
Sleep disorders. *See specific type.*
Sleep pattern disturbance, 227-230
Social interaction impairment codependence and, 230-234
externalizing behaviors and, 327-330
internalizing behaviors and, 330-333
Social isolation dysfunctional interpersonal relations and, 234-236
in geriatric patient, 388-391
homelessness and, 237-239
illness or disability and, 239-243

Nursing diagnoses and related etiologies appear in italicized type.